Keywords for Health Humanities

Keywords

Collaborative in design and execution, the books in the Keywords series bring together scholars across a wide range of disciplines in the humanities and social sciences, with each essay on a single term to help trace the contours and debates of a particular field. Keywords are the nodal points in many of today's most dynamic and vexed discussions of political and social life, both inside and outside of the academy. Providing accessible A-to-Z surveys of prevailing scholarly concepts, the books serve as flexible tools for carving out new areas of inquiry.

For more information, visit http://keywords.nyupress.org.

Titles in the series:

Keywords for American Cultural Studies, 3rd Edition
Edited by Bruce Burgett and Glenn Hendler

Keywords for Children's Literature, 2nd Edition
Edited by Philip Nel, Lissa Paul, and Nina Christensen

Keywords for Asian American Studies
Edited by Cathy J. Schlund-Vials, Linda Trinh Võ, and K. Scott Wong

Keywords for Disability Studies
Edited by Rachel Adams, Benjamin Reiss, and David Serlin

Keywords for Environmental Studies
Edited by Joni Adamson, William A. Gleason, and David N. Pelow

Keywords for Media Studies
Edited by Laurie Ouellette and Jonathan Gray

Keywords for Latina/o Studies
Edited by Deborah R. Vargas, Nancy Raquel Mirabal, and Lawrence La Fountain-Stokes

Keywords for African American Studies
Edited by Erica R. Edwards, Roderick A. Ferguson, and Jeffrey O. G. Ogbar

Keywords for Gender and Sexuality Studies
Edited by the Keywords Feminist Editorial Collective

Keywords for Health Humanities
Edited by Sari Altschuler, Jonathan M. Metzl, and Priscilla Wald

For a complete list of books in the series, see www.nyupress.org.

Keywords for Health Humanities

Edited by

Sari Altschuler, Jonathan M. Metzl, and Priscilla Wald

NEW YORK UNIVERSITY PRESS   New York

NEW YORK UNIVERSITY PRESS
New York
www.nyupress.org

References to internet websites (URLs) were accurate at the time
of writing. Neither the author nor New York University Press is
responsible for URLs that may have expired or changed since the
manuscript was prepared.

Please contact the Library of Congress for Cataloging-in-Publication
data.

ISBN: 9781479808090 (hardback)
ISBN: 9781479808106 (paperback)
ISBN: 9781479808083 (library e-book)
ISBN: 9781479808069 (consumer e-book)

New York University Press books are printed on acid-free paper, and
their binding materials are chosen for strength and durability. We
strive to use environmentally responsible suppliers and materials to
the greatest extent possible in publishing our books.

Manufactured in the United States of America

10 9 8 7 6 5 4 3 2 1

Also available as an e-book

Contents

Introduction: Sari Altschuler, Jonathan M. Metzl,
 and Priscilla Wald 1

1. Access: Todd Carmody 7
2. Aging: Erin Gentry Lamb 10
3. Anxiety: Justine S. Murison 13
4. Bioethics: Lisa M. Lee 17
5. Care: Rachel Adams 20
6. Carrier: Lisa Lynch 23
7. Chronic: Ed Cohen 27
8. Cognition: Deborah Jenson 30
9. Colonialism: Pratik Chakrabarti 33
10. Compassion: Lisa Diedrich 37
11. Contagion: Annika Mann 40
12. Creativity: Michael Barthman and
 Jay Baruch 43
13. Data: Kirsten Ostherr 47
14. Death: Maura Spiegel 50
15. Diagnosis: Martha Lincoln 54
16. Disability: Rosemarie Garland-Thomson 58
17. Disaster: Martin Halliwell 61
18. Disease: Robert A. Aronowitz 64
19. Drug: Anne Pollock 68
20. Emotion: Kathleen Woodward 71
21. Empathy: Jane F. Thrailkill 74
22. Environment: David N. Pellow 78
23. Epidemic: Christos Lynteris 80
24. Evidence: Pamela K. Gilbert 83
25. Experiment: Helen Tilley 86
26. Gender: Gwen D'Arcangelis 90
27. Genetic: Sandra Soo-Jin Lee 93
28. Global Health: Robert Peckham 96

29. Harm: Tod S. Chambers 99
30. History: David S. Jones 103
31. Human Rights: Jaymelee Kim 106
32. Humanities: Sari Altschuler 109
33. Humanity: Samuel Dubal 113
34. Immunity: Cristobal Silva 117
35. Indigeneity: Michele Marie Desmarais and
 Regina Emily Idoate 120
36. Life: Matthew A. Taylor 124
37. Medicine: Sayantani DasGupta 128
38. Memory: James Chappel 131
39. Microbe: Kym Weed 134
40. Narrative: Rita Charon 137
41. Natural: Corinna Treitel 140
42. Neurodiversity: Ralph James Savarese 142
43. Normal: Peter Cryle and Elizabeth Stephens 146
44. Observation: Alexa R. Miller 149
45. Pain: Catherine Belling 152
46. Pathological: Michael Blackie 155
47. Patient: Nancy Tomes 159
48. Pollution: Sara Jensen Carr 162
49. Poverty: Percy C. Hintzen 164
50. Precision: Kathryn Tabb 167
51. Psychosis: Angela Woods 171
52. Race: Rana Hogarth 174
53. Reproduction: Aziza Ahmed 177
54. Risk: Amy Boesky 180
55. Sense: Erica Fretwell 183
56. Sex: René Esparza 186
57. Sleep: Benjamin Reiss 190
58. Stigma: Allan M. Brandt 193

59. Stress: David Cantor   196

60. Technology: John Basl and Ronald Sandler   199

61. Toxic: Heather Houser   202

62. Trauma: Deborah F. Weinstein   206

63. Treatment: Keir Waddington and
        Martin Willis   209

64. Virus: John Lwanda   212

65. Wound: Harris Solomon   215

References   219
About the Editors   267
About the Contributors   269

Introduction

Sari Altschuler, Jonathan M. Metzl, and
Priscilla Wald

Musing, in the first months of a new century, on what he called "Infectious History," Nobel Prize–winning microbiologist Joshua Lederberg (2000, 290) predicted, "The future of humanity and microbes will likely unfold as episodes of a suspense thriller that could be titled *Our Wits versus Their Genes*." Lederberg was instrumental in defining the phenomenon that came to be known as "emerging infections." The term referred to the proliferation of microbes that caused catastrophic communicable disease in humans. For Lederberg and his colleagues, the phenomenon was not an unknowable threat but a predictable effect of a kind of progress: an expanding global population was moving into areas that had been un- or sparsely inhabited by human beings—thus developing those spaces—while improvements in transportation and an increasingly global economy were moving goods and people rapidly around the world. As these microbes encountered a new species—humans, hence a new food source—they also found a new form of transportation, enabling them to hitchhike around the globe, perhaps mutating in the process. Humans are "major engineers of biological traffic," warned Stephen Morse, Lederberg's colleague, referring not only to literal transportation but also to the practices through which humans produce the ideal conditions for biological growth and dispersal (Morse 1996, 24).

When we began our work on this volume, we did not imagine we would soon find ourselves characters in Lederberg's story. But we should have. Lederberg was hardly alone in his prediction. Epidemiologists and other researchers in the field had long been forecasting what the journalist Laurie Garrett called, in her best-selling 1994 book, the coming plague. And in September 2019, the annual report of the World Health Organization (WHO), entitled *A World at Risk*, warned, "The world is not prepared for a fast-moving, virulent respiratory pathogen pandemic" (World Health Organization 2019, 5). Citing the catastrophic effects of the 1918 global influenza pandemic, which killed fifty million worldwide—2.8 percent of the total population—the report predicted that "a similar contagion" would yield "tragic levels of mortality" and likely spur "panic, destabilize national security and seriously impact the global economy and trade" (15).

Although the COVID-19 pandemic certainly added urgency to this project, our original motivations stemmed from the insight that the pandemic made so broadly palpable: that health is a site in which the social and global inequities of the world are writ large. While the morbidity and mortality rates from SARS-CoV-2 speak loudly to racial and economic inequities worldwide, those same inequities track similarly along the lines of a wide range of health issues, communicable and otherwise. Together the persistence of these inequities shows how far we are from the UN's 1978 Declaration of Alma-Ata that health is "a fundamental human right." The 134 nations and sixty-four NGOs that signed the declaration in 1978 committed to working toward the goal of universal access to primary health care worldwide by the year 2000, the very year in which Lederberg marked the lack of preparedness for a future punctuated by pandemics and other illnesses. Neither the United States nor the world has come close to reaching that goal.

Despite this stagnation in health equity, we noted with great interest that when the pandemic struck, many in health care and among the general public turned to the humanities to understand a novel threat to global human health. History and literature became important resources for understanding global catastrophe and addressing our new reality, especially as they instructed us about the racist and xenophobic dimensions of pandemics past. Likewise, ethicists emerged as necessary experts, with hospitals anticipating ventilator, bed, staff, and later vaccine and treatment shortages that would require life-and-death decisions about care, often exacerbating the impact of the pandemic on racial minorities and disability communities. At the same time, medical schools across the US dramatically increased their humanities offerings. "Wouldn't it be interesting," Sarah Wingerter, physician and director of the Boston University Medical Campus Narrative Writing Program, wrote to one of us in the first pandemic months, "if COVID-19 gives narrative medicine/ reflective writing a boost into mainstream medical education?" Then, on May 5, 2020, the *Journal of the American Medical Association* devoted an entire issue to narrative medicine. Primary care physician and writer in residence at Massachusetts General Hospital Suzanne Koven (2020) tweeted, "A whole issue of @JAMA_current devoted to narratives. . . . Who knew interest in storytelling and #medhum [medical humanities] would surge during a pandemic? (We knew)."

Our convictions both that health is and should be a central topic of critical inquiry and that the humanities has much to offer the study of health and the practice of medicine motivate this Keywords volume. As Lederberg observed, our understanding of health and our practices of health care are deeply shaped by the stories we tell, the language we use, the histories we draw on, and the value judgments we bring.

The idea of a keywords volume first emerged in tandem with the field of cultural studies, in which the sociologist Raymond Williams, author of *Keywords: A Vocabulary of Culture and Society*, was a central figure. The project had its origins in Williams's feeling of estrangement on his return to Cambridge University in 1945 after more than four years in the army. It was as though, he and a colleague who had similarly returned from the war agreed, everyone around them was speaking a different language. The insight led to his 1958 field-defining work, *Culture and Society: 1780–1950*, and, later, *Keywords*. Originally intended as an appendix to *Culture and Society*, *Keywords* is a collection of short meditations on words that, Williams explains, had "at some time, in the course of some argument, virtually forced [themselves] on [his] attention because the problems of [their] meanings seemed to [him] inextricably bound up with the problems [they were] being used to discuss" (R. Williams 1976, 15). It grew out of his realization "that some important social and historical processes occur *within* language, in ways which indicate how integral the problems of meanings and of relationships really are," and that new and changing words offer insight into new and changing relationships (22).

Although Lederberg was not a cultural critic, he came to a similar realization. Of the "new strategies and tactics for countering pathogens" that researchers could explore, he believed "our most sophisticated leap would be to drop the Manichaean view of microbes—'We good; they evil.'" "Perhaps," he opines, "one of the most important changes we can make is to supercede [*sic*] the 20th-century metaphor of war for describing the relationship between people and infectious agents" and replace it with a "more ecologically informed metaphor, which includes the germs'-eye view of infection" (Lederberg 2000, 292–93). A new metaphor, he suggests, would lead to a crucial conceptual shift, the effects of which would be immense. Its benefits might range from research into largely ignored symbiotic microbes and a better understanding of the human biome to a more productive relationship with antibiotics and antibacterial products and new, long-term solutions for intransigent epidemic diseases.

By imagining the future of health, health care, and health research as a question of vocabulary, Lederberg underscores the centrality of words to the ways we inhabit the world. When epidemiologists, medical researchers, and practitioners go into the field, their labs, and their clinics, they bring their worldviews and the vocabularies that shape them. Words are tools that affect how we understand a problem and how we approach a solution. Researchers rely on these tools, as does the general public. We hear repeatedly that we are "at war" with SARS-CoV-2—us versus them—but that obscures what the germs'-eye view might clarify: humans' many roles as traffic engineers and the social and geopolitical conditions that create such outbreaks and turn them into pandemics. Ecological metaphors—ones that convey the germs'-eye view—remind us that the planet, as well as the human body, is a biome; living organisms are intricately interconnected. As Lederberg noted in the early years of emerging infections research, "Many people find it difficult to accommodate to the reality that Nature is far from benign; at least it has no special sentiment for the welfare of the human versus other species" (1996, 3).

War is a human, not a microbial, phenomenon. From public health decisions made in the absence of vital knowledge about a deadly new virus to the widespread efficacy of disinformation campaigns, it has never been clearer that the language of health and health care is not simply a method through which we transmit information but a knowledge-shaping instrument—one that must be used with care and deliberation.

Words do not only crystallize and circulate; they are also records of historical change. They are shaped (and sometimes haunted) by their origins, and the permutations along the way offer an account of the changing relationships and environments—the debates, the struggles to make sense of the world—through which they circulated and helped fashion. *Health* derives etymologically from Old Norse meaning "holy, sacred" and from the Proto-Germanic "whole." Its meanings moved generally from a bodily focus to the broader sense of spiritual as well as physical well-being. In 1946, the WHO, in its constitution, offered a definition of the word that marked the most fundamental commitment of the organization: *health* as "a state of complete physical, mental and social well-being and not merely the absence of disease or infirmity" ("Constitution of the World Health Organization" 1946, 1315). This definition was ratified in 1948, along with the adoption of the United Nations Universal Declaration of Human Rights, which included the principle that "everyone has a right to a standard of living adequate for the health and well-being of himself and of his family, including food, clothing, housing and medical care and necessary social services, and the right to security in the event of unemployment, sickness, disability, widowhood, old age or other lack of livelihood in circumstances beyond his control" (UN General Assembly 1948, article 25). That assumption informs the most basic precepts of any social and environmental justice movement. Health discrepancies among populations record the inequities of any given society; they measure what Stokely Carmichael and Charles Hamilton called "institutional racism"—the difference in mortality rates, for example, of white and Black and Brown babies—and what Johan Galtung (1969), following Carmichael, has termed "structural violence" or "social injustice." Galtung writes, "If people are starving when this is objectively avoidable, then violence is committed, regardless of whether there is a clear subject-action-object relation, as during a siege yesterday or no such clear relation, as in the way world economic relations are organized today" (171).

The capaciousness and pervasiveness of *health*—as a broad description of proper functioning, as an intimate term we use to understand our minds and bodies, as a wide-ranging cultural imperative, as a moral judgment, as a word used to describe a set of professions, and as a central element of all life—make it a fundamental keyword for today's world. It has a set of academic, professional, and popular meanings that mark what Raymond Williams calls "the ways not only of discussing but at another level of seeing many of our central experiences" (1976, 15). These linguistic negotiations play out in the home, in the classroom, in the examination room, in the courts, in the press, on the internet, and most broadly, across the geopolitical relations of our planetary biome. This capaciousness and complexity pushed us to title this volume *Health Humanities* instead of *Medical Humanities* and are why we have insisted on *health* in its broadest sense, not a word that is the exclusive purview of medicine and the health professions but a concept fundamental to all life (cf. Crawford et al. 2010; T. Jones, Wear, and Friedman 2014; T. Jones et al. 2017).

The proliferation of keywords volumes in the twenty-first century is, moreover, an indication of changes in the nature of our fields of study. The rapid technological advances and dramatic geopolitical shifts have given rise to new and changing words—for example, the newly coined and shifting terms that have increasingly shaped an English-language lexicon during the COVID-19 pandemic alone, from *Covidiot* and *Zoombombing* to the more nuanced meanings of *white supremacy* and *systemic racism* to debates over the definitions of fundamental public health terms like *mild* and *endemic*. This proliferation, moreover, in turn signals the need for new kinds of knowledge. As older disciplines shift to new fields of study, keywords volumes have surfaced to help negotiate the changing conceptual terrain. Health humanities is one such field.

Because the concept of *health* persistently defies disciplinary boundaries, we believe a keywords project provides the best conceptual architecture for the health humanities. The lexicon that follows invites students, scholars, and other professionals both to interrogate the words we use to frame the central debates in the field and to work toward a shared vocabulary. Through this approach, we begin to address crucial questions for the health humanities: What needs have given rise to this field of study? What are some of the ambitions, struggles, and key debates that are defining the field? What words are surfacing or changing to make sense of the knowledge emerging in this field? How do the definitions or uses of those words interact, collide, contradict, occlude, and generate new understanding? What kinds of work, care, and community do they make possible, and what insights do they foreclose? Are there words that might serve us better?

Just as we recognize the capacious multidisciplinary reach of the term *health*, we are equally committed to the capaciousness—and rigor—of the term *humanities* in the title of our volume. We recognize and embrace the diversity of health practitioners, therapists, social scientists, artists, and humanities scholars who compose the health humanities, from the broad commitment of the medical humanities to humane health care to the social justice orientation of the health humanities, as Erin Gentry Lamb and Craig Klugman (2019) have argued. At the same time, we understand the *humanities* themselves as a set of rigorous ways of knowing and methods of analysis that have a unique and foundational place in the study of health (for more on *humanities* in the health humanities, see "Humanities"). As Catherine Belling has argued, the humanities cannot be reduced to the art or the science of fields like medicine but instead offer a crucial third perspective that questions "the epistemology, ethics, and language of both biomedical science and clinical practice" (2017, 20). Approaches characteristic of the health humanities make both empirical and nonempirical analysis possible as they facilitate movement across scales of analysis. Moreover, humanities-based inquiry offers a flexibility to move between empirical (already central to knowledge making in medicine, the health sciences, and the social sciences) and nonempirical ways of knowing (philology, close reading, cultural analysis and history, philosophical and theoretical inquiry, for example) that holds powerful potential, as Lederberg described decades ago, to shed new light on foundational and critical questions in health and health care. In the spirit of his challenge, we begin from the study of what and how words mean, what they do, and how they have organized knowledge, culture, medicine, science, and society in the past, how they do so in the present, and how they might do so in the future—fundamental questions the humanities prepare us to answer.

1

Access
Todd Carmody

In the broadest strokes, the keyword *access* refers to "the power, opportunity, permission, or right to come near or into contact with someone or something" (*OED Online* 2021, "access"). This definition highlights the spatial or environmental dimension of *access*. As disability activists and scholars have argued, questions of access foreground the body's relation to the built and social environment. Attending to access also highlights the necessity of making public infrastructure—and public life more generally—responsive to a diversity of human bodies and abilities. In architecture and technology, access interventions include wheelchair ramps, widened toilet seats, lever-shaped door handles, Braille lettering, closed-captioning in videos, and universal design. In civil society, policy and legal interventions support equal access to jobs, housing, education, public space, public institutions, art, and culture. In health care, equal access initiatives aim to guarantee all individuals affordable, high-quality, and culturally and linguistically appropriate care, including preventative medicine, emergency care, and mental health support.

While perhaps most notable among disability studies scholars in the health humanities, the issue of access is a central concern across the shifting constellation of disciplines that make up the health humanities more broadly. Whether in anthropology, bioethics, or literary studies, scholars explore the relationship between bodies and built and social environments of all kinds. Many focus in particular on access to health and health care

broadly understood and on the intersectional histories of class and embodiment implicated in long-standing disparities. Indeed, a shared commitment to making health universally accessible is a common aspiration of many scholars in the interdisciplinary field of the health humanities.

And it's easy to see why. In the United States, economic issues have long been at the heart of inequitable access to health and health care. Throughout the early republic and antebellum eras, most medical care was provided in the home by the members of one's family—a burden that fell disproportionately to women—or by private physicians. Only people without financial resources or families able to care for them were treated (or warehoused) in hospitals, which commonly doubled as poorhouses. The professionalization of medicine that began in the early twentieth century did not end this economic segregation or disrupt the gendered division of medical labor. Instead, the gradual emergence of what is often called the "medical-industrial complex"—a system of commodified care managed by business interests, medical professionals, and the insurance and pharmaceutical industries—deepened extant inequalities and further devalued the care work performed by women (Ehrenreich and Ehrenreich 1971). Access to health care became even more tightly and problematically bound to the white middle-class heterosexual family when paid labor—generally by male breadwinners—became a prerequisite for receiving insurance in the mid-twentieth century.

For many socially marginalized people, these economic disparities in access to health and health care have been compounded by the inequitable distribution of both the benefits and the harms of medicine. Historically speaking, certain people have been more likely to interact with health-care institutions as test subjects than as recipients of salutary care. Trans and gender nonconforming people, for instance, were crucial to the emergence of *scientia sexualis* at the turn of the twentieth century but typically could not access supportive health services. More recently, as T. Benjamin Singer writes, the erasure of transgender people from public health settings has been accompanied by a "bewildering profusion of trans-related categories," demographic designations that create new points of access for marginalized individuals while also bolstering biopolitical relations of power (2015, 61).

The history of African American access to health and health care reflects a similar dynamic of erasure and hypervisibility. Running parallel to the long history of experimentation on Black bodies that Harriet A. Washington calls "medical apartheid" is an equally long history of coercive care rooted in chattel slavery (2006). As historians have shown, enslaved people were most likely to receive medical care at the behest of enslavers motivated chiefly to preserve their financial investments. Indeed, the diagnostic category of "soundness" used by physicians, slave traders, and slaveholders equated the health of enslaved people with their capacity for labor (Fett 2002, 20). Such nomenclature and the managerial practices it sanctioned, as Rana A. Hogarth argues, also silenced the claims to authority that enslaved people made on behalf of indigenous healing practices (2017). Enslaved people were thus unable to determine either how they accessed health care or what kind of health care they were given.

Questions of Black access to health and health care were no less vexed after emancipation. Not only did Black veterans of the Union army face sustained discrimination when seeking medical treatment and invalid pensions, but the terms on which freedom itself was imagined under radical Reconstruction were often tacitly ableist. Whether "voting with one's feet" or endeavoring to prove one's humanity at work on "forty acres and a mule," the coming of freedom left many people behind (Downs 2012). In the early twentieth century, a similar segregation took hold in the budding medical profession. Finding their communities excluded from Jim Crow facilities and mistreated by white physicians, many African Americans built on older traditions of mutual aid and club movements to create community-based modes of access. The Black hospital movement channeled this energy into a successful wave of institution building, consolidating a tradition of self-help that the Black Panther Party (BPP) forcefully took up a half century later (Gamble 1995). As Alondra Nelson has shown, the BPP mobilized a range of community-led responses to face down old and new barriers to accessing health care (2011, 183).

Disability activists have also connected access to health care to struggles for civil rights, though often by challenging rather than cultivating medical authority. The disability rights movement, after all, was inaugurated in part as a response to the "medical model" of disability. This phrase describes the long-standing conviction—among medical professionals but also the broader public—that disability is a cognitive or physiological problem in need of medical intervention or correction. The medical model not only dismisses how people with disabilities experience their lives and bodies, but it also enforces a top-down model of health care. People with disabilities, in other words, have historically had little say in how—or even whether—they access resources and services. Beginning in the 1960s, activists associated with the Independent Living Movement in the United States and the Self-Advocacy Movement globally set out to wrest control away from medical authorities (Joseph Shapiro 1993, 51). Ultimately, these movements succeeded not only in creating systems that allow people with disabilities to determine how they access health care but also in challenging the assumptions about individual self-sufficiency often implicit in the idea of access itself. For these activists, in other words, access is less a matter of asserting one's autonomy than affirming communities of care and networks of interdependence.

More recent disability activists have returned to the idea of access not to challenge the authority of the medical establishment but to underscore the limitations of earlier rights-based approaches to social advancement. Organizing under the banner of disability justice, these activists acknowledge the importance of legislation like the Americans with Disabilities Act but argue that framing access as an issue of individual rights leaves too much on the table—and too many in the cold. Movement organizers and leaders maintain that many disabled people, particularly disabled people of color, are unlikely to "achieve status, power, [or] access through a legal or rights-based framework" (Sins Invalid 2019, 14). Emphasizing disability justice rather than disability rights means underscoring that access is not a single-identity issue but rather shaped by disability's intersections with race, gender, sexuality, age, immigration status, and religion, among other categories of identity and experience. Just as consequentially, disability justice paradigms frame access as a collective rather than an individual project. As the activist and performance collective Sins Invalid argues, only "universal access can lead to universal, collective liberation" (14). From this vantage, truly meaningful access to health and health care—essential in many disabled people's lives—cannot be realized without abandoning individualist notions of accessibility and addressing systemic barriers to collective liberation.

Indeed, if *access* first became a keyword for the health humanities as framed by the disability rights movement, contemporary scholars and practitioners might look to the paradigm of disability justice to reconceptualize what Aimie Hamraie has called "the historical project of knowing and making access" (2017, 3). Such a reconceptualization would mean approaching access—to built and social environments but also to health and health care—as a collective undertaking and not an individual right. Doing so would also involve rethinking the field's shared commitment to making, per the World Health Organization's constitution, the "highest attainable standard of health" universally available ("Constitution of the World Health Organization" 1946, 1315). Rather than redress disparities in the systems and structures that currently exist to foster health, promoting access would mean ensuring that everyone has the collective means to reimagine and remake those systems from the ground up.

2

Aging

Erin Gentry Lamb

Aging is the biological, social, and cultural process of growing older. It is a lifelong process, but the word's common usage focuses our attention on later life; we are more inclined, for example, to describe childhood and young adulthood as "growing up." The language and imagery we use to describe aging—from the stair-step images of the Ages of Man to over-the-hill birthday cards—map the life course as a rise and a fall; the progress implied by growing "up" contrasts with the decline narratives we frequently associate with aging (Gullette 2011). Cultural ideas of aging as decline are shaped strongly by the biological process of aging into old age. While individuals have varied experiences of biological aging—invariably shaped by accumulated advantages and disadvantages over the life course—changes in physical functioning are inevitable, and many additionally experience changes in mental capacity. However, our broad associations of old age with physical and mental decline too often dictate the social roles and cultural ascriptions associated with older people. For example, regardless of health or work status, we are likely to perceive any seventy-year-old as a retiree whose contributions to society are limited to volunteering, grandparenting, and consumption—of both commercial goods (a positive) and health-care resources (a negative). Such limited views of older people's social worth and capacities provide the fodder for ageism: stereotypes, prejudice, and/or discrimination on the basis of age. As biological notions

of aging have had an undue and problematic influence on the social practices and cultural meanings around old age, decoupling aging from decline should be a focus for health humanities.

Like many other characteristics American society tends to ground in the body—including sex, gender, race/ethnicity, and bodily ability—age is an identity category that affects an individual's self-concept, place in social hierarchies, and interactions with others. For example, age conditions our expectations of others' appearance and behavior, as indicated by fashion magazine articles on "age-appropriate" clothing and admonishments of those who are not "acting their age." However, age is the one identity category where, if we live to our expected limits, we will all experience the entire spectrum of its identities from young to old. While some individuals may chafe at being categorized as "young" or "middle-aged," "old" is an identity eschewed by most; it is rare to hear "old" claimed with pride. Instead, age denial thrives across many cultures, evident in phrases like "Sixty is the new forty" and in our multibillion-dollar global antiaging market.

One impetus toward age denial is the association of old people with health needs, which has defined many countries' perceptions of population aging. Dramatic shifts in life expectancy during the twentieth century have made this group a larger and more visible portion of our population. Within the United States, people sixty-five and older composed just 4.1 percent of the population in 1900, as compared to 16 percent in 2018 and an anticipated 21.6 percent by 2040 (Administration on Aging 2017). The growing "dependency ratios"—that is, ratios of older (sixty-five plus) to working populations (fifteen to sixty-four)—give rise to panicked warnings about the burden of a growing population of old, dependent people and our unpreparedness to provide them with long-term care; in one global survey, countries with the lowest dependency ratios had the highest percentages of citizens reporting population aging as a "major problem" within their countries (Pew Research Center 2014). Stigmatizing language such as "the silver tsunami" or the hashtag #BoomerRemover, which trended in the early months of COVID-19, dehumanizes older adults by emphasizing the catastrophic care needs anticipated to fall on younger populations and by devaluing older lives (Charise 2012; Kendall-Taylor, Neumann, and Schoen 2020).

As such, the care needs of an aging population are ripe for health humanities intervention. While experts predict a worldwide net shortage of fifteen million health workers by 2030, driven largely by population growth and aging, ageism discourages practitioners from working with older populations (Liu et al. 2017). Currently, approximately 80 percent of US long-term care given at home is provided by unpaid caregivers, typically family or friends—a staggering amount of unrecognized labor (Administration on Aging 2020). One reason for high rates of informal caregiving is that little governmental support exists for long-term care. For example, should someone need skilled nursing home care, Medicare (health insurance for adults sixty-five plus) only covers one hundred days. Most nursing home care is paid for by Medicaid (health insurance for those with low income or disabilities), requiring many to spend down their assets until they qualify (US Centers for Medicare and Medicaid Services 2020). Our federal health systems are built for acute care; they only minimally account for the largely chronic health needs of an aging population, which can be best approached by coordinated care and management (Aronson 2019). Even for those who can afford it, nursing home care is rarely what we would wish for ourselves or loved ones; such facilities emphasize safety and protection at the expense of what matters most: "a life of worth and purpose" (Gawande

2014, 128). To meet the care needs of older people, our current health systems—including insurance and long-term care facilities—need to be transformed, and health humanities can and should provide the vision to shape new policies (World Health Organization 2020b).

Many age-related experiences have also become a more central and problematic focus of health care over the course of the twentieth century; menopause, andropause, baldness, erectile dysfunction, osteopenia, and senility have all come to be defined and treated as the province of medical experts rather than typical experiences along the natural life span (Bell 1987; van de Wiel 2014; Conrad 2007; Larkin 2011; Bond 1992). Scientific and medical voices have increasingly pushed to view aging as a disease more than a natural process, corresponding to the rise of "antiaging medicine" (Bulterijs 2015; Gavrilov and Gavrilova 2017; Balasubramanian 2020). Biotech companies have cashed in on this view; for example, Google's Calico was presented to the public as an effort to "cure aging" (e.g., S. Lee 2014; K. Anderson 2015). Medicalization is a double-edged sword; it legitimizes experiences and frequently provides treatment options while limiting possible interpretations and often creating stigma. Health humanities has a role to play here too in thinking critically about the medicalization of aging and intervening where it may help people feel more positive about their prospective aging.

Ageism is an important social determinant of health that leads to negative health consequences at both individual and structural levels (Chang et al. 2020). In laboratory studies, elders respond to age cues: those primed with negative stereotypes perform worse on a variety of cognitive and emotional tests (Chrisler, Barney, and Palatino 2016, 90–91; B. Levy 2009, 334). Psychologist Becca Levy has shown that negative age stereotypes held by an individual can affect their "memory performance, balance, gait speed, and hearing"; "exacerbate stress"; "predict worse health behaviors over time, such as noncompliance with prescribed medications"; "predict detrimental brain changes decades later"; and predict a greater likelihood of having a cardiovascular event (B. Levy 2009, 332; B. Levy et al. 2020, 175; B. Levy et al. 2009). Conversely, the internalization of positive age stereotypes has been shown to have beneficial health effects, such as a greater likelihood of practicing preventive health behaviors as one ages, a decreased risk of dementia, and—in one study—longevity gains of seven and a half years on average over those with less positive self-perceptions of aging (B. Levy and Myers 2004; B. Levy et al. 2018; B. Levy et al. 2002). This gain—seven and a half years—is nearly 10 percent of the average global life expectancy, which underscores the stakes of how we narrate aging (World Health Organization 2020a).

Structural ageism is most visible in access to and quality of care. A primary mechanism of structural ageism is health-care professionals' ageist attitudes or behaviors, which, even when unintentional, can affect elders' care. Examples include overattributing older patients' symptoms to age; less time spent with elderly patients, especially during follow-up visits; more negative attitudes toward older patients; and clinical decisions that limit patients' access to care due to age rather than health needs (Pasupathi and Löckenhoff 2002; Chang et al. 2020, 14–15). Taken together, the health consequences of ageism can be not only deadly but also expensive: one study, looking at eight of the most expensive medical conditions, estimates that the effects of ageism are responsible for one in every seven dollars spent annually on older Americans' health care (B. Levy et al. 2020).

Countering ageism in health-care practitioners and the population at large would be a valuable focus for health humanities work. Within health professions education specifically, health humanities can add

critical complexity to the received ideas about aging, particularly complicating the medical model of aging as decline. Furthermore, the health humanities can also bring much-needed intersectional analysis to addressing ageism (Ayalon and Tesch-Römer 2018, 8).

The health humanities can promote other narratives of aging. For example, emotional well-being improves from early adulthood to old age, even accounting for declines in physical health (Carstensen et al. 2000). Happiness and life satisfaction across the life span have been found—across 132 developed and developing countries—to map into a U-shaped curve, where people are happiest as children and older adults and experience a midlife low, a shape that is the inverse of our typical stair-step images of the life course (Blanchflower 2020; Carstensen et al. 2000). Subjective well-being in old age remains high even in the presence of physical and cognitive disabilities (Jopp and Rott 2006). Where such data do *not* hold true, as in cases of individuals with dementia, the causes are likely social and medical stigma: supportive social networks and the ability to participate—sources of life satisfaction—are often endangered by diagnosis (C. Cooper, Bebbington, and Livingston 2011; Shakespeare 2014). Thus, dementia is a key area for health humanities to promote alternative narratives to the dominant view of dementia as loss of self. We need to find more complex ways to talk about dementia and to think about selfhood in relation to memory and function loss; we also must invest in creating age-friendly and dementia-friendly environments (Basting 2009; AARP 2020).

While the biological process of aging may exert an unduly negative influence on social and cultural processes of aging, individual and societal views of aging can likewise affect biological experiences of aging. This reciprocity means there is tremendous opportunity to enhance the lives and health of older people, not to mention save billions in health-care costs, by promoting more complex and diverse views of aging for health-care trainees and professionals and for individuals of all ages. Health humanities is "a strongly mission-driven field, united by a shared commitment to social justice" (Klugman and Lamb 2019, 5). Addressing our narratives of aging and manifestations of ageism is an essential part of that work.

3

Anxiety

Justine S. Murison

In the twenty-first century, anxiety has become one of the leading mental health diagnoses for adolescents and adults alike, matched by a rise in prescriptions of antianxiety drugs like Ativan and Xanax (Schnittker 2021, 1–2; Tone 2009, 228–32). Burnout among health-care professionals was already a topic of concern at medical schools and has only increased greatly during the COVID-19 pandemic. Addressing this phenomenon has itself become a publishing boon, with books like *Burnout: The Secret to Unlocking the Stress Cycle* (2020) or *Anxiety at Work: 8 Strategies to Help Teams Build Resilience, Handle Uncertainty, and Get Stuff Done* (2021) promising to help readers relieve anxiety—or, at least, make it work for rather than against capitalist aims. Books on anxiety and burnout as qualities of the twenty-first century or of the millennial generation have also proliferated, including Jonathan Crary's *24/7: Late Capitalism and the Ends of Sleep* (2013) and Anne Helen Peterson's *Can't Even: How Millennials Became the Burnout Generation* (2021).

Considering both the rising levels of diagnoses *and* the rising cultural attention to anxiety—interconnected phenomena, of course—we might be forgiven for thinking that ours is an era uniquely anxious. But what is revealing about the history of anxiety, from a health humanities perspective, is that naming one's era "the age of anxiety" has been a ubiquitous practice since at least the eighteenth century. As this keyword will show, anxiety is knit into the very narratives that we tell about Western modernity.

The contemporary diagnosis of "generalized anxiety disorder" has a long history but one occluded by the fact that the word itself (*anxiety*) was not always the term under which the symptoms we associate with anxiety traveled. The English word *anxiety* comes from the French *anxiété*, meaning "worry, disquiet," and *anxiété*, in turn, comes from the Latin *anxietās* for "worry, solicitude, extreme care, over-carefulness" (*OED Online* 2021, "anxiety"). Classical authors, including in the Hippocratic Corpus and Cicero's writing, for instance, discussed a disorder distinguished from sadness, one that gives the feeling of being "constricted." They also distinguished between a personal trait—being prone to anxiety—and the feeling itself (Crocq 2017).

Unlike some fellow travelers like *melancholia* or *depression*, *anxiety* does not appear as a medical term until the late nineteenth century. Rather, other terms were more often used to diagnose disordered feelings of concern or worry, including several residual terms from humoral theory—"the vapors," hypochondria, spleen, sensibility, and panophobia (a panic terror), or simply just "having the nerves" (Crocq 2017; Logan 1997). Yet the proliferation of these terms in the West, starting in the seventeenth century, suggests an increasing impulse to diagnose an excessive worry that becomes mentally and physically debilitating. Whatever term it fell under, though, anxiety was and continues to be a psychological disorder best known for its somatic traces—fidgeting, sleeplessness, exhaustion, indigestion, and muscle aches and pains. It is therefore a disorder that, after Elizabeth Wilson, we must understand as deeply physical as well as mental (2004, 8).

Starting in the eighteenth century, *anxiety* (and its corollaries like *nervousness* and *neurasthenia*) became associated with the fast-paced life of the urban West and with wealth, whiteness, and femininity. One of its earliest names was the "English malady," coined in 1733 by George Cheyne (novelist Samuel Richardson's physician) to diagnose an ailment caused by aristocratic luxury, a diagnosis transformed into a middle-class phenomenon by Cheyne's medical predecessors, including Thomas Arnold and Thomas Beddoes, at the end of the eighteenth century (Logan 1997; R. Porter 1992). Their focus was on various nervous ailments they perceived as prevalent in the largely urban middle and upper classes, whose new wealth came from England's overseas empire and the early Industrial Revolution.

In tandem with the nineteenth-century professionalization of medicine and a growing medical interest in the nervous system, physicians in the United States, Great Britain, and Europe began to articulate a specific diagnosis medical historians point to as the origins of modern *anxiety*. In particular, two figures—George Miller Beard and Sigmund Freud—would shape the cultural and medical language around anxiety for the twentieth and twenty-first centuries. Beard's 1880 *Practical Treatise on Nervous Exhaustion* (1881) was a major historical shift toward a more narrowed sense of anxiety as a diagnosis. In keeping with his contemporaries, Beard emphasized somatic elements caused by the nervous system. *Anxiety* remained largely a colloquial rather than professional word for such debilities.

Beard's interest was nervous *exhaustion*. He was one of the first physicians, though not the last, to link anxiety to a type of burnout: that the somatic and emotional tension of worry can lead to collapse. Later in the twentieth century, this would be called *nervous breakdown*. Like his predecessors, Beard considered this disease through a national lens, claiming its greater prevalence in the United States: the "chief and primary cause of this development and very rapid increase of nervousness is *modern civilization*, which is distinguished by these five characteristics: steam-power, the periodical press, the telegraph, the sciences, and the mental activity of women" (1881, vi). Neurasthenia thus assumed class hierarchy, but with his invocations of "civilization" (contrasted throughout to "savage" nations), Beard built his diagnosis out of racial and gendered hierarchies as well. As he puts it, nervous exhaustion is due, first, to "a fine organization," prevalent in "the civilized, refined, and educated, rather than of the barbarous and low-born and untrained—of women more than men" (26). Though neurasthenia could be diagnosed in middle- and upper-class white men, those diagnoses marked their *disordered* bodies. Beard implies here that white women's nervousness is slightly different, that it is intrinsic and a sign of "civilization," reinforcing Kyla Schuller's argument that the nervous, impressible bodies ascribed to white women played a role in the stabilization of racial hierarchy (Schuller 2018a, 62). Neurasthenia solidified several cultural aspects that would lead to the modern definition of *anxiety*: that it has to do with the pace of life in modernity, that it has to do with "civilization" and thus whiteness, and that white women are more susceptible to nervous exhaustion because of their embodied nature.

Neurasthenia did not survive as a medical or even cultural term, but some of its main characteristics were amplified and globally popularized by Sigmund Freud. Freud rejected the somatic aspects of studies of the nerves that were the medical focus of the late nineteenth century, but he did expand upon a hint in Beard's work that in modern civilization "the conventionalities of society require the emotions to be repressed" (Beard 1881, 120). Freud's first article on anxiety sought to distinguish what he called "anxiety neurosis" from Beard's theory of neurasthenia, placing anxiety at the center of psychoanalysis. As Jason Schnittker explains, "For Freud, anxiety represented a kind of energy, sometimes discharged in healthy fashion, and sometimes repressed, though providing the fuel for all kinds of affective and

somatic symptoms" (2021, 26). While Freud initially named sexual repression the most elemental cause of anxiety, his broader emphasis on environmental and cultural factors became a focus of psychoanalytic practice in the twentieth century.

For much of the twentieth century, the diagnostic divisions and tools psychologists and psychoanalysts brought to their practices reflected this heyday of psychoanalysis and "anxiety neurosis." That term appeared in the *DSM-II* (1968), and *anxiety* named the general symptom of all neuroses until the 1980 *DSM-III* and *DSM-III-R* introduced the diagnosis still used today: generalized anxiety disorder, or GAD (Crocq 2017). The most recent edition, *DSM-5* (2013), separates GAD from other types of anxiety disorders, including social anxiety, separation anxiety, agoraphobia, and panic disorder, among others. As has been true since the classical era, GAD is characterized most by "excessive anxiety and worry (apprehensive expectation) about a number of events or activities. The intensity, duration, or frequency of the anxiety and worry is out of proportion to the actual likelihood or impact of the anticipated event. The individual finds it difficult to control the worry and to keep worrisome thoughts from interfering with attention to tasks at hand" (American Psychiatric Association DSM-5 Task Force 2013, 222). There are surprising continuities with the rise of nervous disorders in the eighteenth and nineteenth centuries: the *DSM-5* notes that women are more prone to GAD than men and that "individuals from developed countries are more likely than individuals from nondeveloped countries to report that they have experienced symptoms that meet criteria for generalized anxiety disorder in their lifetime" (American Psychiatric Association DSM-5 Task Force 2013, 223). Thus, "generalized anxiety disorder" still carries many of the gendered, racial, and colonial theories that had accrued historically to the ideas of nervousness and anxiety.

The prevalence of psychoanalysis made the terms of anxiety and repression foundational not just to psychological treatment but to the West's colloquial language about mental health, shaping the Cold War era's self-understanding as an "age of anxiety," especially in the United States. While talk therapy was the remedy prescribed by psychoanalysis, the first antianxiety drug, Miltown, was developed in 1955, and since that time, diagnoses of anxiety and pharmacological solutions for it have risen apace. While the midcentury produced a variety of literary and cinematic narratives that showcased male neurotics like the anxious protagonist in Alfred Hitchcock's *Vertigo* (1958), the pharmacological transformation of anxiety was imagined as decidedly white and female. White women were twice as likely to be prescribed benzodiazepines like Valium, which was dubbed "Mother's Little Helper" after the Rolling Stones' hit. The 1970s backlash to minor tranquilizers came both from conservatives, who focused on white homemakers' addictions to them, and from second-wave feminists, who critiqued the overprescribing of women (Tone 2009, 180–85, 189–201).

But just like every nervous or anxious era before it, the Cold War era was soon eclipsed; the twenty-first century has declared itself *the* age of anxiety. Growing income inequality, fast-paced technological changes that have sped up communication, social media, 9/11, climate change, a global pandemic, and the rising tide of illiberalism across the West—these have all combined to spark new claims that *this* is the era of intense and acute anxiety. Still, the list of reasons seems to repeat, with slight differences, George Cheyne's claims about aristocratic luxury and global imperialism and George Miller Beard's concerns about technology and women's intellectual development. In many ways, it is hard to disaggregate the elements of anxiety as a disorder from our understanding of the experience of modernity. Understanding how *anxiety* as a disorder and diagnosis emerged and today dominates so much of Western culture thus requires a health humanities approach: it is cultural and somatic, psychological in the deepest sense (often rooted in childhood experiences) but also epiphenomenal, characteristic of a society, nation, and age. Above all, anxiety (as affective experience and medical diagnosis) is intrinsic to the narratives the West has long been telling itself about its modernity, technological rationality, and racial and gendered hierarchies.

4

Bioethics

Lisa M. Lee

Situated in the applied branch of ethics within moral philosophy, *bioethics* is the study of what we ought to do or ought not to do and why in the fields of science, health, and technology. *Bioethics* arrived relatively late to the health humanities vocabulary. Attempting to bridge science (*bio*) and the humanities (*ethics*), Van Rensselaer Potter introduced the term *bioethics* to the United States in 1971. Without this connection, he feared, our very survival as a species was at risk (Potter 1971; L. Lee 2017). Potter recognized and articulated what was then a novel idea: that we must consider Earth's entire ecosystem as we advance science and technology to improve the quality of our existence. Separately and simultaneously, Andre Hellegers and Sargent Shriver developed what they called a "bioethics institute" at Georgetown University (Reich 1995; L. Lee 2017). Despite creating the same term to describe their new field, their vision differed from Potter's, focusing on health, health care, and practical problems arising in clinical care and medical research (L. Lee 2017).

Although medical ethics (also called clinical ethics) existed before the 1970s, its early iteration consisted of a list of obligations medical doctors had to their patients, such as "First do no harm" (Jonsen 1998). At the time Potter and Hellegers introduced *bioethics* to the United States, two high-profile events captured national attention, drawing the focus of bioethics toward Hellegers's narrower conception of the term. The first was the case of Karen Ann Quinlan, a twenty-one-year-old who,

following ingestion of drugs and alcohol, existed in a persistent vegetative state through the use of various life-support measures for over a decade (Appelbaum and Klein 1986). The Quinlan case highlighted the growing complexity of ethical questions related to medical care, particularly at the end of life. The second event was the public revelation of the unethical, US Public Health Service–funded study of syphilis in poor, Black sharecroppers in and around Tuskegee, Alabama. During the infamous forty-year study, popularly known as the Tuskegee Syphilis Study, US government officials withheld syphilis treatment to observe the already well-described natural history of disease in Black men (J. Jones 1993). This study, along with twenty-two others described in the medical literature six years earlier (Beecher 1966) and revelations of Nazi experiments during WWII, underscored the lack of ethical oversight of researchers and the abuse of vulnerable persons for experimentation.

With clinical and research ethics in the popular press, use of the term *bioethics* as envisioned by Hellegers grew quickly. Following these high-profile cases, the federal government (first Congress, then the president) empaneled a series of bioethics committees to advise government agencies on ethical issues emerging from rapid advances in health care, science, and technology (Brian and Cook-Deegan 2017). With the science and technology added as topics for bioethics committees to study, use of the term *bioethics* surpassed *medical ethics* (Google Books 2021) and became the umbrella term reflecting a conception broader than Hellegers's but narrower than Potter's.

Disciplinary diversity defined US bioethics committees and contributed to what we now consider a defining characteristic of the field. Members of national bioethics committees included philosophers and theologians, as expected, but given the applied nature of the work, lawyers, social and political scientists, patient advocates, physicians, and research scientists also made significant contributions. The diversity of disciplines coming together to solve ethically challenging problems in health, science, and technology prompted growing interest in the professionalization of a new field of bioethics. This growing interest led to the development of degree programs, primarily at the master's level, which offered a credential to persons trained in other disciplines and provided a cadre of diverse experts with training in the application of ethics and moral philosophy to health policy (L. Lee and McCarty 2016).

Additionally, the federal government added funding opportunities related to bioethics for academics with an interest in studying ethical, legal, and social issues (ELSI) associated with scientific advances in the late twentieth century. The US National Institutes of Health introduced competitive grant funding for bioethics in the early 1990s, allocating 5 percent of the extramural Human Genome Project funding for ELSI topics (Langfelder and Juengst 1993). Private funding for bioethics-related scholarship grew from the Greenwall Foundation's growing interest in bioethics in the 1980s. The vigorous response to and interest in Greenwall's bioethics funding prompted the foundation to focus solely on bioethics by 2011 (Greenwall Foundation, n.d.).

The combination of research funding and degree programs legitimized bioethics as a field of study, and professional organizations emerged. Bioethics was firmly set as a field, although there remains a robust debate about whether it has or ever will mature into a discipline (L. Lee and McCarty 2016). One critique of calling bioethics a discipline is a lack of consensus about exactly what composes the field and what tasks a professional bioethicist performs.

Debate continues about what the evolving field of bioethics includes and how to categorize its components. Many bioethicists use the term *bioethics* as an umbrella term to capture study and practice in four broad focus areas. Each area, with its different centers of concern, has developed grounding theories, principles, and values to drive its work.

The first area, biomedical ethics (also called clinical ethics), situates the individual patient at its center. Its grounding principles include individual autonomy, compassion, protection, and individual dignity. The second area, research ethics, places research subjects (human and nonhuman animals) at its center of concern. Its grounding concepts include informed consent, risk reduction, and equitable distribution of burdens and benefits. The third area, public health ethics, places communities at its center and emphasizes such values as solidarity, inclusiveness, human rights, and equity. The fourth area, environmental ethics, places human interaction with the biosphere at the center. It grounds its work in the intrinsic value of nature, the moral standing of nonhumans, and connectedness. Within these broad areas, specialty subfields have emerged to address the particular nuances of complex technologies, including nanoethics, genetic ethics (genethics), artificial intelligence and machine learning ethics, data ethics, and reproductive ethics.

As the field of bioethics has evolved since the introduction of the term fifty years ago, so have the tasks bioethicists perform. Bioethics practitioners perform a variety of tasks depending on the setting in which they work, the funding available to support their work, and their own professional interests. Though not mutually exclusive, most bioethicists work in three settings: academic, clinical, or research.

Academic bioethicists conduct normative and empirical research on a broad spectrum of topics related to their academic interest. Often these topics relate to science and technology, as well as to other topics in the humanities. These broad topics of interest, often funded through private foundations, reflect a more Potteresque approach to bioethics. Federal funding for academic bioethics tends to relate to specific health, science, or health technology research, which limits somewhat the scope of the work to a more Hellegers-Georgetown approach.

Clinical bioethicists generally practice bioethics through a mechanism called health-care ethics consultation (Aulisio, Arnold, and Younger 2000). In 1992, the US hospital accreditation body required that patients have access to a mechanism to address ethical conflicts with the health-care team (McGee et al. 2001). Nearly all hospital systems have developed in-house ethics consultation services composed of a team of individuals, some of whom have bioethics training (McGee et al. 2001). Clinical bioethicists assist patients, families, and health-care teams in resolving ethical disagreements about care plans.

Research bioethicists provide ethics advice and consultation in research settings, including academic medical centers, universities, and independent research organizations (M. Cho et al. 2008). The role of a research ethicist varies, but a leading practice is to engage research ethicists early in the research development process to ensure that ethical dimensions across the project are identified and addressed (Jongsma and Bredenoord 2020). Research bioethicists often serve as members of governmentally mandated research compliance boards such as the Institutional Review Board (IRB), Research Ethics Board (REB), or Institutional Animal Care and Use Committee (IACUC), providing ethics expertise in the context of regulatory requirements.

Regardless of focus, subspecialty, or practice context, bioethics reflects a practical and applied interpretation of the broader field of moral philosophy. Bioethicists depend on theories of moral philosophy and ethics, including deontology, consequentialism, virtue ethics, divine command theory, feminist and care ethics, and justice and social contract theory, among others. To make decisions about what we ought to do, bioethicists employ various methods, including principlism, casuistry, narrative ethics, and pragmatism (Arras 2017). Bioethicists with public policy responsibilities often engage in democratic deliberation to solve bioethical problems using a pluralistic approach that encompasses empirical information, values, and lived experiences of affected communities (Gutmann and Thompson 1997; PCSBI 2016).

In its first fifty years, contemporary bioethics has expanded in some respects and contracted in others. The initial vision for the field was to consider what we ought to do in order to live in harmony with our ecosystem as science and technology rapidly expanded. The practical implementation of that vision resulted in a narrower focus on health and medicine with a number of areas of specialization and subfields of practice. Over the next fifty years, untenable inequities in global health, wealth, and opportunity in an increasingly diverse world; growing zoonotic threats resulting in novel infectious diseases; and the impact of climate change on human health will lead bioethics to consider a larger remit, pushing the field closer to Potter's expansive vision of bioethics as the study of what humans ought to do to live harmoniously as one part of Earth's complex ecosystem.

These macro issues will be considered by bioethicists in addition to, not instead of, the individual-level, ethically complex topics in health. The ability to capture terabytes of digital information, including personally identifiable sensitive health data, raises questions about health privacy and information autonomy. The introduction of artificial intelligence, machine learning, and other technology-assisted methods into medicine and public health raises questions about agency, informed decision-making, and professional accountability. Rapid advances in genomics, including germline editing, raise questions about the very essence of life, what it means to be human, and what kind of life is worth living.

As bioethicists approach these questions, it will be critical to create space for previously unheard voices to contribute to the discourse. Women in all societies, people across the globe with less economic and social power, people of color in predominately white cultures, people with disabilities, and people of sexual and gender minorities increasingly and rightfully demand a role in bioethics and policy decision-making that has been left too long to men with social and economic privilege. While some progress has been realized—as demonstrated by a growing number of such subfields as queer bioethics (Wahlert and Fiester 2012), disability bioethics (Garland-Thomson 2017; see "Disability"), and Black bioethics (K. Ray 2021)—in most of the developed world, a traditional white, Christian, heterosexual, highly educated, male perspective has shaped the theoretical and rhetorical norms of bioethics. One of the most important tasks for the field of bioethics will be to continue to open its aperture to incorporate perspectives of all persons and groups affected by its policies and decisions about some of the most fundamental existential questions we face as inhabitants of the planet.

5

Care

Rachel Adams

Care is so frequently paired with health that *health care* is often used as a fixed compound word. Yet, paradoxically, health and care have become increasingly detached from each other, comprising different activities, professions, and ethical principles.

Care is work, an attitude toward others, and an ethical ideal. In most societies, the majority of care work is done by women, who are seen as more naturally predisposed to caring virtues like nurturance, generosity, and empathy and also obligated by their social statuses as daughters, wives, and mothers (Kittay 1999; Glenn 2010; Noddings 1984; Ruddick 2002; Tronto 2015). The idea that care is "given" complicates its association with work, paid or unpaid, and care is largely absent from Marxist theories of labor. However, feminists observe that economically productive activity recognized as "work" is subsidized by the uncompensated labor of numerous others, mostly women and people of color (Bonnar 2006; Fineman 2004; Kittay 1999). Recognizing care as work draws attention to unpaid labor within the family but also paid caregivers like nannies, home health aides, and elder companions, who are among the most poorly compensated and unappreciated of all workers. Many work in private homes, where they are isolated from one another, and may develop emotional bonds with dependents. Moreover, care work requires patience, restraint, and generosity that cannot be documented on a time sheet. These qualities have made it difficult for care workers to self-advocate or to organize, as have workers in other professions (Boris and Klein 2012; Glenn 2010).

While care has a longer association with sorrow, concern, and burden, its meaning as "charge, oversight, attention, or heed with a view to safety and protection" first arose in the 1400s (Wald 2008). In monarchial societies where most people were subjects rather than citizens, dependence was the norm. Powerful men understood themselves to be interdependent with their subordinates. Care work was distributed according to gender, with women tending to children and household chores and men engaging in more physically taxing activities like farming and building. By the eighteenth century, *independency* referred to owning property, a status that freed men from the need to work and granted them political rights. To be dependent meant to engage in wage labor rather than belonging to the owning classes. The radical innovation of the American Revolution was to declare all white men independent, regardless of whether they owned property (Fraser and Gordon 1994). At the same time, radical Protestantism advocated an independent and individualized relation to God. Dependence was redefined from a social relation to a status identity assigned to women and non-white people, including slaves and Native Americans (Glenn 2010).

The era of industrialization reinforced the separation and gendering of public and private, work and domestic life, care and labor. The validation of wage labor made *dependency* an increasingly pejorative term linking economic need to moral qualities of weakness, inability, and poor character (Fraser and Gordon 1994). Caregiving activities were increasingly separated from understandings of meaningful work. It was also during the era of industrialization that many European countries developed nationwide social welfare programs to care for the poor, sick, and disabled. In the US, new workers' compensation laws obligated employers to pay for medical care and lost wages of sick or injured employees, and in 1935, the Social Security Act provided a basic safety net to the unemployed and elderly. Its definition of protected workers excluded domestic and agricultural laborers, occupations dominated by African Americans and other people of color, laying the foundations for racial bias that shapes welfare policy to the present day (Boris and Klein 2012; Fraser and Gordon 1994; Glenn 2010).

The history of care is also shaped by the professionalization of medicine and rise of institutions. Until the late nineteenth century, most health care occurred at home, where women tended to sick and disabled family members, sometimes advised by spiritual healers or doctors. The professionalization of medicine shifted authority for treatment of the sick and disabled to credentialed doctors, whose knowledge had priority over that of family and more traditional healers. Although hospitals had existed since the Middle Ages, their primary mission was containment of infectious disease and care of the poor. Only in the nineteenth century did medical institutions shift toward treatment and rehabilitation of the ill. Rising numbers of hospital patients and the professionalization of health care increased demand for nurses, an occupation dominated almost exclusively by women. As hospitals took on treatment of the sick and disabled, home was reserved for the care of children, elderly relatives, and dependents with illnesses and disabilities that did not require more technical medical support.

Technological developments played an equally important role in the history of care. Hospitals were ideal places for bulky, complicated medical equipment, but extended hospital stays were expensive (Risse 1999; Starr 1982). During the Great Depression, the US government sought to save money and create jobs by hiring more nurses to visit elderly and chronically ill patients at home (Boris and Klein 2012; Glenn 2010). As the century wore on, complex medical devices became more portable and user friendly. New equipment allowed hospital management to economize by discharging patients who were sicker and more medically involved to their homes or outpatient facilities for care (Arras 1995). Once a small movement, home hospice became an industry that promised to cut costs for hospitals while providing support and equipment to comfort the dying and their families (Braswell 2019). Many patients and families who welcomed the thought of dying at home found the resources inadequate to meet their needs. The current system relies heavily on the unpaid labor of family, who rarely anticipate the time, effort, and emotional toll of caring for a dying person (Braswell 2019).

Care for dependent people with disabilities followed a similar historical cycle from home to institutions. Traditionally, disabled people who survived childhood were cared for by their families and communities. In the nineteenth century, the same institutional culture that gave rise to hospitals also developed massive facilities for housing people with disabilities. Early institutions aspired to educate and uplift their clients in preparation for their return to their homes and communities. But as optimism about the possibilities of reforming the "feebleminded" waned, more clients became permanent residents, abandoned by their families to the care of the state (Trent 2017). New understandings of heredity made it a shameful secret to have a disabled relative, and the function of residential facilities shifted from education and reform to warehousing (D. Cohen 2013). Hidden from public view, conditions of institutional life deteriorated for staff and clients, who endured rampant crowding, abuse, and neglect (Carlson 2010; Carey 2009; Trent 2017). Not until the 1970s did journalists expose a vulnerable population living in a kind of squalor rarely seen in modernized countries. Widespread public outrage fueled the movement for deinstitutionalization, which called for closing facilities of mass confinement and shifting residents into smaller facilities and community settings (Carey 2009).

Deinstitutionalization is an important chapter in the history of care, one that has made people with disability-related dependencies more visible, autonomous, and integrated than at any time in the past century. A new generation of people with disabilities has been empowered by the new climate of inclusion. Refusing the role of passive bystanders, they claim to be consumers and citizens entitled to determine the circumstances of their own care (Charlton 2000; Joseph Shapiro 1993). Deinstitutionalization changed the nature of care for people with disability-related dependencies in the US and Europe; however, the movement was incomplete. Shuttering large institutions was a momentous step, but the money it saved has not been channeled into adequate resources to relocate formerly institutionalized people, provide them with care, and uphold the rights of home care workers (Carey 2009; Ben-Moshe and Carey 2014).

The chronic underfunding of community-based care has been amplified by a disability rights movement reluctant to acknowledge dependency (Kittay 1999; C. Kelly 2016). Calling for independence, advocates denounced the image of disabled people as vulnerable and needy (Charlton 2000). Many early activists in the US were college students who received care from friends or classmates in a spirit of communal generosity. These idealistic relationships emphasized the quality of life and dignity of the disabled consumer rather than the pay or working conditions of the care provider (Boris and Klein 2012). As such, they obscured the needs of the most dependent disabled people, as well as the rights of care workers. The struggle to reconcile the autonomy of disabled people to dictate the circumstances of their care and the well-being of paid providers—usually women and people of color—continues into the present (Boris and Klein 2012).

This entry focuses on the Global North, where changing demographics and social conditions have created rising demand for paid caregivers; however, the impact of those changes is planetary. Because of its low status and pay, care work has increasingly fallen to immigrant women from regions of the world plagued by exploding foreign debt, shrinking state welfare, and the decline in traditional occupations such as subsistence agriculture. Workers from the Philippines or Tibet are prized by a global elite because their cultures are reputed to value superior caregiving, and the economies of these nations and others like China, Mexico, and India rely heavily on remittances from women workers abroad, creating a "global care chain." Migrating workers leave behind their own dependents, creating a deficit of care in their home countries (Boris and Parreñas 2010; Ehrenreich and Hochschild 2003; Kittay 2005; Parreñas 2001).

Care is often high on the list of unsustainable practices looming on the horizon for the next generation to resolve. Journalists sometimes describe a mounting "crisis of care" that risks casting dependent groups like the elderly and disabled into the familiar position of being a costly burden. A more productive approach to the changing demographics of care would require a dramatic reconsideration of how we define and value work, personhood, and a good life for both caregivers and receivers. To do so will require not just changes in education, policy, and social organization but also cultural shifts in how dependency is understood and how providers are valued. Health humanities is a field well positioned to orchestrate difficult conversations about how to make "health care" more than a hollow signifier, imagine better ways to sustain our fragile systems, and recognize the exchange of care as a source of value, meaning, and creative possibility.

6

Carrier

Lisa Lynch

Carrier has its origins in *carricāre*, the Latin word meaning "to cart." In medical parlance, disease is "carted," a freight transmitted by one individual, often unwittingly, to one or many others. Disease might be transmitted through viruses or bacteria shared between bodies or through a piece of genetic code passed on to an unborn child. In both cases, carriers of disease are socially maligned and stigmatized. Scholars in the health humanities have studied the causes and effects of such stigmatization, especially as race, class, gender, and disability often determine perceptions of and responses to disease carriers.

The contemporary notion of the infectious disease carrier—a person who poses a health risk to others whether or not they show symptoms of disease—was first established by the bacteriologist Robert Koch in the early twentieth century (Mendelsohn 2002; Leavitt 1997; Wald 2008). Twenty years after his groundbreaking work on the infectious transmission of tuberculosis refocused scientific attention on the germ theory of transmission, Koch further established that typhoid could be spread by individuals who showed no symptoms, so-called healthy carriers (Akkermans 2014).

Koch's research established as scientific fact a concept freighted with a long history of fear and suspicion. Western contagionist thinking began as early as the Renaissance, when Girolamo Fracastoro described human transmission of syphilis through "fomites," or tiny particulars activated in certain circumstances (Karamanou et al. 2012). Likewise, practical measures to isolate ill individuals date back to the Middle Ages with the quarantining of people with what was then known as leprosy and plague as well as sea voyagers and, later, victims of yellow fever and cholera (Tognotti 2013). By ending the debate between the contagionists and miasma theorists about whether disease could be blamed on "unclean" environments or "unclean" individuals, Koch allowed scientists to assign blame to the latter camp, cloaking social marginalization of sick and poor people in the guise of medical necessity (Cook 2002). And by proving that healthy individuals could carry disease, Koch's work stoked fears that marginalized individuals might harbor disease in secret.

These associations and fears have continued through the present, shaping how we understand the concept of the healthy carrier. Scientific, cultural, and popular representations of human disease carriers since the 1890s have been largely adversarial, depicting carriers as liminal figures with innate or acquired moral deficiencies that are incorporealized as infectious illness and who infect others through self-involved or even predatory behavior. Carrier narratives (Wald 2008) have been not only a powerful cultural touchpoint but a powerful political tool; around the world, carrier narratives play a role in public health policy, immigration policy, and national security policy.

In the health humanities, discussion of the carrier has often focused on the discursive and actual othering of those who are identified as carriers. The most familiar carrier in the history of the term is Mary Mallon, or "Typhoid Mary," an Irish-born cook whose actions and their consequences have inspired some of the more significant works of humanities scholarship on the carrier as a concept. Mallon is believed to have infected over fifty people with typhoid in New York City in the early twentieth century. After she was identified as a source of infection, she was arrested as a public health threat and quarantined. She never believed herself to be a source of infection, and when she was released, she returned to work as a cook. After some sleuthing by public health officials, she was identified as a typhus source a second time and quarantined until her death.

Health humanists identify in Mallon the cultural and social roots of public health as well as the balance between individual liberties and public safety. Her case resonates not only because of the dramatic nature of her story but also because the drama that unfolded around her coincided with the popularization of the notion of the healthy carrier and the instantiation of early twentieth-century "medical policing" (Mendelsohn 2002), public health that positioned healthy carriers as threats to be managed in the interest of public safety, which often mapped on to the desire to police particular populations and behaviors. Wald argues Mallon's case inaugurated a narrative about disease transmission that had broad cultural implications for "the medical pathologization of social disorder and the reconceptualization of social responsibility" (1997, 210).

As scholars have noted, Mallon's pathologization also set the stage for the treatment of other healthy carriers like HIV-positive individuals (Leavitt 1996; Wald 2008). Indeed, the stigmatization of so-called AIDS carriers powerfully reinforces the circular relationship between fear of the healthy carrier and social marginalization. HIV/AIDS was initially identified in Euro-American culture as a disease affecting mainly gay men, feeding into the pathologization of homosexuality and the portrayal of gay men as alternately monstrous/predatory or feminized/weak (Redman 1997). Early intervention around HIV/AIDS in the US thus was hampered by moral opprobrium; it took nearly a decade of activism to motivate research funding for the disease (Epstein 1996). Furthermore, the overrepresentation of white, gay men during the early phases of the AIDS epidemic led some to stigmatize AIDS transmission as related to masculine and predatory behavior. At the same time, men who contracted HIV were seen as effeminate, even within the gay community (Kruger 1996). Thus, in the early years, men with HIV were represented as at once aberrantly masculine and aberrantly feminine (Redman 1997).

A decade later, HIV became less associated with the gay community as more people contracted the disease (Higgins, Hoffman, and Dworkin 2010). To some degree, a more sex-inclusive understanding of HIV infection had positive public health outcomes, debunking the dangerous myth that because mostly men had been infected, women were somehow immune (Treichler 1988). But as a discourse around women with HIV emerged, it was overdetermined by medical discourse that had for centuries maintained the normativity of the heterosexual male body and inherent "pollution" of the female body (Gilman 1987), identifying women—especially prostitutes—as the primary carriers of venereal disease (Spongberg 1998), with "Typhoid Mary" replaced by "HIV Jane" (Chan and Reidpath 2003).

In the Global South, where women's rates of infection outpace their male counterparts, women are imagined as primary carriers. Throughout sub-Saharan Africa and in Haiti, HIV-positive women experience stigmatization, violence, and ostracism, which can interfere with their ability to seek treatment (Rankin et al. 2005; Santana and Dancy 2000). While existing gender inequality is a main driver of this stigma, feminist research highlighting the vulnerability of women to HIV, filtered through public health discourse, has also sometimes negatively reinforced the role played by women in transmission (Ngwira 2017). These narratives of AIDS have been perceived in the Global South as extensions of the imperial legacy of North-South relations, and they are countered with blame deflection (the stigmatization of women) and outright denialism (Mbali 2004).

In fact, the colonial and imperial legacy of contemporary medicine is a persistent concern of health humanities research on the carrier concept (Kumagai and Naidu 2019). Gradmann (2015) points to the influence of tropical medicine on Koch's notion of the carrier, suggesting carrier narratives are thus overdetermined by a racialized discourse that sees indigenous populations through the lens of the risk posed to colonialists. The collision of bacteriology and tropical medicine had effects on the latter field as well, shifting emphasis away from locating disease in "streets, swamps and sewers" to locating it in the racialized body (Honigsbaum 2016). This allowed for an understanding of disease transmission that slotted comfortably into preconceptions about racial superiority and the threat posed by intimate contact with the colonial or postcolonial other (W. Anderson 1998). The mid-1990s Western panic over an Ebola outbreak in Zaire demonstrated the persistence of these stereotypes; as Schell and I (Schell 1997; Lynch 1998) have written, during the initial panic over a potential global outbreak of Ebola, the xenophobic racialization of the carrier narrative manifested as a concern for protecting the West from African carriers in the name of "biosecurity." Like narratives about typhus or HIV, Ebola stories are inherently stories about the fear of outsiders, who are marked as both different and threatening and who are embedded in complex discourses of power and marginalization.

"Genetic carrier" narratives are also predicated on fear of difference. The term *genetic carrier* is used to refer to people who pass on disease or disability not through infection but through genetic transmission—for example, parents who are carriers of Tay-Sachs, Huntington's, or sickle cell disease. In health humanities scholarship, such genetic carriers are seen as having a distinct set of representational and ethical concerns. While genetic counseling is now commonplace for newly pregnant women and those seeking fertility treatment and presented largely as an unquestioned good, disability scholars have uncovered links between prenatal genetic screening and the history of eugenics (Shakespeare 1998). Such screening and the selective abortion that can follow, some argue, is a form of discrimination that poses a threat to the personhood of children with genetic disabilities (Parens and Ash 2000, 23). Writing about genetic screening in the context of assisted reproductive technology like IVF, Karpin and Mykitiuk (2020, 23) suggest such testing is related to "neoliberal rationality and biomedical conceptions of normalcy that are based on values and practices about who is marginalized in the present," elucidating how this rationality pressures both doctors and prospective parents to see their genes as risks to be eliminated. Karpin and Mykitiuk's work is typical in that they look at genetic screening through the lens of the clinical encounter. Little research has emerged thus far on how the recent popularization of home-based carrier screening, which allows prospective parents to screen for genetic risks via mail-order kits, might change how such parents understand and navigate their choices.

Just as home genetic testing has the potential to change narratives around so-called genetic carriers, the emergence of the global COVID-19 pandemic upended the representation of the idea of the healthy or asymptomatic carrier around the world. In the US in particular, this representation has been shaped by the populist political debate around the virus's pathology. At the beginning of the pandemic, the idea of the so-called Chinese carrier echoed earlier xenophobic associations between disease and racial others (including associations between Asians and the global SARS outbreak of 2003) and led the US to focus early containment strategies on foreign travel restrictions that did little to stop COVID's spread. Globally, COVID denialism has been rampant in populist countries, engendering suspicion about the very existence of healthy carriers of the virus. This populist conception of COVID's reach limited the ability of such countries to test and trace the disease. Competing narratives about the spread of the virus during a historic moment that could ill afford uncertainty resulted in a public health crisis with few precedents in modern times.

7

Chronic

Ed Cohen

What makes an illness "chronic"? When does illness begin to be chronic? Does *chronicity* refer to the unfolding of a disease process, or does it constitute a temporal convolution that might entirely change one's "lifetime"—that is, one's awareness of life as both temporal and temporary? In ancient Greek myth, Kronos (whose name *chronic* immortalizes) was the leader of the Titans and the ruler of time, especially time viewed as violent and devouring (Marini 2019, 59). The myth itself invokes a chronological concept of time in which the past overtakes and consumes the present, if not the future, such that the "cause" of the present necessarily lies "behind it" somewhere in the past. Chronological time has always governed medicine, ever since it first began to be medicine around the fifth century BCE. In part, that's because both disease and healing are processes and as such only unfold in time. They make time matter in the most material of senses. Thus, from the moment medicine entered the therapeutic marketplace 2,500 years ago, time has been of its essence. Since antiquity, medicine has promised to help us know what happens to us when we fall ill in the hope that such knowledge can reduce the time during which we suffer, if not help us recover. Indeed, medicine first defined itself as "medicine" when it distinguished itself from competing therapeutic modes (e.g., magicians, root cutters, temple priests, doctor-prophets, purifiers, drug vendors, herbalists, and the like—not to mention the gods) by insisting that its knowledge—and only its knowledge—offered the best shortcut to recovery (Holmes 2010).

Medical knowledge has thus always been "timely" by definition, as ancient physicians underscored when they invented the two technologies that still delimit medicine's domain: diagnosis and prognosis. Both of these strategies of medical knowing (*gnosis* means "knowledge" in ancient Greek, hence *diagnosis* means "by way of knowledge" and *prognosis* means "knowing in advance") situate temporality at their root insofar as the ability to predict, if not affect, future outcomes depends on a careful attending to the present moment—to what medicine still calls our "presenting problems." Of course, as part of medicine's raison d'être, diagnosis and prognosis could never be effectively separated, as the author of the Hippocratic text *Prognostic* explained more than 2,200 years ago:

> It seems to me best for a physician to try to understand things in advance. For if he knows them in advance and predicts in the presence of his patients what is happening, what has happened, and what will happen (to the extent that these things were left out of the patient's original account), the more he will be believed to know his patients' real situations, so that people will dare to place themselves in the doctor's hands. What's more, he will give the best treatment if he knows in advance what will happen on the basis of present symptoms. (W. Jones 1931, 8–9)

As this Hippocratic author reveals, from its inception in ancient Greece, temporality has always informed medicine's knowing capacity, which has in turn constituted its stock-in-trade.

The key temporal moment of medicine during antiquity was that of crisis. *Crisis* described a transitional phase in the process of a disease in which the physician had to either intervene or refrain from intervening in order to encourage its natural resolution. In Greek, *krisis* (κρίσις) means (1) judgment, decision, or separation; (2) choice, election, or interpretation; and (3) event or issue to be decided. Subsequent to the emergence of medicine, it also metonymically came to mean a turning point or sudden change in a disease. In other words, crises call for—and call forth—medical interpretation. They designate moments of urgency that demand decisiveness and judgment. This governing orientation accords with medicine's original ethos: the *med-* in *medicine* derives from an Indo-European root that means "to govern," "to judge," or "to cure" (Benveniste 1945, 5). While we might think contemporary medicine abandoned its ancient roots long ago, this early imperative nevertheless continues to guide its present practice. This is why modern medicine continues to function best in a crisis. Unfortunately, it is far less equipped to address conditions that endure over long periods of time with no easily discernable turning points—in other words, those we call "chronic."

Consider some of the terms that contemporary medicine uses to describe its levels of intervention (a.k.a. "care"): emergency, intensive, acute, palliative, rehabilitative, hospice, and occasionally preventative. While there are plenty of medical specialists who consider themselves "critical-care doctors" and "intensivists," none of them call themselves "chronicists," and there's no medical subspecialty called "chronic care." (In medical terms, chronic care would almost be an oxymoron and hence frequently gets outsourced to rehabilitation or long-term care facilities [Kaufman 2005].) As the list of its main modes of intervention suggests, modern medicine mostly continues to situate crises at the center of its financial and epistemological enterprise, and as many of us who have lived through such critical events

can attest, when we're "in crisis," medicine is often at its best.

One reason why medicine has gotten good at operating in crisis mode derives from a decisive turn in medical thinking that occurred in the middle of the nineteenth century that shifted the structuring metaphor of medicine from crisis to war. At that time, the experimental physiologist Claude Bernard definitely broke with the Galenic/Hippocratic tradition that had informed medical doctrine for the preceding two thousand years and introduced an entirely unprecedented way to think about the living organism (Canguilhem [1968] 1994, 131). Instead of imagining that an organism only exists as part of a coupling of organism and environment, as humoral medicine had held for the previous two millennia, Bernard claimed that the only scientifically relevant "environment" was the "internal environment," or as he named it, the "milieu intérieur" (Bernard [1867] 1947). This doctrine made experimental bioscience epistemologically feasible, and it continues to underwrite all the laboratory-based bioscience on which contemporary biomedicine depends. In light of his "scientific" redefinition of medicine's primary locus of concern, Bernard proposed that medicine should henceforth strive to weaponize the human organism's vital project of self-defense. Thus, he argued that medicine should aspire to provide "arms" and "weapons" in the organism's ongoing war against disease (Bernard 1865, 123).

Bernard's aspirational militarization of medicine continues to characterize modern medicine's métier, which thrives on addressing the acute. Ample evidence for this bellicose tendency appears in the multiple declarations of war that the COVID-19 pandemic evoked from politicians and physicians around the world, which underscore that medicine's default mode is military—not to mention the many other declared "wars" on cancer, heart disease, AIDS, and so on.

Unfortunately, this rhetorical call to arms does not help much when it comes to illnesses that can't be "defeated," illnesses with which we have to learn to live instead. In principle, the temporality of war is bounded by a declaration and by a cessation, and peace prevails in the intervals between periods of war. Chronic conditions confound such neat temporalizations, sometimes continuing unabated over the course of an entire life. They don't readily succumb to armed interventions, often requiring instead long periods of negotiation, détente, and if we're lucky new modes of coexistence. In such cases, *peace* cannot refer to the absence of struggle but at best refers to living well amid the struggle. While medicine obviously does recognize the persistence of "chronic diseases" as an increasingly prevalent empirical problem in most industrialized economies, especially in relation to the increasing costs of "managing" them, it might be more helpful to think about chronicity in terms of illness rather than disease—that is, in terms of what people experience rather than in terms of what medicine supposes it knows (Kleinman, Eisenberg, and Good 1978).

Distinguishing between illness and disease helps us recognize that chronic illnesses often trouble medicine's preferred narrative arc in ways that confound the very notion of disease. Many chronic conditions—autoimmune illnesses, for example—belie medicine's epistemological and financial investments in ontological theories of disease, if only because their "causes" remain steadfastly unknown and their "cures" elusive (E. Cohen 2017). Thus, in medical terms, chronic *disease* refers to conditions that medicine diagnoses as pathological but for which it cannot establish reliable plotlines or resolutions. It names conditions that disrupt medicine's capacity to create a confluence between diagnoses and prognoses (which the author of *Prognostic*, quoted earlier, proposed as medicine's key selling point

more than two millennia ago), since chronic disease does not submit to a dependable denouement. Chronic *illness*, on the other hand, refers to the experiences that those of us diagnosed with chronic diseases live through. Because there are by definition no cures for chronic illnesses, they present enduring experiences that challenge us to innovate new modes of going on living. From this perspective, what makes an illness chronic is not merely its medical irresolvability but also the fact that it disturbs our capacity to synchronize our bodily tempos and flows with the temporalities demanded by the political and economic milieux within which we live. Of course, all illness indicates a disruption of the ability to engage in activities that we consider valuable (Canguilhem [1966] 1991). That is what prompts us to seek medical attention in the first place. In the case of nonchronic and nonterminal illnesses, this temporal orientation entails "taking up an interrupted activity or at least an activity deemed equivalent by individual tastes or the social values of the milieu" as quickly as possible (119). One of the main obligations of the "sick role," according to Talcott Parsons, is to get better and return to those value-producing activities as soon as possible (1964, 312). Alas, for those of us who live with chronic conditions, such temporal resynchronizations often prove difficult, if not impossible. What makes an illness chronic, then, is not any specified pathology—since there are now a multitude of possibilities—but rather the extent to which it reveals that for us "time is out of joint" (to invoke Hamlet's observations about the "rotten" state of Denmark).

Today the list of conditions considered chronic expands rapidly with no appreciable way to define any physiological commonalities. Illnesses that were once considered death sentences—AIDS, for example—have been transformed into chronic ones. Other conditions that are considered chronic may not be medically validated as "diseases" at all (such as post-treatment Lyme syndrome, chronic fatigue, and fibromyalgia). New potentially chronic conditions appear unexpectedly, like the so-called COVID "long-haulers" (a metaphor that transforms time into space). As different as these conditions might be, however, what unites them into a common category is not only their indefinite temporal durations but also the ways they disrupt medicine's normative chronologies of disease resolution, which privilege definite endings, primarily cure or death.

Chronicity emphasizes a different understanding of what it means to be a living organism. It reminds us that as living beings, we are not things called "bodies" but rather ongoing events, transformations of matter and energy localized in time and space. We are processes, not substances. Modern medicine primarily addresses us as substantial beings whose existence can be reduced to biochemical or biophysical phenomena that are temporally specific. Of course, this can be helpful in many cases, but what persistent or indeed irreducible pathologies reveal is that our lives do not always conform to medicine's preferred temporalities. Chronic conditions thus challenge us to reimagine what we take illness to mean beyond what medicine offers. Medicine certainly has much to offer those of us whose conditions refuse tidy medical resolutions; nevertheless, chronicity's temporal convolutions call upon us to reimagine life and health beyond medicine's tidy temporal narratives.

8

Cognition
Deborah Jenson

The Latin roots of the term *cognition* pertain to knowing or recognizing. Although all world traditions engage with knowing and recognizing, use of this specific term and a related lexicon date from the medieval period (Chaney 2013). Cognition became central to Western philosophy when the seventeenth-century French philosopher René Descartes proposed that the constitution of knowledge depends on methodic doubting, an act that in turn produces an experiential consciousness of existence: cogito, ergo sum, or "I think, therefore I am" (Cottingham 1978).

Anatomical study of the brain and the nervous system in the nineteenth and twentieth centuries subsequently led to the founding of the subdiscipline of cognitive science, focused on the study of mind and mental processes. At the same time, Descartes's intellectualistic privileging of the *res cogitans* (the "thinking thing") over the *res extensa* (the "extended thing," often understood as the body) was garnering criticism for its implicit segregation of mind from body. Indeed, inquiry into how the body "matters" in cognition had taken on urgency in numerous disciplines. In 1991, the Latin American scientist Francisco Varela merged biology and Western phenomenological philosophy with world "mindful" meditative traditions, including Buddhism, in the influential model of "embodied cognition." In this concept, as his collaborator Evan Thompson later summarized, "a cognitive being's world is not a pre-specified, external realm, represented internally by its brain, but is rather a relational domain enacted or brought forth by that being in and through its mode of coupling with the environment" (E. Thompson 2016, xxvii). The body in this context serves as "an adaptively autonomous and sense-making system" in which the world is enacted or brought forth rather than processed (xxvi).

Embodied cognition arguably is foundational to the health humanities' exploration of bodily agency and rights. And yet the health humanities resist referring to the body's knowledge and meaning making as "cognition" per se. After all, cognition is featured in modern biomedical health care primarily in relation to perceived deficits, delays, disorders, and impairments and in terms of diagnostic, treatment, legal, or forensic contexts. Such assessments have long relied on measurement and scoring, using problematic tools such as intelligence testing. The related term *mental* also is linked to conventional touchstones of mental health and deviations contextualized as illness. Normative understandings of cognition are deeply problematic, and a central challenge of the health humanities is to explore critical approaches to normative ideas of cognition and their application without replicating either the ideas themselves or the ways of knowing from which they arise. The health humanities integrate artistic, performative, community-engaged, and scholarly approaches that privilege nonnormative, diverse, socially just notions of cognition. They challenge the empirical and unquestioned framing of able-bodiedness/able-mindedness as empirically measurable, natural, and meritocratic (A. Taylor and Shallish 2019; Sandel 2009). Likewise, philosophers such as Mark Fisher (2009) have uncovered the turn toward mental illness as a biochemical phenomenon unfolding simultaneously with the depoliticization of mental illness's social causes, which inform advocacy around the concept of diverse brain structures known as neurodiversity (see "Neurodiversity"). The health humanities take on the structural mechanisms of marginalization and bias that make cognition not only a descriptive concept but one that determines opportunity and status.

Embodied cognition applies not just to patients' experiences and perceptions of their health and health care but also to health-care providers' clinical performance, use of medical technologies, and educational practices. Clinical cognitive studies reveal how cognition is embodied in scenarios like the following, where a clinician-educator demonstrates a visualization of a kidney while inserting a drain and observing a patient's breathing: "First, the kidney, as visualized by Irene, is not really seen or physically contacted, but is observed on a screen and imagined when touching the patient. This 'image' of the kidney, as well as Irene's knowledge about the drain and the patient's breathing pattern, facilitates her motor activities. . . . Action and perception are interrelated and constrained by factors in the clinical environment in the moment (e.g., the patient, colleagues, instrumentation and trainee)" (van der Schaaf, Bakker, and Cate 2019, 219). The radiologist in this anecdote from the emerging field of clinical cognitive studies demonstrates what Lambros Malafouris (2013) calls "thinging," where the visualization technology serves as a kind of extension of the health-care provider's perceptual apparatus. This cognitive/sensory outsourcing to technology in health care is not fundamentally different, in such a perspective, from the disabled blind person's navigation of the environment with a cane. Malafouris cites the "blind man's stick" analogy: "Where do we draw . . . as Gregory Bateson asks, a delimiting line across the extended cognition system which determines the blind man's locomotion? At the tip of the stick? At the handle of the stick?" (Malafouris 2008, 4). Medical technologies and the use of a cognitive extender or prosthesis like the "blind man's stick" both exemplify the situated quality of cognition: "the extent to which we all depend on physical and social environments to think" (Savarese 2015, 40).

The term *neurophenomenology*, with clinical as well as philosophical meanings and applications, was also developed by Varela as an extension of the concept of embodied cognition for consideration of the body's organs as sites and structures of cognition themselves. The "gut-brain," for example, which is represented by the millions of nerve cells lining the gastrointestinal tract, communicates with the central nervous system, sending as well as receiving signals that register in shifting mental and emotional states. Here the gut microbiome, shaped by diet, is implicated in cognitive health: to some degree, you "think what you eat." Such approaches have been extended to the conceptualization of the cognitive roles of multiple organs, including the heart and blood vessels' roles in triggering or registering the sympathetic ("fight or flight") nervous system or the parasympathetic ("rest and digest") nervous system and the overall response to homeostasis (a state of equilibrium) or to disturbance or danger. Depraz and Desmidt (2019, 493) explore the cardiovascular basis of the "bodily-emotional heartsystem" as intrinsic to mammalian cognition. Organs are not the only focus of this approach: Varela also explored cognition at the cellular and systems levels through the theory of autopoiesis, or the system-wide dynamic in the organism that "allows cells to configure their own relevant world" in the self-realization of the living, as opposed to the use of external materials to create something other than self (Varela 1995, 210).

Neuroscientific research from the 1990s onward into phenomena such as the mirror neuron system, in which an individual's motor neurons fire both upon execution of action and upon observation of another's action, deepened understanding of the role of motor systems in cognition (Jenson and Iacoboni 2011). From the notion of embodied cognition, a field of "4E cognition"—embodied, embedded, enacted, and extended—further highlights cognition outside of intellectual performance (Newen, de Bruin, and Gallagher 2018).

The idea of cognition itself is, of course, culturally and linguistically specific. The French designation of "mind" employs the word used in religion for "spirit" (*esprit*), which also overlaps with the concept of "wit"—both awkward bedfellows for the brain's symbolic representation of the cerebral subject. Martinican psychiatrist Frantz Fanon and his Algerian colleague Jacques Azoulay note that cognition is a culturally contextual value: designing a social therapy program in a ward for men in Algeria required first asking, "What were the biological, moral, aesthetic, cognitive, and religious values of Muslim society?" (Fanon and Azoulay 2015b, 364). Also, because cognition is subject to the judgment and cultural values of health practitioners, it risks closed feedback loops in the understanding of cognition itself. As Fanon and Azoulay explain, the cultural framing of a statement such as "The genies [*djnoun*, or 'spirits'] are what produce madness" means one thing "on the lips of a Maghrebi Muslim, because in Algeria such belief is normal and adapted," and something else entirely "in Paris, where nothing justifies it, it does not agree with standard ideas" (Fanon and Azoulay 2015a, 384).

In considering these cultural and linguistic dimensions of cognition, we must bear in mind global health humanities critiques of the colonial history of science and medicine. The prominence of the cerebral subject in scientific and medicalized cultures can be aligned with white supremacist dominance over Global South identities and patterns of thought and knowledge, called "epistemicide" by activists in cognitive justice (Santos 2018). Caribbean and Latin American philosophers have worked to decolonize concepts of cognition by focusing on situated somatic and social perception. Jamaican philosopher Sylvia Wynter (2015), for example, proposes finding a lived and collective ritual or "ceremony" for the decolonial emancipation of knowing. Andean indigenous models of organic interdependence in *vincularidad* (relationality) provide one area of alternatives to Western cognition and participate in the communities and heritage of "decolonial thought" (Mignolo and Walsh 2018), informing paradigms of cognitive justice.

Finally, the notion of brain plasticity offers another avenue of health humanities engagement with the problem of the limited view of cognition too often held by health-care practitioners. Neuroplasticity, often celebrated as the modeling of the individual through experience and memory, can also occur as "destructive plasticity," in which through brain injury or neurodegenerative disorders, people may become other to themselves (Malabou [2009] 2012). Imagining cognition outside of developmental and linear frameworks exposes a radical contingency in the very production of selfhood delegated to the brain in cognition.

In summary, the brain is both everywhere and nowhere in health humanities today. Embodied cognition underlies current artistic and scholarly health humanities explorations of the body clinical, yet new generations of health humanities have much to gain by deepening post-Cartesian understanding of cognition in pursuit of integrated and socially equitable conceptions of body and mind.

9

Colonialism
Pratik Chakrabarti

The term *colonialism* is derived from the word *colonial*, which in turn is derived from *colony*. Each of these terms reflects the different meanings inherent in the word *colonialism*. The *Oxford English Dictionary* describes *colony* as a "settlement in a new country; a body of people who settle in a new locality, forming a community subject to or connected with their parent state" (*OED Online* 2022, "colony"). The term *colonial* signifies much more than a settlement by a foreign power; it refers to the "principle, policy, or practice" of forced occupation and exploitation of a country, its people, and its resources by another country (*OED Online* 2022, "colonialism"). The term *colonialism* has an even broader scope; it denotes a system that appears colonial, or reflects similar forms of practices or principles of exploitation, which may or may not refer to the specific historical phenomenon of colonial exploitation by European and North American counties.

The history of modern colonialism began in the sixteenth century when western European countries ventured across the Atlantic and the Indian Ocean in search of new trade routes to Asia, and from its beginnings, it structured Western medicine. Between the seventeenth and the twentieth centuries, these nations expanded their colonies in Africa, Asia, Australia, and the Americas. Colonialism defined modern medicine and medical cultures by providing new medicinal ingredients, drugs, and therapeutic practices (Chakrabarti 2014, 1–19). Colonialism also shaped the development of several specific disciplines, including race science, tropical medicine, and epidemiology.

There are two parallel trajectories in this history of colonialism and medicine. On the one hand, there is the history of the introduction of Western biomedicine in the colonies in the form of hospitals, pharmaceuticals, vaccines, epidemiological studies, and sanitary measures. Introduced primarily for European settlers and the colonial armed forces, these institutions and provisions were subsequently extended for the local population. Most of the colonial epidemic eradication or control measures, such as for malaria and smallpox, were authoritarian and heavily driven by technology, which extended the hegemony of Western biomedicine in the colonies and alienated indigenous populations from colonial health policies (Packard 2007, 150–76; Arnold 1993, 116–58). Modern hospitals and other primary health facilities were introduced in the colonies at very limited scales, often located near European settlements or commercial interests and largely inaccessible to the larger population. For example, at the time of independence (1947), India had virtually no established rural health-care system, while 90 percent of India's population lived in villages (Dutta 1955). These engendered the inequitable nature of public health facilities in several postcolonial nations. At the same time, colonial hospitals became the main sites of medical training. In India, for example, various medical colleges—such as the Madras Medical College; the Grant Medical College, Bombay; and the Lahore Medical College—taught Western biomedicine exclusively. The doctors and nurses who trained there served in various parts of the British Empire (Greenwood and Topiwala 2015).

On the other hand, the "colonial bioprospecting" (Schiebinger 2004, 73–104) of indigenous medicinal plants and therapeutic traditions led to massive transformations in European drug markets and therapeutics and subsequently contributed to the growth of Western pharmaceutical industries in the nineteenth century. From the seventeenth century, large-scale importation of drugs to western Europe from Asia and the New World transformed European medical catalogs and therapeutics, incorporating new plants, herbs, and healing traditions (R. Porter and Porter 1989). The colonial bioprospection of African medicinal herbs from the nineteenth century took place at the time of the rise of pharmaceutical industries in Europe and North America. European interest in African medicinal products and the appropriation of African ethnobotanical knowledge for modern pharmaceuticals led to the use of herbs such as the *Strophanthus*, traditionally used in Africa both as a poison and as a drug, to produce the strophanthin drug for cardiac diseases. At the same time, the colonial governments banned the use of the plant by traditional healers due to its association with poisoning (Osseo-Asare 2014).

These changes in medical practices were accompanied by major structural transformations in the colonies. The establishment of industrial mining, modern farming, plantations, and railways and the growth of new urban centers in Asia, South America, and Africa led to the clearing of forests, the building of dams, and large-scale labor migrations, causing famine, floods, epidemics, and the breakdown of traditional economic and social practices. The intervention of Western biomedicine in the colonies was part of the broader marginalization of traditional practices—including traditional medicine and institutions—and the general loss of agency. European colonial officials often misunderstood African medical practices as signs of African primitive culture and viewed them as witchcraft, magic, or superstition. They often instituted laws that banned these practices, forcing the people to act in covert and subversive modes. The attacks on traditional healers by colonial forces—such as in the suppression of Obeah in the West Indies, Shona spirit mediums in Zimbabwe, and the Aro oracle in Nigeria or the German persecution of healers in Tanganyika—were not just attempts at introducing European scientific ideas and practices but also designed to destroy their traditional political authority. The practices nevertheless survived, often as clandestine and hybrid traditions. As Africans were brought to the Caribbean and American plantations as slaves from the seventeenth century, a diverse blending of diseases, medical systems, and plant-based pharmacopoeias took place between the Old and New World. For example, in Brazil, African slaves adopted the use of indigenous medicinal plants from the Amerindians. At the same time, Africans had carried many West African plants and weeds with them, which entered the medical practices of the indigenous populations, and African healing systems often flourished in the Americas. In those processes, African-based ethnomedicine traveled to and survived in various parts of the Caribbean islands and America. Healers in Africa too incorporated New World plants and spirituality in their therapeutic corpus (Voeks 1993).

These alternative and often subversive medical practices survived in the twentieth century, and hybrid medical traditions were sustained in postcolonial Africa, imitating modern biomedicine practiced in Western-style hospitals and dispensaries, standardizing medical dosages, using technologies such as X-rays, and serving contemporary social, cultural, and economic realities (Digby and Sweet 2012). Fusions of African healing and biomedicine have continued particularly in response to HIV/AIDS (Schoepf 1992). These experiences have been essential to postcolonial alternative healing practices. Indigenous medicine in Asia and Africa engages and negotiates with contemporary themes as well as draws from colonial experiences to define the current trajectories of health humanities (O'Brien 2001; Marsland 2007).

These two historical trajectories of the expansion of Western biomedicine and the marginalization of traditional medical practices prepare us to understand how the broader remit of the term *colonialism* is particularly relevant to health humanities. As a discipline, health humanities incorporates the voices of a range of caregivers, such as allied health professionals, nurses, patients, and caretakers (Crawford et al. 2010). Colonialism provides the context to these diverse experiences of contemporary health and well-being. Immigrant doctors, nurses, and emergency respondents, often trained at the erstwhile colonial medical institutions, form a significant part of health-care services in the Global North. The history of migrant doctors and health workers of the National Health Service in Britain, for example, has been linked to the history of colonialism and postcolonial immigration (Bivins 2015). At the same time, COVID-19 has exposed the inadequate health-care infrastructure in several postcolonial nations in Asia, Africa, and South America, many of which bear the footprints of the lopsided nature of colonial public health, where large sections of rural populations have been left without primary health care.

Contemporary approaches in health humanities have recognized the significant role alternative cultural and social practices play within biomedicine. These have referred to colonialism in generating that critique of Western biomedicine as well as the search for lost and marginalized healing traditions and practices. Broadly speaking, when health humanists refer to *colonialism*, they do so to trace both the instances of marginalization and the voices of the marginalized groups within modern biomedical culture. For example, critical theory, which is a key theme in health humanities, has sought to understand critical and cultural healing, "to comprehend the cultural scripts, counternarratives, and performances that have strengthened individuals and communities and healed wounds caused by biomedicine itself" (Garden 2019, 2). In this endeavor, the colonial and postcolonial experiences of biomedicine—as marginal, deviant, and counternarrative—have been vital. These also refer to colonialism to expose the dominant and hegemonic narratives of Western biomedicine in terms of curative and preventive practices, sexuality, corporeality, and insanity. Queer theory, which critiques the dominant ideas of sexuality and gender in Western biomedicine, has identified some of the roots of these normative approaches in the history of colonialism. Colonialism provided, scholars argue, the scope to impose and practice the mainstream ideas of sexuality and race as modes of control. A particular example is HIV/AIDS in Africa, where remnants of homophobic colonial laws were adopted by postcolonial nation-states transcribing sexual and moral stigmas on the AIDS sufferers. The spread of HIV/AIDS in Africa in the 1980s was often explained by the colonial stereotypical ideologies of "unchecked, unbridled sexuality amongst indigenous Africans and amongst blacks in general" (Spurlin 2018). Such references to the history of colonialism and its legacies in postcolonial health have been formative in the establishment of the discipline of medical humanities in Africa.

The contemporary relevance of colonialism in health humanities and in modern societies is also redefining *colonialism* as a keyword. Just as Raymond Williams was captivated by changes in the word *culture* after World War II (1976, 9–11), the contemporary experiences of COVID-19 exposing the deficiencies of global public health provisions, along with the public displays of racism and xenophobic nationalism across the world, have shifted our understandings of *colonialism*. The word is now also useful to recognize contemporary corporeal

and cultural marginalization and suffering. In that context, *decolonization* has added new immediacy to understandings of colonialism. Within historical scholarship, *decolonization*, which originally referred to the political processes of withdrawal of European nations from their colonial power, has acquired significant political and cultural momentum as a category of decentering discussions on "evidence, agency, authorship, temporality, and structure" (W. Anderson 2020, 369).

Decolonization signifies the need to politicize and historicize contemporary economic, social, and cultural inequalities through the history of colonialism. Similarly, "decolonization of health" is a significant part of social activism, intellectual deliberation, and academic curriculum in health studies (London School of Hygiene & Tropical Medicine 2022). These identify and situate the structural inequalities in global health as part of the historical legacies of colonialism in histories of slavery, racism, and colonial health systems (Büyüm et al. 2020). Decolonization has provided the necessary critique of postcolonial medicine and health care that Randall Packard has shown to be otherwise lacking (2004, 97). In health humanities, decolonization and, in turn, colonialism represent contemporary health inequalities as cultural and social effects of colonialism and the urgency to "repoliticize" and "rehistoricize" health (Büyüm et al. 2020). The two terms are now inseparable from each other.

10

Compassion

Lisa Diedrich

In the introduction to the edited volume *Compassion: The Culture and Politics of an Emotion*, Lauren Berlant describes the project as "seeking to understand the concept [compassion] as *an emotion in operation*" (2004, 4). "In operation," Berlant explains, "compassion is a term denoting privilege: the sufferer is *over there*" (4). Berlant's volume explores how compassion operated culturally and politically in a particular time and place—the United States in the 1990s and early 2000s. In the volume's opening essay, also called "Compassion," literary critic Marjorie Garber offers an extensive genealogy of the word, concept, and practices of compassion. Garber's essay and Berlant's introduction historicize the term in relation to political discourse around the turn of the new millennium. Garber argues that the two most recent US presidents at that time—Bill Clinton and George W. Bush— "sought to associate themselves, at least rhetorically, with the concept of compassion" (18). She cites Clinton's "compassionate catchphrase" ("I feel your pain") and Bush's "compassionate conservatism" as attempts to operationalize compassion politically.

Neither Berlant's volume as a whole nor Garber's essay in particular addresses compassion in operation in medicine or in its allied fields, including the field of the health humanities. Nonetheless, the cultural politics of compassion and the genealogies of the concept and its multiple practices as presented in the volume are useful for looking at compassion in operation in

health care and health humanities. I will discuss two rhetorical shifts in the use of the term that might help us diagnose the condition of the health humanities and health care in late liberalism. The shifts in usage are (1) from compassion to compassion fatigue (compassion as modified by a feeling of tiredness) and (2) from care to compassionate care (compassion as added as a modifier to the practice of care). I argue that these shifts in usage are signs, or what we might call an etymological structure of feeling (R. Williams 1977), of the condition of the health humanities and/in health care in late liberalism—that is, the way we can discern forming and formative processes of health-care provision in the shifting language of compassion.

The first definition for *compassion* in the *OED* is this: "Suffering together with another, participation in suffering; fellow-feeling, sympathy" (*OED Online* 2021, "compassion"). However, this usage is now obsolete. The current use shifts the emphasis from *suffering with* another to *feeling for* or *being moved by* the suffering of another. Fellow feeling disappears from the definition and is replaced by a dichotomous and unequal relationship between the one who suffers and the one who is moved by the suffering of another—this is what Berlant highlights when she notes that "compassion is a term denoting privilege" (2004, 4). Yet even more recently, the etymology of the word moves us, paradoxically, from feeling (with or for) to an absence of feeling or "compassion fatigue," a phrase first used in the US in 1968 and defined as "apathy or indifference towards the suffering of others or to charitable causes acting on their behalf." Garber cites Susan Moeller's 1999 book *Compassion Fatigue: How the Media Sell Disease, Famine, War, and Death* as detailing the "commodification of compassion" and "its use and misuse" in the media (Berlant 2004, 19). The most frequent early use of the term referred in particular to the numbed response of people in countries with a large and seemingly sudden influx of refugees. Here, a geopolitical phenomenon becomes about the capacity (or incapacity) for individual feeling. The term was added to the definition of the word *compassion* in March 2002 and currently stands at the end of the entry (*OED Online* 2021, "compassion"), almost as if all compassion burns out, leading to compassion fatigue. Thus, compassion fatigue signals a millennial structure of feeling that has become concretized in the present moment as a willful numbness to the suffering of others. We might even go so far as to say that a Trumpian politics of cruelty is a hardened ideological formation against the social expectation of the performance of compassion. Writing at the dawn of the new millennium, Berlant seems to anticipate Trumpism as reaction formation, noting that she was "struck by an undertone accompanying the performance of compassion: that scenes of vulnerability produce a desire to withhold compassionate attachment, to be irritated by the scene of suffering in some way" (9). Considering this political shift, it seems necessary to ask, What is the work of the health humanities in the face of such cruel disregard for the suffering of others as ideology in our contemporary moment? Is compassion an adequate response to cruelty?

The other related rhetorical shift in the use of the term *compassion* that I want to address briefly is the increasingly frequent use of the phrase *compassionate care* in the present moment, especially in healthcare settings where care does not necessarily require compassion as a component of treatment. Regarding the phrase *compassionate conservative*, Garber notes that the phrase conveys "in its insistent and alliterative adjective, traces of an intrinsic uneasiness," and she asks what the alternatives might be, presciently arriving at "a *cruel* conservative" (Berlant 2004, 18) as one possible outcome. I contend that the phrase *compassionate care* similarly suggests an uneasiness about our practices of care in the current moment, and "its insistent and alliterate adjective" also brings alternatives to mind, including callous care, abstract or distracted care, cruel care, and even careless care. In the past, care could be good or bad, but when and why did we come to emphasize that our care is or should be compassionate? Doing a Google Ngram search of the phrase, we discover that this shift happened around 1980, which is also the same time that the phrase *compassion fatigue* became increasingly popularized and health care was becoming increasingly neoliberalized.

What does the rhetorical redundancy of the phrase *compassionate care* tell us about how we care now? I argue that the redundant phrase is a sign of what we might call, paraphrasing feminist anthropologist Elizabeth Povinelli, the culturalization (and depoliticization) of care in late liberalism (2011, 26). It also suggests an individualistic rather than structural approach to the problem of the delivery of good care. In an article about calls for compassionate care in the UK, Roberta E. Bivins, Stephanie Tierney, and Kate Seers note that appeals for compassionate care policies have been made "in the wake of high-profile accounts of negative health services experiences" (2017, 1023). They describe recent attempts to measure the quality and efficiency of compassionate care, a process that focuses on nurses as the individuals responsible for delivering compassionate care (or not). As an alternative to this individualistic and gendered model, Bivins, Tierney, and Seers recommend instead an approach that includes structural analysis, significant resources, and transformative leadership. They assert that "practising compassion requires a facilitating social architecture promoting norms of trust, concern and empathy, in which compassion is treated as a collective responsibility, rooted in well-defined practices across the whole range of staff roles" (1025). For me, this institutional analysis of what is required for practicing compassion, as distinct from an individual being compassionate, links to discussions about best practices in the health humanities. In *Communicative Biocapitalism*, Olivia Banner presents "a mode of analysis attuned to structures" (2017, 28) in place of an emphasis on interpersonal skills and cultural competency. Citing Jonathan M. Metzl and Helena Hansen's (2014) structural competency along with cultural competency in medical education, Banner offers a critique of the "empathy hypothesis" in operation in medical and health humanities that individuates compassion. Recall Berlant's formulation: "the sufferer is *over there*."

Like Banner's work on empathy, my work seeks to consider these shifts of compassion in operation in relation to the emergence of the health or medical humanities as a new discipline—a feeling discipline—in medicine in the late 1960s and early 1970s and the attempts to institutionalize practices of feeling in medicine in the four decades since (Diedrich 2015). I am interested in this phenomenon in relation to the emergence around the same time of the hegemony of biomedicine and evidence-based medicine. The logic of biomedicine maintains an illusion of separate spheres between science/medicine and art/feeling—that is, compassion as supplemental to rather than internal to medicine.

Thus, I argue in general that compassion has become the "disciplinary imperative" (Wiegman 2012, 53) of the health humanities. In conclusion, I offer three problematizations of the field in relation to this disciplinary imperative as a provocation for further institutional analysis of emotions in operation in medicine and health care: health humanities (1) is a spatial and temporal repository of feelings in and for medicine, (2) participates in rather than challenges the instrumentalization of care in medicine, and (3) promulgates

a negative disposition toward theory and abstraction that suggests that theory hurts. I propose an alternative that is *against* compassion not in the sense of being opposed to feeling in general and compassion in particular but in the sense of being close to and affected by feeling. Such a position helps avoid the trap of health humanities as the soft place where doctors get to feel good about themselves as feeling human beings rather than a hard place of thought about the practice of medicine.

11

Contagion

Annika Mann

For the health humanities, *contagion* arrives as a term already contested. Contagion first appears as the Latin *contagio* or *contagium*, meaning "to touch together." As a loose theory of transformational, contaminating contact, contagion has a long history of use beyond communicable disease. From about the second century BCE, these terms, along with *inficere* and *infecto*, were used across the Mediterranean to refer to a variety of phenomena that could be negative or positive; religious or folk; inter-, intra-, or extrahuman (Nutton 2000; Pelling 2001). These included the practices of animal husbandry, winemaking, and dyeing; the communication of corrupt morals; and the progress of certain diseases. Contagion more narrowly defined as a specific kind of communicable disease is more recent, at least in the West. The *Oxford English Dictionary* dates contagion as "The communication of disease from body to body by contact direct or mediate" to the early sixteenth century. This belated sense of contagion as communicable disease reflects changing conceptions of disease pathology in medieval and early modern Europe. While the Black Death (*Yersinia pestis*) decimated much of Asia, North Africa, the Middle East, and Europe during the thirteenth and fourteenth centuries, it was only during the sixteenth century that natural philosophers in Europe and England first began to theorize that certain diseases might be generated primarily by elements outside the body (Carlin 2005). During this same period, in contrast, modes of inoculation were already being practiced in the Ottoman Empire, China, and India (Needham 2000; Sudan 2016).

Debates about the proper use of *contagion* as a term for contaminating contact illustrate a range of ethical and practical cruxes in the health humanities. For during the first decades of the AIDS crisis, humanists debated whether the term ought rightly to belong to biomedicine—defined by physicians and epidemiologists. Susan Sontag (1978) argued that contagion stigmatizes those who are ill by collapsing disease and carrier. For Sontag, the job of the humanist is thus to demystify contagion and delimit its use. Other theorists pointed out that preventing the contaminating operations of metaphor by enforcing the boundary between "literal" contagions and stigmatizing language is an impossible and indeed undesirable task. Lee Edelman (1994), for example, argued that beliefs about conceptual difference and ideational purity are themselves shot through with homophobia and genocidal impulses from Plato to the present. These insights have been borne out by more recent scholarship that has illuminated just how inseparable stigmatizing narratives about contagion have been from those of medical discovery. Priscilla Wald's (2008) *Contagious* demonstrates that contagion has since at least the 1880s been understood via an "outbreak narrative," a formulaic plot that locates viruses first within foreign, dehumanized patient zeros, only to be contained by heroic epidemiologists acting in the national interest. Today, health humanities scholars continue to point out the dual, equally embodied dangers that attend deployments of the term *contagion*, whether that be the violence encouraged by Donald Trump's repeated, racist epithet "the Chinese virus" for COVID-19 (Herrera 2020) or the ways contemporary biomedicine defines diseases so as to commodify, individuate, and delegate responsibility for health (Elliott 2010).

As a term for the ability to "touch together" what should be held apart, *contagion* also affects contemporary disciplinary territories and divisions of labor. Their mingling is both an opportunity and a problem for the health humanities. Contagion frustrates attempts to separate biology or epidemiology from the study of what has been identified with culture rather than nature: language, emotion, technology, and the production of art. Hence, contagion licenses the health humanities as a field that takes that very inseparability as its origin. But contagion also causes difficulty because it is so often used to stigmatize and so useful for describing the effects of communication. Contagion has functioned as a central paradigm for theorizing how language and community formation operate in fields like sociology, anthropology, cultural studies, and postcolonial studies (O'Connor 2000; Wald 2008; P. Mitchell 2012; K. Nixon and Servitje 2016). But, as scholars of disease have noted, using contagion as a means to explain the transmission of culture risks confusing a scholar's methodology and her object of study. This confusion can erase the particularities of bodies and their ecologies (rendering all bodies, like all carriers, the same) and obfuscate the structures of power through which contagion always operates and simultaneously reveals. For, as plague writers from Thucydides to Defoe have attested and as the following example aims to illustrate, contagion highlights the normally invisible relations that make up our shared worlds—from the movement and containment of certain bodies, to the quality of air, to the mechanisms of data collection and dissemination. In so doing, contagion renders visible the means by which we are already intimately connected to one another. That sudden visibility is provoking. For the health humanities, that provocation might be an opportunity to contest and remake unjust systems.

Contagion's ability to disrupt systems of power might best be exemplified by the Enlightenment, when taxonomy ruled supreme. During the seventeenth and eighteenth centuries, writers in western Europe and what would become Great Britain aimed to create enduring hierarchies of difference that would license and bring order to their nation's growing empires. The revaluation of contagion forms part of this attempt, as natural philosophers, experimentalists, and physicians named and defined its operations more rigorously than before. In England and Scotland, contagion was frequently understood via the experimental work of chemist Robert Boyle: as dangerously invisible yet material corpuscles that could spread by either immediate or mediated contact, including touch, breath, saliva, clothing or other soft objects, and general atmosphere. But though its means of spread were various, contagion was usually posited to arise first from either crowded, unventilated spaces or the operation of heat on stagnant water, especially that containing rotting vegetable or animal matter. As such, contagion was placed within the period's environmental medicine, in which the health and sickness of populations was argued to be primarily determined by the impact of climate, with hot, moist climates the most dangerous and damaging (Jordanova 1978; R. Porter 1995; Cantor 2002). Throughout the eighteenth century, university-trained physicians circulated a hierarchical climatography that habitually argued contagious diseases move from east and south to west and north—from what Robert Markley (2010, 107) has termed *biohazards* like the West Indies and India to the metropole—via the cramped holds of ships (Golinski 2007; Janković 2010).

The taxonomies of the seventeenth and eighteenth centuries may not have wholly hardened into claims of essential racial or sexual difference, yet environmental medicine operated hand in glove with imperial extraction, tying the health and sickness of populations most directly to geography. These hierarchies were bolstered by a "science of man" that aligned permeability—vulnerability to contagion—with whiteness and progress (H. Thompson 2016; Hogarth 2017; Seth 2018; Schuller and Gill-Peterson 2020). Physicians and philosophers like John Locke, David Hume, and Adam Smith regularly argued that white, upper-class bodies were more permeable and sensitive. Further, they made the human body's sensitivity, its capacity to be moved, central to the production of knowledge. For Hume in particular, the passions of others operate as communicable contagions that move the self. He writes, "Hatred, resentment, esteem, love, courage, mirth and melancholy; all these passions I feel more from communication than from my own natural temper and disposition" (1739, 72). He also says, "Emotions disturb and displease us: we suffer by contagion" ([1751] 1998, 64). But these affective contagions, even if displeasing, are productive because they prompt the voluntary operations of the mind. Ultimately, for these entwined Enlightenment projects—environmental medicine, the science of man, colonization, and the slave trade—vulnerability to contagion, rather than impermeability, forms the starting place for improvement, differentiating the civilizable human from the not.

And yet even as contagion was deployed as a means to mark out geographic difference and bodily superiority on behalf of Western physicians and philosophers, contagious phenomena continued to reveal connections across orders intended by those authors to remain distinct, particularly metropole and colony and British self and foreign other. For example, fears of plague led to the 1721 passage of the Quarantine Act in England, which allowed for cordon sanitaires around any town thought to be infectious and more strictly regulated quarantines for vessels and their contents (including crew) returning from countries thought infectious (M. Healy 2003). Yet, as Travis Chi Wing Lau (2016) has argued, even as those boundary-enforcing measures were being passed, medical experimentation suggested that the health of the British state came from its incorporation of foreign bodies. Encouraged by Lady Mary Wortley Montagu, physicians in 1721 conducted the Royal Experiment, infecting six inmates of Newgate Prison with smallpox in exchange for their release, or death (all survived). For Lau, this first clinical trial and the debates that followed highlighted how British health could be generated from foreign technology and foreign matter, as the self is best healed by incorporating, rather than policing, the other. Thus, if fears of contagion originating outside England prompted procedures of identification and restriction, the Royal Experiment encouraged instead technologies of quantification and inoculation, designed to increase the health of certain populations (Runsock 2002).

Contagion during the seventeenth and eighteenth centuries thus incited what Foucault has termed both *disciplinary powers* and *biopower* on behalf of the state (Foucault 2003). But, importantly for the health humanities, contagion also occasionally upended professional and aesthetic hierarchies by licensing new and radical interpretations of the world. *Contagion*, as an infectious corpuscle that might heal or a communicable passion conjured first by one's imagination, traversed minds and bodies, material and immaterial realms (Shuttleton 2007; A. Mann 2018). Those crossings offered opportunities for persons up and down the social scale, including radicals, Methodist preachers, Grub Street writers, women writers, and Quakers, who deployed contagion so as to claim for themselves the capacity to produce productive, healthful infections of the body, the soul, or even the body politic (McDowell 1998; M. Anderson 2015). These writers did so via recipe books that promoted alternative therapies and artistic productions meant to incite and inflame, as well as in essays, manifestos, and philosophical treatises. Erupting most virulently during the Great Plague of 1665 and the period of French and Haitian revolutions, these writings took contagion as the opportunity to propose new political systems—like theodicies—that were often argued to begin as contagion but subsequently bring about cure (Hammill 2010; Barney and Schrek 2010).

Ultimately, what this historical discussion aims to illustrate are the difficulties and risks of using contagion as a keyword in the health humanities. As metaphor, virus, or feeling, contagion brings pain, suffering, and death; it reveals but also instantiates inequity. Contagion incites attempts to further confine and police, to further systematize eugenic policies that guarantee the health of the few. But the possibility remains that the connections contagion brings to visibility and the complex responses it provokes can germinate new understandings of risk, new communities of care, and new social organizations.

12

Creativity

Michael Barthman and Jay Baruch

The budding medical student examines the patient, exploring every symptom and recording every detail. The abdomen is . . . kind of tender? The story is just as ambiguous. The patient's account disorients her: he dodges questions, forgets answers, and at times, prickles. The patient says too much or too little. Nothing lines up. Each piece of information generates more uncertainty. Being a doctor seemed like it would depend on commanding a vast knowledge. She is finding that in the practice of medicine, knowledge alone is inadequate.

Taking care of patients necessitates creativity, as physicians have long known. The word traces its etymological roots to the Latin verb *creare*: to bring something forth or to make or produce. The word *creativity* had a more religious meaning—one connected to divine creation—until the second half of the twentieth century, when it evolved to refer to the *imagination* and new ways of knowing the world (Kristeller 1983; R. Williams 1976). For centuries, doctors have recognized the need for creative thinking beyond observation and empirical data alone to make sense of ambiguous or difficult problems in research and care (Altschuler 2018). Apollo is, after all, god of both medicine and poetry. Contemporary poet Dean Young (2010, 14) echoes past understanding, describing imagination as "what we appeal to and rely on when our empirical data has proved insufficient to the case."

Today definitions for creativity include elements of originality and value, the act of bringing something into the world that's original and appropriately useful given the constraints of a task (*OED Online* 2021, "creativity"). Creativity is also making order out of chaos and finding unexpected connections. For us, imagination finds purchase in the world as creativity.

Despite the appearance that medicine is solely a data-driven field, our student discovers that a physician is lucky when empirical data alone can guide her. Clinical medicine requires physicians to be responsive to unique patients and dynamic situations. Critical choices are made in the process of gathering and interpreting subjective and objective clinical evidence. Creativity might go unrecognized, but it is fundamental to the practice of caring for others.

Ambiguity and Uncertainty Necessitate Creativity

While medicine claims to be an evidence-based practice where each clinical decision is supported by methodologically rigorous research, the reality is that ambiguity and uncertainty remain the norm, which is why creativity is essential to medical practice (Luther and Crandall 2011). Ambiguity means inexactness, that which is not explicitly defined. Uncertainty applies to situations where information is unreliable, unknown, or difficult to predict (Stevenson and Lindberg 2010). Navigating these inherent and often unacknowledged conditions of clinical medicine requires shrewd and adaptable thinking.

In 1989, Jerome Kassirer, former *New England Journal of Medicine* editor, wrote, "Absolute certainty in diagnosis is unattainable, no matter how much information we gather, how many observations we make, or how many tests we perform" (1989, 1489). It is unsurprising this is detrimental to patient care. Physicians unable to tolerate uncertainty are prone to excessive diagnostic testing, which, in turn, puts patients at risk for adverse events

(Simpkin and Schwartzstein 2016). They're less likely to include uncertainty in conversations with patients or to engage in shared decision-making (Politi and Légaré 2010). An inability to tolerate uncertainty and ambiguity is harmful to the clinician and associated with psychological distress in medical students (Hancock and Mattick 2020; Lally and Cantillon 2014).

In reality, certainty cannot be bestowed, nor can students or health-care practitioners be rescued from ambiguity. A healthier approach is to treat uncertainty as a starting point for inquiry. Mark Doty's (2010) remark about the process of writing applies equally to clinical care: "In any process of inquiry, our uncertainty is our ally; it's a good thing for a poet, being in a state of not-knowing. . . . The longer we can stay in the state of uncertainty, of unfolding possibility, the better." Creativity provides footing to push beyond what is known to what is possible.

Medicine Is a Creative Act

Consider creativity as the use of imagination to bring something meaningful and novel into the world. Just as a person seeks to make original, evocative paintings or poems, one seeks diagnoses, prognoses, treatments, and connection. Each attempt informs the next, drawing attention to new details, shaping sensibilities, and inspiring fresh approaches. This iterative process, common to any creative endeavor, is *practice*.

As in artistic practice, problems and solutions propel medical practice. Sometimes the goal is clear, but how to achieve it is not. A diagnosis or solution may be apparent, but the path to reach it is uncertain. Other times, the diagnostic workup is obvious, but the final diagnosis is not. This is unsettling for physicians who are trained to expect concreteness or rely only on deductive reasoning. Still, the physician is left to deliver their best assessment and plan. Embracing creativity in practice can equip a physician for these situations. The creativity of practice is learned primarily by exposure to senior practitioners, though deliberate instruction in thinking differently is finding inroads in medical education (Helmich et al. 2018; Auerbach and Baruch 2012; Liou et al. 2016; Eichbaum 2014; Kumagai and Wear 2014; Schaff, Isken, and Tager 2011).

Self-compassion and resilience accompany a deeper understanding of creativity in practice. Practice does not make perfect—it makes better. A constraint implies a form of restriction or limitation. While constraints can be troubling, creativity helps us approach them as inspiration, a way to shake off the familiar and force new connections. A poet writes in the parameters of a *ghazal*. A musician plays within a key. Physicians abide by the wishes of patients. They also practice with limited time, hospital beds, medications, blood products, and staff. A physician may be forced to choose who does or does not receive these resources. Deeper comfort with creativity's role in medicine lets a physician embrace constraints as formative.

However, medicine isn't puzzle solving; it's constructing meaning from messiness. Even the best research studies are interpreted and applied to individual patients. Each is a complex character in a narrative driven by hopes, fears, responsibilities, and struggles. Each ailing body is tangled in a unique web of social, economic, and relationship challenges. Tod Chambers (1999) proposes that storytelling doesn't simply recount events; it produces knowledge and shapes experience (see "Harm" and "Narrative"). Practitioners must think with stories.

But which details are relevant in a patient's story? What is the patient saying? What's left out? What vulnerabilities—embarrassing or frightening details— shape the story? Patients work through meaning in tandem with the clinician. In the face of uncertainty and ambiguity, the best clinicians apply their experience, know-how, and creativity. Still, too often physicians dismiss symptoms that don't line up with biomedical causes (Seaburn et al. 2005). When this happens, they're not building understanding through creativity but listening with a particular end in mind.

When faced with uncertainty, clinicians often shut down creativity, searching for more fitting information or forcing misfit data into a recognizable diagnosis. The opportunity to think openly and become aware of the choices we make is a powerful function of creativity in medical education (Baruch 2017). Physicians can and should be trained for conditions of ambiguity and uncertainty (Helmich et al. 2018). Medical education can prepare students by deploying them into the clinical space earlier and using arts-based practices. The purpose isn't to turn clinicians into artists but to cultivate the methods and habits of creatives who are skilled at framing problems differently. This approach forges opportunities for clinician-educators to bridge creative thinking and medical practice (Auerbach and Baruch 2012; Liou et al. 2016; Schaff, Isken, and Tager 2011). This type of curriculum necessitates an intentional focus on how we think (Eichbaum 2014).

Creativity Is an Inclusive and Emergent Act

Creativity is an *inclusive* act. One's experience and knowledge are invited by the imagination to create a new mode of understanding and doing. For example, a person brings her pertinent knowledge (interview questions, exam maneuvers, science, and clinical evidence) into a task like caring for a patient and invigorates it with her broader knowledge and experience (whether or not, at first, it seems to apply). The result can be a poem, a diagnosis of interpersonal violence from a series of vague medical complaints, a song, comfort amid a grave illness where physical complaints hide loneliness, or even a well-timed joke. The inclusive nature of creativity is vital to a physician's ability to adapt to unique patients and situations. Physicians do this through improvisation, which architect Kyna Leski (2015, xvii) describes as necessary "in any situation without a plan, script, or map, and when you find yourself in the unfamiliar. Improvisation is needed in a crisis when on the spot . . . decisions are made and actions taken." To leverage creativity, we have to realize its function on a practical level in medical practice, which can be achieved only if we understand its inclusive and emergent nature.

The emergent nature of creativity is its most extraordinary quality, when mundane ingredients jolt to life as something greater than what they are. Most people have held an instrument and know that even with instruction in the mechanics of playing, rarely can music be made on the first go. Given time, though, something special occurs: music. This is what we mean by an *emergent* act. Creativity makes the practice of clinical medicine emergent. Clinical medicine is not just knowledge and checklists. In a few years, revisit the student we first introduced. You will find her knowledge and skills have coalesced into a comfort with messiness and willingness to accompany patients into difficult experiences. The whole that emerges is a unique way of being, connecting, and caring for patients that exceeds what is expected from the constituent parts. It isn't always perfect, but it is better than mechanistic thinking alone. Sometimes, it's a diagnosis. Often, it's an assessment and plan that doesn't necessarily provide answers but dignifies the patient with a thoughtful and caring encounter.

From Creativity Emerges Connection

Our creativity arises from our environment and those around us. Dean Young explains, "I always tell my students not to worry about originality; just try to copy the manners and musics of the various, the more various the better, poetries you love: your originality will come from your inability to copy well: YOUR GENIUS IS YOUR ERROR" (2010, 48). Our creativity is a collage of those who came before and shapes those who come with us and after us. We are made better by those who work alongside us.

The inclusive and emergent nature of creativity opens the physician to recognizing more and different meanings in patients' experiences, which has the makings of connection. Acknowledgment of another person's experience as having meaning preempts the bias and bigotry that divide people into arbitrary categories—and it is rooted in creativity. For a physician, few faculties are more valuable than the ability to honor the meaning of a patient's experience, regardless of how incomprehensible or unfamiliar it might be. The opportunity to come into close proximity with our thinking process and to train our minds to work more openly is a powerful function of the arts and creativity. For medical education, this requires a reconceptualization of the traditional educational model to include medical disciplines, humanities scholars, artists, and designers (Baruch 2017).

This connection between the doctor's understanding and the patient's is arguably the most powerful thing to emerge from the practice of clinical medicine. It is the bedrock of empathy. In no other field is empathy more necessary than for the patient and physician. To return to Dean Young, "THE HIGHEST ACCOMPLISHMENT OF HUMAN CONSCIOUSNESS IS THE IMAGINATION AND THE HIGHEST ACCOMPLISHMENT OF THE IMAGINATION IS EMPATHY" (2010, 14).

13

Data
Kirsten Ostherr

Data is the plural form of *datum*, a noun that refers broadly to "an item of (chiefly numerical) information, esp. one obtained by scientific work, a number of which are typically collected together for reference, analysis, or calculation" (*OED Online* 2021, "datum"). *Data* is also widely used in the context of computing to designate "quantities, characters, or symbols on which operations are performed by a computer, considered collectively. Also (in non-technical contexts): information in digital form" (*OED Online* 2021, "data"). In these two uses of *data*, we find a cluster of entangled connotations arising from the intersections of scientific work, quantification, and computation, which shape the meaning of this term for the field of medical and health humanities.

A defining epistemological distinction between the practice of medicine and the scholarly field of medical humanities lies in the divergent forms of evidence and interpretive methods used for research in these domains. While the phrase *the art of medicine* has historically sought to capture an intangible aspect of doctoring that relies more on clinical intuition than on scientific training, various branches of medicine have sought to define themselves as scientific undertakings for centuries, especially since the late nineteenth century (Bynum 1994; J. Warner 1995). In contrast to the art of medicine, the science of medicine has sought to develop systematic methods that produce quantitative data to establish causal relationships that guide diagnosis and treatment. The increasing use of computational methods since World War II further solidified the role of data across all fields of medical practice. The emergence of the randomized controlled trial as the gold standard for "evidence-based medicine" in the late twentieth century enshrined the centrality of data to the science of medicine (see "Evidence").

Data thus functions as the privileged form of evidence for medical knowledge creation, while for the health humanities, that role has most consistently been filled by *narrative* (see "Narrative"). In the presumed data-narrative dichotomy, several important attributes emerge. Data in medicine is assumed to be objective, neutral, standardized, precise, replicable, subject to quantitative analysis, and generalizable on a population scale. Narrative is considered to be subjective, situated, individualized, ambiguous, unique, subject to qualitative analysis, and nongeneralizable, drawn from a single case or a collection of singular cases. In this formulation, data is a building block of science, while narrative is not (Bleakley 2005). Thus, the patient's story may hold important clues to the history and likely trajectory of a disease, but it is rarely incorporated into the medical record (beyond minimal fragments) or in clinical trials.

A major contribution of health humanities has been a critique of the data-narrative dichotomy. As health humanities scholars and others have demonstrated, commonalities between data and narrative include how they are structured by contextual specificity and social construction as well as the role of interpretation in making both forms of evidence meaningful. While illuminating how quantitative data are themselves the products of situated values and priorities in scientific research and technology development, critiques of this dichotomy also highlight how data function in medical and health contexts to validate normative perspectives and concerns and marginalize or pathologize others (Gilman 1985; Benjamin 2019b).

Nevertheless, two recent developments have entrenched the role of *data* as the preeminent form of medical evidence and as a critical site for humanities engagement. First, the adoption of electronic health records (EHRs) by US clinical practices dramatically increased because of financial incentives offered by the HITECH Act of 2008 (Adler-Milstein and Jha 2017). This shift led to the digitization of patient records, which rendered formerly handwritten, analogue notes into the form of data and reduced the availability of unstructured narrative documentation. EHRs played an important role in constructing patients as *data subjects*, fully available for computational analysis and intervention. Health humanities researchers have analyzed the implications of this shift, as EHRs fragment the patient's illness narrative, dehumanize the clinical encounter, and expose patient data to privacy breaches and exploitation by third-party data brokers (Ebeling 2016; Tanner 2017).

Second, around 2010, *big data* became a keyword for a phenomenon shaping both the business and the aspirations of health care. The availability of extremely large health and medical data sets led to the emergence of new fields of research and new models of patient care, including personalized and precision medicine (see "Precision") that were built upon computational approaches to health. While the term *big data* had been used since the 1990s, it entered the popular lexicon with the publication of Mayer-Schönberger and Cukier's eponymous book in 2013. Soon thereafter, *big data* and the resulting *data-driven medicine* (Nigam Shah and Tenenbaum 2012) began to displace *evidence-based medicine* as the premiere signifier of rigorous, research-based, quantitative decision-making for diagnosis and treatment of patients. In recognition of the growing body of research in this field, *big data* became a Medical Subject Headings (MeSH) term in 2019, with its scope defined as "extremely large amounts of data which require rapid and often complex computational analyses to reveal patterns, trends, and associations, relating to various facets of human and non-human entities" (US National Library of Medicine 2019).

The emergence of big data was facilitated both by the widespread adoption of EHRs in medical practices and by the development of high-speed mobile web technologies that expanded the consumer market for smartphones (Ross, Wei, and Ohno-Machado 2014; Purswani et al. 2019). Personal smartphone use provided vast quantities of data to app developers, internet service providers, and cloud storage vendors that facilitate digital "signal traffic" (Parks and Starosielski 2015). The notion of a digital (or quantified) "self" emerged through these practices, lending credence to the idea that the social and behavioral data produced through the activities of twenty-first-century daily life might contain health-relevant insights (Neff and Nafus 2016). The practices that enabled the perpetual generation of *big data* have come to be understood as "datafication," or "rendering into data aspects of the world not previously quantified" (Kennedy, Poell, and van Dijck 2015, 1). This development has meant that aspects of illness experience that may previously have been understood as comprehensible only through narrative are now being presented as quantitative data. The "datafication of clinical and self-care practices" resulting from widespread personal tracking of behavior has produced asymmetrical power relations, as governments, credit rating agencies, insurance companies, and consumer technology companies collect and mine those data (Ruckenstein and Schüll 2017). In this exchange economy, *data* has become a commodity ripe for exploitation and corporate profit.

Marketers of self-tracking devices (step counters, heart rate monitors, sleep trackers, etc.) claim to democratize and personalize access to health by giving individuals greater control over their own health data. Yet doing so requires that users share extensive personal information with the third parties who provide the apps, devices, and analytics that capture, store, and interpret the data. When these data exchanges occur in medical settings, laws such as HIPAA and the Common Rule are in place to limit exposure of personal health information (PHI) and protect the patient's privacy (although EHR data remains vulnerable to exploitation, even with these policies in place; G. Cohen and Mello 2018). In contrast, technology companies are not subject to any comprehensive data privacy law that would restrict their dealings with users' PHI, with some exceptions due to Europe's General Data Protection Regulation and California's Consumer Privacy Act (Price et al. 2019). Consumers must agree to the terms of use that, in turn, allow technology companies to mine users' data. These contrasting scenarios of health data regulation in clinical and metaclinical settings (Ostherr 2020b) raise significant ethical concerns due to the lack of uniformity around the treatment of data sharing, privacy, and consent (Ostherr et al. 2017; Zook et al. 2017). Moreover, health humanities researchers have warned that this framing of data-enabled patient autonomy lends itself to a neoliberal logic of individual accountability that misdirects responsibility for the effects of systemic and structural factors leading to poor health outcomes (Lupton 2013).

The issues of privacy related to the expanded traffic in health data have led some researchers to utilize the term *dataveillance* to describe "the monitoring of citizens on the basis of their online data" (van Dijck 2014, 205). A critical distinction between *surveillance* and *dataveillance* is the emphasis on ubiquitous, continual tracking of all digital network activity for potential future exploitation. As technology companies become more involved in health care, their vast data sets of consumer activity, generated through practices of dataveillance, are mined for the purpose of predicting patients' future health risk profiles (Price and Cohen 2019). These predictions tend to replicate existing patterns of bias and inequality in health care, treating the social determinants of health—such as race, class, residential zip code, education, and other types of data—as proxies for health (Obermeyer et al. 2019). For the field of health humanities, the emergence of health dataveillance underscores a shift away from the ontological primacy of the patient's health narrative. Under conditions of dataveillance, "what your data body says about you is more real than what you say about yourself" (Critical Art Ensemble, quoted in Raley 2013, 121).

The *data self* that results from health datafication may bear little relation to a patient's narrative self, yet this data-driven health identity now plays an outsized role in shaping many patients' encounters with healthcare systems. Critiques of the influence of the data paradigm in medicine have highlighted the absence of contextual nuance when only measurements amenable to quantified sensing are included in diagnosis and treatment. As Lisa Gitelman has observed, "When phenomena are variously reduced to data, they are divided and classified, processes that work to obscure . . . ambiguity, conflict, and contradiction" (2015, 172). Overreliance on data paradigms can likewise further atrophy necessary clinical skills such as "tolerance of ambiguity." In response, health humanists have offered narrative competence to cultivate this essential skill (Charon 2006; Baruch 2013).

Yet the overall trajectory of health care points toward increased use of data-driven tools such as predictive algorithms, artificial intelligence systems, precision medicine, and patient navigation bots that privilege quantitative interpretation of health and illness data over narrative framings that better negotiate the ambiguities of patient experiences. Future health humanities contributions should include developing new research methodologies dedicated to examining the intersections of data and narratives and more humanities-based research on the development of natural language processing tools for analyzing unstructured health narratives (Zolnoori et al. 2019). Likewise, we must evaluate the social and ethical implications of using artificial intelligence in patient care (Ostherr 2020a). Finally, health humanities must contribute more robustly to the design and development of digital health technologies such as smartphone apps and wearable devices and collaborate with legal scholars seeking to influence the emerging regulatory landscape around health data privacy and sharing.

14

Death
Maura Spiegel

Death can awaken us to the ways we, as individuals and as a culture, create meaning. The health humanities gives practitioners a context in which to locate or rediscover meaning and deepens our capacity to approach end-of-life issues with dying persons and their families with alertness and sensitivity to individual and cultural dynamics. It offers clinicians opportunities for reckoning with guilt and feelings of failure that can accompany the unpreventable losses and for honoring and grieving the dead. Reckoning with historical and current racial and caste inequities in life expectancy can move clinicians to work for change.

In the face of death, the health humanities, like ritual, has the potential to restore a sense of human connection and meaning. In some sense, the health humanities returns death to medicine.

Medicalization of Death

Death, from Old English *deaþ*, which in turn came from Germanic *dauthuz*, is a cognate with Old Frisian *dāth*, *dād*, *dāt*; Old Dutch *dōth*; Old High German *tōd*; Old Icelandic *dauðr*; Old Swedish *döþer*, *döþe*; and Old Danish *døth* (*OED Online* 2022, "death").

The word *death*, meaning the permanent cessation of life, has remained constant across borders and over time, at least among Euro-American cultures. Its medical definition, however, continues to evolve. For much of Western history, death was determined by the cessation of the heartbeat. Following the development of artificial respirators and the early success of heart transplantation, a 1968 Harvard report urged a new medical definition of death: brain death, for unconscious respirator-dependent patients with irreversible brain stem damage ("Definition of Irreversible Coma" 1968, 339). Brain death was eventually accepted across the US, clearing the way for organ transplantation from persons sustained by artificial means deemed dead by brain stem criteria. The concept of brain death remains controversial, however, with groups including Native Americans, evangelical Protestants, and Orthodox Jews rejecting it on religious grounds. Since organs designated for transplantation can now remain viable outside the body for longer periods, medicine may revert to the heart-lung definition of death.

Medicine's confidence in its ability to forestall death has grown with the proliferation of machines and medicines. Invasive procedures can become the default as physicians face dilemmas of discontinuing life-sustaining treatments or interventions. For doctors, fear of legal repercussions, time constraints, and institutional culture can play a part in prolonging a life, along with family pressure, guilt, or fear of failure.

Hospitals' institutional routines often frame a patient's final days. As death approaches, physicians who have run out of treatment options absent themselves. As Sandra Gilbert puts it, doctors "put on their roller skates" (2006, 192), and patients and families often experience a sense of abandonment. These patterns take a toll on doctors too. Because most hospital deaths occur at night, the protocols around death are performed by doctors in procedural isolation: calling the code, telephoning the family, and filling out the death certificate. Some argue that the lack of ritual and sense of failure contribute to physician burnout.

"I learned about a lot of things in medical school, but mortality wasn't one of them," writes Atul Gawande.

"The way we saw it—and the way our professors saw it—the purpose of medical schooling was to teach us how to save lives, not how to tend to their demise" (2014, 1). Studies show a need and desire among medical students and trainees for further training in end-of-life care. They recognize the special obligation to individualize care; to attend to patient and family preferences, values, beliefs, and cultures; and to create a process of shared decision-making.

Health humanities has made some strides toward intervening in how hospital deaths are managed, facilitating the close reading of literary texts with the aim, in part, of helping clinicians turn their focus back to their own current practices and norms with a critical eye. Gawande shows how this can help. He recalls reading Tolstoy's *The Death of Ivan Ilyich* as a medical student and noting that at the time he and his classmates did not connect it in any way to their own experiences; they saw it as written in a "primitive time" with little reference to the end-of-life practices of contemporary health care (2014, 6). Gawande's understanding changed as an intern, when, tending to a patient nearing death, he opted for an eight-hour surgery that successfully removed a tumor but led to a grievous ICU death days later. All the doctors on this case—oncologists, radiation therapists, and surgeons—had understood for months that their patient would die of his cancer, but Gawande says, "We could never bring ourselves to discuss the larger truth about his condition or the ultimate limits of our capabilities, let alone what might matter most to him as he neared the end of his life. . . . We offered no acknowledgment or comfort or guidance" (6–7). Reconsidering Tolstoy's story with more experience—and more attentively—Gawande reflects, "We did little better than Ivan Ilyich's primitive nineteenth-century doctors—worse, actually, given the new forms of physical torture we'd inflicted on our patient" (7). Richard

Selzer likewise observes, "It will do your patients no harm to have their doctor feel fraternal about dying" (1982, 200).

The shift within health care from paternalistic to shared decision-making has expanded the bioethical principle of patient autonomy; in addition to providing sufficient information before obtaining consent for treatment, the principle now includes telling patients the truth about their diagnoses and prognoses. Seeking to protect their loved ones, family members might plead with a doctor not to disclose a dire prognosis, putting the clinician in a difficult position. Here again, health humanities has a role to play in preparing clinicians for end-of-life discussions, developing the skills of remaining present, listening closely, responding to a patient's values, recognizing that a patient's information preferences can be ambivalent, and creating a shared sense of trust. These discussions do not call for "truth dumping," which Willard Gaylin calls a "derogation of the complexity of human relationships" (Harden 1982). Neither, however, should clinicians avoid end-of-life discussions that can postpone palliative care until only the last few hours or days of life.

Medicine is slowly shifting from prolonging life by any means to foregrounding quality of life. The concept of the "good death" is not universal but deeply contextual. For those wishing for a home death, for example, end-of-life doulas supplement medical care. The modern hospice, which began in the 1960s, and, more recently, palliative care both aim to meet physical, emotional, and sometimes social and spiritual needs.

Amid a growing concern that death has been outsourced to medicine, a scattershot movement has arisen to encourage people to confront the inevitable, to normalize it, to share fears and philosophies, to speak openly about how we end our lives, and to plan for it. Informal "death dinners" and "death cafés" have begun to sprout up around the world. They address questions about do not resuscitate (DNR) orders and other end-of-life preferences. Many believe such conversations are salutary; one's views about how to live should determine how one dies.

These conversations include the topic of "medically assisted dying" or "physician-assisted suicide," which has long been a point of contention. US proponents of legalization prefer the former term, calling the latter term misleading in that the person in the process of dying is seeking not to end an open-ended life span but to find dignity in imminent death. Arguments in favor of legalization cite respect for patient autonomy and relief of suffering. Those opposing fret over a slippery slope—the possibility of "suicide contagion"—and concern for patients suffering from depression. Many disability activists oppose the practice on the grounds that physicians—as gatekeepers—can misjudge quality of life. In 1997, the US Supreme Court ruled that there is no constitutionally protected right to die; they left the decision to the states. Nine states and the District of Columbia have decriminalized or legalized the right to die.

Death is also increasingly medicalized through the use of cadavers in contemporary US medical education. While a central practice in Western anatomy instruction, acquiring bodies has always been a challenge. In the eighteenth and nineteenth centuries, human dissection itself was frowned upon and in many places illegal (Garment et al. 2007, 1000–1005). Officially, it had been almost exclusively limited to executed criminals, viewed as added punishment, but it was an open secret that "resurrection men" stole bodies from fresh graves to sell to medical schools. In many places, the theft of the body was not itself a crime, but the public was often horrified. In 1788, a "Doctors' Riot" broke out in New York City, where doctors and King's College (later Columbia University) medical students were dragged into the street to answer for the stolen bodies (Hulkower 2011, 24). By the mid-nineteenth century, most US medical schools followed French educational practices, requiring a course in anatomy, which increased the demand for cadavers. Race and poverty typically determined which bodies ended up on dissecting tables. The bodies of Black people, many of whom had been enslaved, were used, and in the nineteenth and twentieth centuries, white medical students sent postcards of themselves posing with Black corpses propped in undignified positions. To avoid some of these abuses, states offered all unclaimed bodies, mostly from almshouses and prisons, to medical schools (Hulkower 2011, 25). In 1912, to address the stigma of dissection, two hundred New York physicians publicly pledged to donate their own remains.

Today medical schools use personally donated cadavers, and more prestigious schools receive them in greater numbers. At many schools, memorial services are held for the donors, and sometimes remains are returned to families for burial. Although virtual cadavers are used in some medical education, dissection of a human body remains an initiating rite of passage.

Death, Ritual, and Health Humanities

Mortuary practices, in their great variety throughout history and around the world, carry an outsize importance in tracing the emergence of human uniqueness; anthropologists associate them with the very foundations of the distinctly human symbolic order (Kujit 2008, 171–97). Customs and procedures for tending and disposing of the dead have taken many shapes in human history, from the dismemberment of the dangerous dead to propitiation of deceased royalty with richly appointed tombs containing people and goods for use in the next world. With the rise of Judaism, Christianity, and Islam, simpler burial customs arose for even the high and mighty, with graves typically marked by a headstone with a simple inscription.

Across the globe, funerary rites differ dramatically. Buddhists in Tibet and Mongolia practice sky burials, in which the body is placed where vultures can consume it. In the United States, churchyard burials and family gravesites were replaced in the nineteenth century with sprawling parklike cemeteries. Embalming and open-casket funerals came into vogue at the time of the Civil War and with it a lucrative funeral industry. In place of cremation, which has an outsized carbon footprint, a growing movement in the US is promoting "green burials," placing the shrouded body in the soil directly so as not to inhibit decomposition. At the other extreme are "space burials," with options including having your ashes orbit the earth or launched into deep space. Placed in the ground, laid in a tomb, deposited in outer space, or burned on a pyre, mortuary practice marks for family and community the final transfer of the body to another state of being.

The ritualized handling of the dead and the shared acknowledgment of loss are missing from the medical sphere. One Harvard physician proposed that a bell should sound throughout the hospital whenever a patient has died.

Health-care delivery for people nearing the end of life in the United States has changed significantly in the past two decades because of increasing numbers of elderly Americans, structural barriers in access to care, and a fragmented health-care system. As medical trainees continue to report feeling underprepared to navigate end-of-life issues or to manage their own feelings about death and dying, biomedicine is turning more and more to the global repository of historical, contextual, and creative knowledge and skill that reside in the humanistic disciplines.

The health humanities cultivates a critical, historically and culturally contextualized engagement with the subjects of death. It equips learners with an awareness of the upstream social determinants of ill health, the multifactor causes of inequity and "social suffering," diverse cultural understandings of loss, and the lived, subjective experience of suffering. Philosophy and the arts call on us to question the nature of our "knowing." Poet Tracy K. Smith writes, "I think my work is motivated by a wish to connect to something outside of what we can see and understand. Something that might help us to deal with what we're confronted with—the real" (Hond 2018).

15

Diagnosis
Martha Lincoln

Every medical system features processes for assessing a patient's complaint, distinguishing one pathological state from another, and attributing manifested symptoms to specific causes. In other words, every medical system trains practitioners in its protocols for diagnosis. From the Greek διαγιγνώσκω (distinguish, discern), diagnosis is a practice for determining "the nature of a diseased condition" (*OED Online* 2021, "diagnosis"). To make a diagnosis is to comment on the very nature of disease and health—if only indirectly—and diagnostic systems tacitly advance strong normative claims about states of "illness" and "health." The ontological, sociolinguistic, sociological, anthropological, and comparative aspects of diagnosis—both entity and practice—have compelled research for decades.

Broadly speaking, diagnoses do ideological work by designating certain bodies and states of being as abnormal while leaving a residual category of bodies that are considered normal and nonpathological. A diagnosis provides a name for an abnormal state of health, often adding commentary on causes and probable outcomes. Diagnoses are also typically further ordered into categories, coming to make up a taxonomy. The abstract principles that organize a diagnostic taxonomy reveal the ways of thinking common to the medical paradigm in which they are used. Recurrent questions about these abstract principles of diagnosis include the following: Are diseases species of their own, unvarying over time and between patients, or do they manifest only in the given symptoms of ill individuals (Temkin 1977)? Should diagnoses weigh causes or symptoms more heavily? Is diagnosis more powerful if it joins similar pathological conditions under broad descriptors or if it names many distinct conditions (Featherstone and Atkinson 2013)?

Systematized practices for identifying diseases and their causes began in the ancient world. Documentary evidence suggests that diagnostic protocols were practiced in ancient Egypt, Mesopotamia, Greece, Rome, and Persia. "The earliest known scientific writings on rational observations in medicine" appear in the Edwin Smith Papyrus, copied circa 1600 BCE from a yet older source (van Middendorp, Sanchez, and Burridge 2010, 1815); the papyrus delineates different types of injuries and fractures. In the fourth century CE, the Greeks used dreams for their prognostic significance, understanding them to be messages sent from the soul as it observed the sleeping body (Askitopoulou 2015). In ninth-century Persia, scientist and polymath Abūbakr Mohammad-e Zakariyyā ar-Rāzī described diagnostic categories in *Kitab al-Hawi* and *Kitab al Judari wa al Hasbah*, disambiguating smallpox from measles (Amr and Tbakhi 2007).

Diagnostic categories and practices of a given historic moment are often perceived in later historic periods as surprising, even counterintuitive. Surviving documents from Europe's early Middle Ages describe particularly heterodox diagnostic practices, such as wiping a sick person with a piece of lard, throwing the remainder to an unfamiliar dog, and observing the dog's actions to discern the patient's fate (Horden 2011, 2). In the later Middle Ages, European medicine was more informed by scientific and logical reasoning; diagnostic practices included examining urine, blood, and the pulse (Riha 1996; Wallis 2000). Still, fourteenth-century

physicians diagnosed leprosy in patients who exhibited "melancholic, bad, and crafty habits" and "terrifying melancholic nightmares" (Demaitre 1985, 337–38), suggesting the lingering influence of less scientific paradigms. Nonscientific diagnosis remained in the Renaissance and early modern period; physicians primarily understood disease to have natural causes but also recognized "the role of the devil" (Gevitz 2000, 8). European efforts to identify and order diseases in more scientific ways appeared with Jean Fernel's *Universa Medicini* (1554) and Thomas Sydenham's *Opera Omnia* (1685; Moriyama, Loy, and Robb-Smith 2011, 9). Beginning in the mid-nineteenth century, biomedical practitioners classified disease in more uniform and standardized fashion and were increasingly able to aggregate statistical data on the prevalence of different diseases and causes of death (Moriyama, Loy, and Robb-Smith 2011).

Diagnoses in other historic periods or other cultural settings appear strange in part because we do not inhabit the social milieu that produced them—but "our" familiar biomedical diagnostic practices and systems are also unsystematic and contingent. Diagnosing mental illness is particularly complex, as this requires a diagnostician to make a secondhand assessment of a patient's internal experiential and perceptual world and to fit this assessment to a set of standardized diagnostic criteria (Lakoff 2005). "No blood tests, no X rays, no urine samples" assist in psychiatric diagnosis, apart from tests that measure levels of drugs or alcohol (Luhrmann 2001, 34). Observing the process of diagnosing mental illness during hospital grand rounds, medical anthropologist Emily Martin (2007) found that students and faculty had difficulty assigning consistent diagnostic labels to psychiatric patients presenting with complex histories and ambiguous symptomatology—an observation that undoes the impression of a totalizing psychiatric nosology (or taxonomy of diagnostic categories). As Martin's ethnographic account reveals, the racial and class background of psychiatric practitioners and trainees strongly conditioned their diagnostic evaluations—such that culturally normative behaviors in minority patients were interpreted prejudicially as signs of either pathology or malingering (see also Metzl 2009).

As these findings suggest, diagnosis can function as a form of social control, enforcing norms for "healthy" behavior, identity, and personhood and pathologizing people who deviate from these expectations. In societies where medicine is controlled by elites, diagnostic categories and practices often reify elite perspectives. Medical sociologists, medical anthropologists, and historians of medicine have inquired into diagnosis as a form of cultural hegemony, showing many forms of human variation have been constructed—often tendentiously—as medical problems to be identified and treated. In this perspective, controversies over diagnostic labels can function as proxy conflicts for broader social and political struggles (Charles Rosenberg 2003, 498).

While medical systems see the diagnoses they recognize as objectively real, scholars have shown that diagnoses also construct illness socially; diseases are, in ways, produced by classification (P. Brown 1995). The classification of disease varies significantly across contexts: comparative studies of diagnostic systems reveal that bodily states considered to be bona fide pathologies in one medical system can appear nonproblematic or even nonexistent in another (cf. Lock 1993; R. Smith 2002). As diagnostic categories are not self-evident descriptors of natural phenomena, some of the work of diagnosis is persuasive. Technologies for visualizing the body are often used as supporting evidence for a diagnosis, although they are likewise not neutral means of representation and may further contribute to indeterminacy about a patient's state (cf. Dumit 2004; Mol 2005; B. Saunders 2008).

Scholarship in health humanities and social sciences further reveals the variability of diagnostic categories. Researchers have observed how diagnostic categories change over time—particularly in schemata for classifying psychiatric illness, as alluded to above. This can take place when diagnoses are renamed and reconceptualized. For example, the nineteenth-century diagnosis "soldier's heart" was reframed over the twentieth century successively as "shell shock," "battle fatigue," "combat exhaustion," and "post-traumatic stress disorder" (Chekroud et al. 2018; A. Young 1995). Diagnostic variation can also take place when existing diagnoses lose their explanatory power. The mental disturbances hysteria and neurasthenia have both been delisted from the *Diagnostic and Statistical Manual* and are no longer considered legitimate psychological disorders, though they were once commonly diagnosed "women's complaints" (Micale 1993; Kleinman 1986; Tasca et al. 2012). Finally, new diagnoses can be discovered—or invented—in a process called *diagnostic expansion*. Diagnostic expansion reclassifies mental or bodily states that were previously considered normal or nonmedical (Conrad and Potter 2000) as pathological conditions, creating new patients and new disease regimes (Klawiter 2008). Diagnostic variation over time suggests that the advent of new diagnoses and the retirement of "outdated" diagnoses is not simply the artifact of scientific progress and also shows that the perceived legitimacy of a medical label is partially contingent on social mores and prevailing "common sense."

While diagnoses may not be unproblematically "real," their effects on patient experience are often very significant. Diagnosis remains "a prime site for the expression of medical authority" that affects patient lives for good and for ill (Heritage 2005, 90). Emily Martin describes the pronouncement of a diagnosis as a type of performative "ritual of disclosure" (2007, 113) in which the patient receives a new social identity. Productively, diagnosis can resolve a situation of indeterminacy, making legible an inchoate experience of suffering and "legitimating [the patient's] ailments and validating their concerns" (Filipe 2015, 391; see also Killingsworth et al. 2010). It can also relieve a patient of feelings of personal failure, as in the case of addiction and certain mental health diagnoses. Nevertheless, in the case of serious or stigmatized disease, diagnosis can have significant consequences for personhood and identity (Willig 2011). For example, as technologies for genetic and genomic diagnosis become more sophisticated and regularly used, they create new populations of "at-risk" subjects, such as "previvors" of "protodiseases" (Charles Rosenberg 2003, 503) whose symptoms have yet to manifest.

The interactional, social, and symbolic dimensions of diagnosis are highly consequential for patients and populations, and a diagnosis may also spell a wide range of material effects for the diagnosed (N. Rose 2013b). Diagnosis can facilitate or impede the authorization of future medical care and insurance reimbursement, it can furnish or withdraw the grounds for the redress of injury (Jain 2006), it can certify or invalidate a bodily incapacity as legitimately disabling (Petryna 2002), and it can exculpate or convict the perpetrator of a crime on the grounds of their mental state (Parzen 2003). Adriana Petryna has documented high-stakes struggles for diagnostic validation in postdisaster Chernobyl, where exposed individuals pursued diagnoses that would confirm their status as "sufferers" of the nuclear accident and entitle them to state support; as one physician stated, "The diagnosis we write is [like] money" (2002, 105).

Diagnosis is also a form of social capital. It can legitimize a patient's need for care and relieve them of social obligations for the duration of their illness (Parsons 1964). Sociologist Annemarie Jutel notes that "because of its power to confirm status and allocate resources, the diagnosis is also an important site of contest and compromise" (2011, 5). For this reason, patients who suffer from controversial, unexplained diagnoses like Lyme disease, fibromyalgia, and chronic fatigue syndrome often encounter challenges in receiving not only medical but social validation of their symptoms that could help them live more comfortably with their illness (Dumes 2020; Dusenbery 2017; Ramey 2020). Moreover, diagnosis has the potential to pathologize anatomy, physiology, behavior, and culture, particularly when specific disorders become associated with marginalized populations. As Charles Rosenberg explains, "The intelligibility that comes with disease categories . . . comes at the cost of objectification" (2003, 504).

Future health humanities research on diagnosis will likely continue to investigate how and why diagnostic systems change and how these changes—in the form of new diagnostic categories and powerful new diagnostic technologies, for example—can create bioethical quandaries (cf. Gammeltoft 2014; Rapp 1999). One curiously understudied phenomenon is the rise of artificial intelligence technologies such as IBM Watson that supplement or replace the diagnoses made by human doctors (Beam and Kohane 2018). Automated and algorithmically generated diagnoses will likely have profound consequences for the practice of medicine, the distribution of diagnoses across populations, and the experience of patients.

16

Disability

Rosemarie Garland-Thomson

Nowhere is the concept of *health humanities* more filled with contradictions than when it considers the human variations we call disabilities. While we might think of *disability* as the antithesis or lack of ability, the concept is, in fact, a historical invention born in the nineteenth century. There were and are other ways of thinking about disability, and when it comes to conceiving of disability, the goals and practices of *health* and those of the *humanities* are, at times, divergent if not conflicting. The conflict is generative.

The aim of medical science is to convert human variations it classifies as disease, disability, or defect into a state it considers *health*. To do this, medical science sorts human variations into the categories of pathology or normalcy. Disease, disability, and defect are abstract categorical descriptions, interpretive taxonomies or templates fit over distinctive individuals to develop a clinical treatment plan. Modern Western medicine does this by pathologizing human differences (Hacking 1990; L. Davis 1995; Baynton 2016; Garland-Thomson 1996; Kafer 2013).

Over the last twenty years, the humanities have offered another way of understanding disability. One significant way of understanding disability differently through the humanities has been to identify and explicate cultural narratives of human variation. The humanities go beyond social constructivist theories of disability by bringing the knowledge tools of narrative, rhetorical, and semiotic analysis to explicate the cultural work of representation. Cultural representation gives us the meaning-making systems that shape our understanding of disability and how we respond to it as individuals and communities. Medical and cultural understandings of disability have fundamentally different origins. Most professional health contexts view disability as a problem, an acute deviation from a norm. In contrast, disability studies in the humanities emerged from the disability rights movement's framing of disability as a social problem.

The human variations we think of as *disabilities* have changed—semantically and narratively—in the English language since the mid-eighteenth century from understanding grounded in religious narratives toward those produced by medical science, such as the shift from descriptions like *lame* and *halt* to diagnostic categories such as *quadriplegia* and *multiple sclerosis*. These shifts, the humanities reveal, affect knowledge making, institutional practice, and policy. Broad civil rights legislation in the second half of the twentieth century began a process of civil and human rights advocacy that changed the meaning of *disability* once more. Federal laws and policies, such as the 1964 Civil Rights Act, initiated a decades-long process of desegregating public spaces and the built environment through laws requiring that buildings and institutions be made accessible to people with disabilities. Policies such as the 1968 Architectural Barriers Act and the Individuals with Disabilities Education Act (IDEA) also worked to reimagine people with disabilities as citizens, providing equal access through provision of services and a newly accessible built environment. This transformation of the public sphere to accommodate people with disabilities culminated in the United States with the Americans with Disabilities Act (ADA) of 1990 and 2008. Of course, these policies and laws are aspirational and rely on implementation and enforcement, but they nonetheless lay out the reconceptualization of people with disabilities—a previously legally and politically unrecognized group now understood as a protected minority whose rights to equal treatment were historically denied. Through this series of laws and the changes they required, people with disabilities moved from being understood and treated as *patients* to being recognized as full *citizens.*

Still, the modern understanding of human bodies through medical science, which classifies people with disabilities largely as *patients,* works to relieve them of human differences we think of as disabilities. This follows a long history of medical science's commitment to improving humanity. Nevertheless, limiting disability to a condition of health risks making it a eugenic target, marked for elimination from our human community. Eugenics was a worldwide initiative and a way of thinking understood as progress and technological development that aimed to make a better world, improve the species, and alleviate human suffering. Beginning in the late nineteenth century, eugenics proposed social and political policies to increase ideal and valued citizens while minimizing or eliminating people understood as defective. By the early twentieth century, eugenic ideology gave us involuntary confinement and sterilization almost everywhere in the world, and later, the Holocaust, which emanated from a totalitarian regime, committed to eliminating people considered defective from the national community (Stern 2015; Stern 2021; Friedlander 2000; A. Cohen 2016; Comfort 2018; Kevles 1995; Herzog 2018).

A humanistic, especially a narrative and historical, approach to eugenic thought and practice reveals eugenics is a narrative of human variation underpinned by the authority of objective measurement. Eugenic thinking began from newly ascendant practices and knowledges of measurement and calculation to justify shaping human communities through the modern technologies of medical science. Nevertheless, seeing eugenics as a narrative allows us to see it as one historically contingent choice—a choice to privilege certain ways of knowing and telling a story above others. In fact, we know that eugenics is a deeply historically specific way of narrating biological variation that, like what we think of now as *disability,* is a historically specific understanding of human life and being. Both in historical narratives of eugenics and in current eugenic and antieugenic narratives, we need to attentively search for what we now understand as disability and to recognize the relationship between the cultural narratives and semantics of human variation in the past and in the present. In other words, what we think of now as *disability* was present in the eugenics era, but it had not been inflected by the meanings and history that define the word *disability* now (Garland-Thomson 2020).

Expressed as a semantic and rhetorical transformation, the civil and human rights movements of the mid-twentieth century countered eugenic ideology and practice. This sociopolitical shift from eugenic logic to disability rights logic is a narrative of how the feebleminded, idiots, morons, insane, defectives, cripples, sick, weak, helpless, savages, barbarians, coloreds, aliens, foreigners, criminals, prisoners, homosexuals, work-shy, useless eaters, and all people whose lives were unworthy of life were transformed into people with disabilities, people of color, BIPOC, gays, transgendered people, economically disadvantaged, socially excluded, and other designations of dignity and equality.

If we seek to use the humanities to intervene in covertly and overtly eugenicist health narratives that continue to frame disability as a so-called problem for human health and flourishing that would be best eliminated, we could do no better than committing to *disability bioethics* (Garland-Thomson 2012). Bioethics is an applied field of study that grew out of a recognition that, following the Nazi regime and Holocaust, scientific research needed monitoring and revision, especially when informed by religious studies and ethics (see "Bioethics"). *Disability bioethics* begins from the idea that bodily diversity is good for a population—that is, that diverse abilities, bodies, and minds enrich the human experience and population and that, contra eugenics, they must be not only preserved but allowed to flourish. The project of disability bioethics is to bring the cultural history of the sociopolitical category *disability* to what has been until recently an altogether medicalized category. Along with the principles of assuring autonomy, avoiding harm, and supporting benefit that can be applied in medical and health-care practice, bioethics charges us with the more abstract aspiration to uphold justice. Justice invites us to consider the political promise of equality fundamental to modern liberal social orders. Disability bioethics challenges us to develop and practice a radical understanding of equality that recognizes body-minds considered disabled as equal in moral and social value to body-minds that meet the medical threshold of normal. Disability bioethics further challenges health care as an ideology and practice to provide medical treatment that will increase quality of life and remediate suffering without normalizing the human variations we think of as disabilities. This is an enormous and in many ways counterintuitive challenge that the health-care industry must continue to take up in this twenty-first-century era of recognizing and honoring disability as a form of human diversity and a sociopolitical identity category. Disability bioethics can thus counter eugenic ideologies that value human beings differentially. This bioethics of justice cultivates an attitude of humility toward human biodiversity in imagining another's life and how any of us live. It requires health care to resist a notion of technological progress that continually categorizes human diversity in terms of

diseases to be identified and eliminated. This narrow version of health regularizes human minds and bodies according to concepts of advantage or disadvantage, part of a commercially incentivized growth industry of pathological diagnosis and notions of individual liberty at the expense of the common good.

The health humanities should also encourage the idea of disability cultural competence. Developed as a curriculum and set of practices within health-care settings, disability cultural competence can be designed with the goal of implementing justice and autonomy. Achieving disability-competent care will require physicians, patients, and prospective patients to unlearn attitudes and assigned roles that interpret human variations we think of as disabilities primarily as diseases or departures from normalcy. Disability cultural competence is more closely related to structural competence than to current understandings of ethnic or racial cultural competence. This is because disability is a sociopolitical and cultural category that everyone, from patients to health-care workers themselves, can and will enter into sometime over a lifetime. Thus, knowledge of disability as a shared human experience is necessary for everyone. The cultural practices that underpin competence in disability culture are those that support diverse ways of human flourishing and civil and human rights–based understandings of disability encoded in legislation such as the ADA and broader initiatives such as the United Nations Treaty on the Rights of People with Disabilities, which aim to integrate people with disabilities as full citizens (Garland-Thomson and Iezzoni 2021).

Disability cultural competence identifies and develops supports for people living with disabilities without changing their lives to live according to others' expectations. Its content includes (1) biomedical decision-making, (2) disability culture and history, (3) accessible technology and design, and (4) disability legislation and social justice. Its competencies draw from disability culture, arts, literature, history, design, technology, bioethics, and law to expand the medical and rehabilitation knowledges that now address living with disabilities. It promotes quality of life, dignity management and maintenance, access and accommodation requests, self-determination, resilience cultivation, relationship management, community and leadership building, and cultural proficiency for people living with disabilities and their families. It also promotes awareness about disability rights, disability protections, and the benefits of identifying as disabled—such as how to request accommodations in health-care settings and the provisions of the ADA and Genetic Information Nondiscrimination Act for health-care workers, patients, and future patients. Disability cultural competence benefits everyone. These competencies are grounded in the disability principles of nondiscrimination, full and effective participation of people with disabilities in society, respect for difference, and accessibility we find in disability principlism, epistemology, and critical theory (Ouellette 2011; Scully 2008; Garland-Thomson 2017).

Disability bioethics and *disability cultural competence* are just two examples of how the productive friction between medical and humanistic ideas of disability can generate new frameworks and orientations. Health humanists would benefit from such perspectives and knowledge that recognize the full potential of disability to produce more ethical, humane, and just ideas and practices in health and health care.

17

Disaster

Martin Halliwell

Disasters invariably reveal the frailty of human health. Derived from the Middle French word *désastre* and from the Italian *disastro*, *disaster* is an emotive noun that signifies an unfortunate event that is calamitous and distressing in character. Disaster can strike at an individual or family level: a shock diagnosis of cancer, for example. But it is more often used to refer to a large-scale event that devastates a community or a country, raising profound questions not only about life and livelihood but also about who is responsible for curbing public health threats and for protecting the health of a country's citizens.

In terms of its long historical arc, the epidemiological transmission of disease is one of the most visible forms of public health disaster. The transmission of smallpox and bubonic plague among migrating communities emerged historically alongside the development of agricultural economies during the Bronze Age, a two-thousand-year period in Europe, Africa, and Asia (Armelagos et al. 2005; Norris 2016). In early modern history, mass deaths among indigenous communities in the Americas were caused by European travelers and colonists taking smallpox to the New World. Smallpox not only contributed to the displacement of native tribes, but it linked disease transmission to the dynamics of colonialism as well as to the violence of warfare and servitude.

In modern history, a similar confluence between war and epidemic disease also amplified public health threats during the influenza pandemic of 1918–19, which not only contributed to injury and loss of life but arguably became more virulent because of the conditions of warfare in Europe. These examples suggest that warfare is invariably disastrous for public health. Mass deaths, such as the 620,000 lives lost during the American Civil War (1861–65), are unparalleled among national disasters. However, warfare typically leaves lasting scars for survivors and "a new relationship to death," which, as historian Drew Gilpin Faust argues, in the mid-nineteenth century challenged "fundamental assumptions about life's value and meaning" (2008, xviii).

Environmental disasters also implicate these "fundamental assumptions," prompting a range of deleterious short-term and long-term health implications, although there are multiple determining factors, both social and natural, that shape the public health emergency that often ensues (Halliwell 2021). For example, the major ecological disaster in the United States during the 1930s was due to a sequence of droughts across the Midwest and South enflamed by the economic depression in the wake of the 1929 Wall Street Crash. More than fifty dust storms hit Colorado, Kansas, Oklahoma, and Texas between 1932 and 1935, and the flat semiarid landscape and high winds of the Great Plains meant that residents constantly inhaled airborne topsoil, leading to the growth of bacteria in the nose and throat. Dust was only half of the equation; the other half hinged on anxiety and despair triggered by a loss of home and employment. It is tricky to determine to what extent such psychological distress was pathological because of a lack of comprehensive medical data at the time. However, the displaced sharecropper Muley Graves in John Steinbeck's Depression-era novel *The Grapes of Wrath* illustrates this loss of selfhood: he sees himself as an "ol' graveyard ghos'" living in the shadows of abandoned buildings on his former land

(1939, 69). Although President Franklin Roosevelt's New Deal of 1933–39, as an example of "the sympathetic state" in action (Dauber 2013), brought economic relief to farmers across the Plains, bronchial complications, lower rates of fertility, and lingering depression were lasting legacies of the Dust Bowl.

Disaster by flooding is another profound environmental threat to human societies. While drought can often lead to wildfires, as experienced by Californians and Australians in the late 2010s, flooding is a perennial danger for coastal communities. The unpredictability of floods is a regular threat to human health around the globe, from storm surges in Haiti caused by Hurricane Matthew in 2016 to the tsunamis that battered Sri Lanka and Indonesia in 2004 and 2018. The level of vulnerability of a population made homeless, forced to evacuate, or experiencing injury, disease, and death as consequences of flooding often depends on the affected community's access to sustainable aid and medical supplies. Inland floods can be as devastating as coastal floods, as is evidenced by deadly flooding in Pakistan in 2022 following a heavy monsoon.

It is clear that some regions are more vulnerable to natural disasters than others, such as southern coastal states of the United States, but this is often due to a confluence of environmental and human factors (Wald 2022, 612). The Great Mississippi Flood of 1927, for example, was due to heavy rain that fell between August 1926 and April 1927. The flooding saw 640,000 displaced and homeless people from Illinois down to Louisiana, leading to between 250 and 500 deaths as well as many cases of typhoid, smallpox, diphtheria, and pellagra across southern states. The fact that the US federal government was slow to offer support to Delta communities gave weight to the view that the flood was a human-made disaster due to decades of private investments carving up the Mississippi River into local interests rather than a national plan that treated the river as an integrated waterway.

The massive flooding in Louisiana and Mississippi caused by Hurricane Katrina in August 2005 is another instructive case, both for its damage to urban and coastal communities and for the economic and racial divisions it exposed. Winds and floods caused close to 1,600 recorded fatalities in Louisiana, yet residents of New Orleans, many of them African American, experienced complex physical and mental health symptoms relating to infection, trauma, and displacement. Over 1,800 lives were lost overall, and 1.5 million were homeless. The major reason why the damage was so profound in New Orleans was that its flood protection system experienced major malfunctions when the levees were reconstructed after the 1927 Mississippi Flood failed in over fifty places (C. Hartman and Squires 2006). That the relief effort was neither immediate nor carefully coordinated compounded the distress of locals, particularly in the predominantly black Lower Ninth Ward, a residential area that was vulnerable to storm surges and without easy access to health services, revealing deep inequalities along class and racial lines (Rivera and Miller 2007). Overall, an estimated 50 percent of New Orleans residents required mental health support months after the floods, while symptoms of post-traumatic stress disorder were detected in 30 percent of residents in the New Orleans metropolitan area five months later (Kessler 2006).

The mental health toll of environmental disasters is often harder to calculate than the physical needs of affected communities. However, this psychological impact is just as profound, giving weight to the argument that there are similarities in the "human reaction" to different types of natural disasters, whether the crisis is "a toxic spill, an oil spill, an earthquake, [or] a cloud of radioactive fallout" (Erikson 1976, ii; 1994).

The emphasis on commonalities between natural and human-made disasters diverges from a focus on the sociological variants of disaster, a countertrend that is critical of media reports of "panic flight reactions at disaster sites" and pays careful interdisciplinary consideration to the causes and consequences of disasters for particular communities (Tierney and Balsden 1977, 1). Enrico Quarantelli (1998), founder of the Disaster Research Center at the University of Delaware, locates the beginnings of disaster research in the 1950s and 1960s. In contrast, Francis Adeola (2012) links disaster research to the rise of risk studies in the 1980s, together with more recent trends relating to structural inequalities and environmental justice, a view that aligns with Anthony Carrigan's argument that the "capitalist exploitation of natural resources" has amplified debates about the causal determinants of health (2015, 117).

Disasters often raise classificatory and epistemological questions, especially for small-scale events. These events can prove devastating for local communities, but they may not resonate on a national level, such as the 1972 Buffalo Creek Flood in West Virginia (Erikson 1976) or the lack of health and safety protections for coal miners through much of the twentieth century (Derickson 2014a). The rhetorical construction of "disaster" means that it often carries ideological freight for authorities seeking to place or deflect blame with respect to legal liability or when media outlets frame misfortune in dramatic terms in search of headlines. These instances can easily lead to what Timothy Clark calls "derangements of scale" (2012, 148), making it difficult to distinguish the scale of a disaster from belief, rumor, or folklore, which links to the etymology of the term *disastro*, meaning "ill-starred." The idiomatic impulse to use "disaster" in everyday discourse, no matter the scale of events, can obscure the reality of a public health emergency and can result in an echo chamber effect that repeats misinformation until it becomes dogma. This trend pushed the World Health Organization in 2020, during the early months of the COVID-19 pandemic, to tackle "infodemics" and "media-borne viruses" that often accompany disease outbreaks (Rothkopf 2003).

In recognition that international accords are necessary to mitigate large-scale disasters, the United Nations has called on countries to significantly reduce disaster mortality by 2030 and observe the goals of the biennial Global Platform for Disaster Risk Reduction, which began in 2005 as a forum for sustainability strategies (UN General Assembly 2017). However, cross-border and global approaches to disasters need to be balanced by interagency cooperation and by structures that can enhance health citizenship at regional and local levels. This understanding has led the World Health Organization to recognize that disaster health plans cannot be a one-size-fits-all approach because recovery procedures need to be attuned to the specifics of locality and to ensure that communities retain their sense of agency.

18

Disease
Robert A. Aronowitz

For over twenty years, I have taught an undergraduate seminar whose central question has been, "What is disease?" In the first class, I often evoke the parable of the visually impaired and the elephant. Depending on which parts they touch, each person perceives something different. Similarly, what disease *is* depends on when, where, and with what tools and preconceptions you encounter it.

As a framework for understanding the range of disease meanings, it is hard to improve upon Temkin's (1977) philosophical and historical reflections on the tensions between *ontological* and *physiological* conceptions of illness. By "ontology," Temkin meant how *specific diseases* impact different individuals in similar ways, while the physiological view captured the multiple and idiosyncratic ways individuals are sick. Depending on the types of suffering most prevalent in any era and place, ontological or physiological conceptions might have the upper hand. The arch-ontologist Thomas Sydenham (1624–89) practiced in London during plague years, and plague, Temkin quipped, did not distinguish much among individuals.

Temkin also weighed some of the advantages and disadvantages of these ideal types. Sigmund Freud's physiological, dimensional approach to the human psyche in the early twentieth century placed the self-evidently sick and the possibly well on a continuum. It is a small leap to believing everyone is potentially ill. Creating discrete specific diseases from the discovery of microbial agents of disease starting in the late nineteenth century and the elaboration of inborn errors of metabolism starting in the early twentieth century (later understood as arising from genetic variation) can be an engine for making an unlimited number of diseases, some of which might not be suffered (symptomatically, at least) by any actual individual.

The late twentieth-century appearance of AIDS underscored the tensions between ontological and physiological conceptions and catalyzed interest in the social history of disease. The identification of a new etiological retrovirus (HIV) gave ontology an upper hand over a competing physiological, "lifestyle"-influenced, "gay" disease. Yet the divergent and highly visible societal responses to a new, deadly, incurable infectious disease—spread by sex, needle sharing, and blood products—sparked renewed interest in social aspects of disease. Susan Sontag, for example, extended her 1978 argument about countering the stigma and attitudinal baggage enshrouding tuberculosis and cancer to AIDS in 1989.

The rediscovery of the iconoclastic work of Ludwik Fleck (1979) was emblematic of the renewed interest in the sociology of knowledge generally and about disease specifically. Fleck, a Polish-Jewish physician writing in German in the 1930s under the influence of Gestalt psychology and a contemporary Polish philosophy of science (Löwy 2012), emphasized the archeology of disease concepts (part of a more elaborate system of scientific "thought collectives"). For Fleck, the modern concept of syphilis and the development of blood tests to diagnose it, for example, were built, like overlapping transparencies laid on top of one another, from older therapeutic, carnal "disease of the blood" and other conceptions of the disease.

Historians and sociologists in the ensuing decades examined the different medical and social constructions of disease in case studies (e.g., the American medicalization and demedicalization of homosexuality). Such analysis was especially attentive to the construction of mental illness and often inspired by Michel Foucault's emphasis on the role of discourse and power and the labeling of deviance as disease by powerful interest groups such as doctors and pharmaceutical companies. Unfortunately, like any analytical framework, the terms *social construction of disease* and *medicalization* are at times overextended, signaling an author's loyalties in ongoing culture wars more than a method or a process. Charles Rosenberg's (1989a) alternative "framing" formulation—one that emphasized that the recognition, definition, and categorization of disease were necessarily social processes—attempted to refocus scholarship on the insights of specific sociohistorical studies of disease (inviting criticism that the political bite of social constructionist arguments had been defanged; see Cooter 2004).

Philosopher of science Ian Hacking (1999) emphasized that social constructionist accounts of disease got their oomph from unmasking the hard, realistic assumptions of others. It made little sense to argue for the social construction of the Federal Reserve, whose meaning everyone had already accepted derived from social and political developments. Eschewing the short-lived benefits of unmasking someone else's naive assumptions, most sociohistorical accounts of disease in the past few decades have stayed within the familiar boundaries of an enlightened realism and a cautious relativism. A frightening new symptom, an incidental finding on a diagnostic test, or even a news report of a new disease will send most scholars, regardless of their social and political commitments, on a Google search of a specific disease keyword without much epistemological angst. At the same time, there is a broad revulsion to pharmaceutical companies' aggressive selling—and sometimes creation—of disease and risk targets (e.g., premenstrual syndrome, erectile dysfunction, prediabetes) along with the drugs to treat them.

Hacking (2006) also contributed some conceptual clarity to the social dynamics by which diseases are constructed or framed with his concept of the "looping effects of human kinds." People are not just given disease or other labels, he argued; being categorized one way or another changes them and, in time, also the meaning of the category. Knowledge produced by medical investigations and interventions changes patient behavior and the ways clinicians diagnose and treat people, which in turn can transform the epidemiology and clinical profile of disease itself. Epidemiologists and others spoke about "looping effects" without knowing it—for example, the so-called popularity paradox (Raffle and Gray 2007) used to explain the way more diagnoses of screening-detected cancers can lead to apparent improvement in survival rates, leading to more screening, further improvement in survival, and so on. Fleck had already noticed a similar phenomenon (comparing the clinician diagnosing disease to an investor inside a market bubble, unaware that he is helping create, not just respond to, a changed reality), as did Robert Merton (1948) and others in different aspects of social life.

In clinical practice and medical education, Arthur Kleinman and Leon Eisenberg were the most visible promoters of the related distinction between *disease* and *illness*—the former highlighting the objective, biological, and mechanistic aspects of being sick, the latter the individual's subjective experience. This distinction contributed, as Kleinman would later regret, to a simplistic move within medical education to study and teach cultural competency, the putative culture-specific explanatory frameworks for illness. Later correctives such as the move toward structural competency (knowledge of structural racism, "caked in" disadvantage, and the

complex mediation of how social realities get "under the skin") by physician–social scientists Jonathan M. Metzl and Helena Hansen (2014) partly righted this excess. Relatedly, others have questioned the focus on disease per se in social studies of health and argued for more focus on disability (e.g., Linker 2013), debility (e.g., Julie Livingston 2005), and social suffering (Feierman 1985), often resulting from detailed historical and ethnographic accounts of sickness in non-Western places.

Anthropologists—in particular, Margaret Lock (1993)—have also argued for the different ways that cultural factors might materially shape disease, most vividly presented in the contrasting "local biology" of menopause in Japan and North America. Other studies that mix social and materialist histories of disease, often non-Western or comparative, have been part of a larger scholarly move to complicate simple narratives of culture-bound syndromes and medical pluralism (see especially Mukharji's 2016 concept of braided medical traditions).

Clinicians have, in turn, offered parallel criticisms and innovations. Alvan Feinstein (1967) railed against the role atemporal, narrow disease concepts played in diagnostic practices and therapeutics. He pointed out the harms of not considering, especially in clinical research, the entire spectrum of disease and the diverse trajectories of individuals labeled with the same diagnosis and rekindled some clinical and epidemiological interest in the importance of prognostic knowledge and the powerful role of illness behaviors—and especially the ways patients encounter the health-care system—in shaping prognosis.

A related tension in what disease means animates the fields of social epidemiology and population health. Geoffrey Rose's seminal 1985 paper contrasted disease in individual versus population terms. At a population level, average height is highly correlated with life expectancy (e.g., the modern Dutch are the tallest and live longest), but there is no reason to despair if you are born short in Holland or anywhere else; the association is only operative at the population level. A hung jury does not mean that individual jurors are conflicted—it's a description at another level. We could and do screen populations to find individuals with the highest blood pressure or serum cholesterol and bring their values back to normal with medications. But this individual strategy is an entirely different one from intervening in the population-level causes of ill health—for example, the political economy of tobacco consumption (by raising taxes on cigarettes) or the societal norms that sustain inactivity (via educational campaigns). However, the population approach does not necessarily preclude medicalizing an entire population. We can give everyone a polypill against heart and other diseases and perhaps move the entire population distribution of risk in a better direction. Less controversial medicalized population interventions are mass vaccination and water fluoridation, although few interventions are without their critics.

Critics within and outside medicine have pointed out that people increasingly suffer from chronic diseases while our medical institutions and health-care resources remain focused on more acute ones (McKeown [1976] 1980). However, the major historical transformations are more complex than more people living with diseases that last a long time and that are more resistant to quick fixes. Instead, many diseases have been transmuted—radically transformed—by our interventions. Feudtner (2003) pointed out how insulin treatment of diabetes allowed diabetics to survive longer but with new vision, cardiac, renal, and cardiovascular problems. The experience of identifying, anticipating, and managing risk has become central to the chronic disease experience (Aronowitz 2015). Diseases have also

been bureaucratized (Charles Rosenberg 2002); diagnosing them may trigger entitlements to disability or denial of health insurance coverage, and diagnoses have become indispensable to hospital management.

The modern medical focus on individual risk factors of disease has lately morphed into one for highly specific individual biomarkers that might be targeted for intervention. We now have precision medicine, personalized medicine, and individualized genomic diseases (see "Precision"). In some ways, we have come full circle. Temkin himself pointed out that ontology could be molecular—there could be a "specific disease" approach to the individual. Yet some skeptical epidemiologists remind us that a science of the individual remains elusive, for generalizable clinical knowledge implies a pattern with some regularity, for which we need a group, even a small one (G. Smith 2011).

Will our experience of the COVID pandemic have an enduring impact on the way we resolve tensions about what disease means? Almost everything about COVID has been widely debated in both the clinical literature and the lay (and social) media. It has become common to speculate on what suffering means in places that have little capacity to test and give effective supportive care. A positive result on a precise COVID PCR test creates a compelling case for a commonsense ontology, while the person with asymptomatic COVID and the long-hauler challenge it: What are the legitimate boundaries of CO-VID disease? Which symptoms of long COVID are due to persistent infection or some individual-influenced factor? What suffering do we attribute to the virus and what to the individual's psychic makeup and predispositions? And how might we ever agree on such distinctions? Clinicians and patients attuned to the complexity of ill health are generally predisposed to view any one individual's suffering as legitimate, even if with current diagnostic concepts and tools there is only "illness" and not disease.

COVID has made esoteric epidemiological concerns over detection bias, comorbidity, diagnostic sensitivity and specificity, and case fatality everyday lay ones. There is widespread angst about medical ignorance over why some individuals get sick and not others and over who will live with and who will die from this disease. These and other pressing unanswered and often unasked questions stem in no small measure from medicine's failure to fully integrate ontological and physiological concepts of disease.

19

Drug
Anne Pollock

Whether licit or illicit, drugs are richly material-semiotic objects: this means that they carry both matter and meaning. Even as drugs are concrete objects with the capacity to reorder our bodies on a molecular level, that is never all that they do. For their consumers—and also for their makers, distributors, and even observers—the physiological impacts of drugs are inseparable from meaning making.

The word *drug* is both a noun and a verb. As a noun, it refers to a substance with transformative physiological effects. The effects are typically divided into licit and illicit, as in the following: "(1) any natural or artificially made chemical that is used as a medicine" and "(2) any natural or artificially made chemical that is taken for pleasure, to improve someone's performance of an activity, or because a person cannot stop using it" (*Cambridge English Dictionary* 2022, "drug"). As a verb, the word means "to administer a drug," although "to drug" is rarely used in a neutral way and usually has nefarious connotations.

The most prominent licit sense of *drug* is in the context of the pharmaceutical industry, as in *drug discovery*. The most prominent illicit sense of *drug* is in the context of street-level recreational drugs, as in *drug dealer*. Concerns about "drug pushers" are pervasive in both domains, which points to the intertwined character of the licit and illicit spheres. Drugs frequently travel across il/licit boundaries—for example, historically, cocaine was a recommended treatment for alcoholism, and currently, OxyContin users turn to heroin, while heroin users turn to methadone maintenance.

The word *pharmaceutical* has a more neutral valence than *drug*. *Drug* comes from the fourteenth-century Middle English *drogge*, in turn thought to derive from Middle Dutch for *droge-vate* (dry barrels) because herbs used as medicines were typically distributed that way. Yet the power of the word *drug* can better be appreciated through the etymology of its sometime synonym *pharmaceutical*, which originated in the Greek word *pharmakon*. In his influential essay "Plato's Pharmacy," Jacques Derrida (1981) illuminates the polyvalence of the word *pharmakon*, a term that has often been mistranslated as "remedy," pointing out that *pharmakon* also means "poison." Derrida argues that "Plato is suspicious of the *pharmakon* in general, even in the case of drugs used exclusively for therapeutic ends, even when they are wielded with good intentions, and even when they are as such effective. There is no such thing as a harmless remedy. The *pharmakon* can never be simply beneficial" (99). The inseparability of remedy (desired effect) and poison (undesired side effect) has made the *pharmakon* a valuable analytic for ethnographically informed consideration of pharmaceuticals (Martin 2006; Persson 2004). Bringing side effects into the analytical foreground helps push beyond the banal acknowledgment that drugs can be harmful if they are used inappropriately and shows that even and indeed sometimes especially for the most compliant of patients, drugs can be beneficial and harmful to the same person at the same time.

There are also additional ways in which suspicion of the *pharmakon* is illuminating with regard to broader apprehension of the drug as an object, whether the pharmaceutical or the recreational drug. For Derrida, Plato has two concerns: first, "the beneficial essence or virtue of a *pharmakon* does not prevent it from hurting," and second, more profoundly, "the pharmaceutical remedy is essentially harmful because it is artificial" (Derrida 1981, 99). The *pharmakon* is a risky supplement that subverts the natural. Taking drugs is cheating.

Sport is the most prominent site in which drugging is cheating, especially anabolic steroids that are proscribed as "an unnatural form of embodied masculinization" (Henne and Livingstone 2019, 13). Student use of pharmaceuticals as study aids is also often normatively characterized as cheating, even as a robust body of research suggests that more moral complexity is at play, both because drug consumption by individuals is situated in social and regulatory landscapes and because their subjective experiences can include not only rationalist motives but also enjoyment of focus on work (Pickersgill and Hogle 2015). Pharmaceuticals can also reinforce unfairness in broader society, as when anti-addiction drugs are provided to privileged people but denied to others, a "pharmaceutical prosthesis" that props up racial privilege (Hansen 2017, 325).

The very notion of an anti-addiction drug reminds us of an additional element of danger in drugs: dependence. We turn to drugs to produce a desired effect—medicinal, performance enhancing, or pleasurable—but in doing so cede control to the drug, and many drugs are taken because the person "cannot stop using it" (*Cambridge English Dictionary* 2022, "drug"). While the nefarious infinitive *to drug* connotes intent to control, once consumed, drugs can take their own course of action. In slipping a roofie or administering an anesthetic, the drug is a means of the subversion of the person's control. Institutions can abuse drugs in this way, as when schools push the use of attention deficit disorder drugs to make children easier to manage and when prisons use psychotropic drugs to keep prisoners quiet (Hatch 2019). Yet the phenomenon of addiction makes obvious that with or without a drug pusher, drugs themselves can exert compulsion.

Self-determination in the realm of drug use is an inadequate solution to the problem of drugs' capacity to control us, and moreover, the imperative to be in control is itself ideologically laden. In many contexts, for example, recreational drug use in moderation is socially sanctioned—*temperance* no longer means "abstinence" but instead "social drinking"—and medication should be taken as correctly prescribed, no more and no less. This worldview privileges vigilant maintenance of prudent moderation. And yet it is generally considered to be morally superior to forswear over-the-counter or prescription drug use if at all possible. Follow a good diet and exercise to limit the need for cardiovascular risk-reducing drugs such as statins, practice good hygiene and safe sex to avoid acquiring infection, and use antibiotics and painkillers sparingly. Alcohol may be a good social lubricant, and antidepressants may be a good way of managing chemical imbalances in the face of life's challenges, but drug use can provoke defensiveness, since drugs are often derided as the "easy way out." It is conventionally held that lifestyle change should be the first solution for individual medical problems and that social change would be a fundamentally better solution for broader social problems because drugs are imagined as shortcuts or stopgaps that can distract from or even get in the way of more fundamental transformation (Pollock 2012, 177–78). At the same time, we live in an age of polypharmacy and consumer culture. It is normal to be on "drugs for life" (Dumit 2012), so why *not* have better living through chemistry?

In market-based medicine, patient-consumers take control with drugs, but they do so in a saturated ideological landscape in which desires do not precede social existence. There has been rich health humanities critique of the way that pharmaceutical advertisements not only sell diseases but also sell social identities. For example, psychotropic treatments from Deprol to Valium to Prozac have long been imbricated in reinforcing normative ideas about ideal femininity by "selling sanity through gender" (Metzl 2003), and Viagra's promotional materials can be read as scripts that rearticulate the psychological or relational category of "impotence" into biomedicalized "erectile dysfunction" and offer normative masculine users "potency in all the right places" (Mamo and Fishman 2001).

And yet alternative readings of gender scripts are never completely suppressed. Queer theorists have been particularly perceptive about the fraught but generative potential of drugs' stories. Drugs in general are "re-creational" (Race 2009, 9): objects that facilitate the re-creation of ourselves and our world. Normative gender is operating on the supply side, with particular forms of masculinity idealized in narcotrafficking that queer theory problematizes (Núñez Noriega and Espinoza Cid 2017). Normativities also shape drug taking, most evocatively in the consumption of exogenous hormones, whether for birth control or for trans/gender expression (Preciado 2013). None of that is a reason to Just Say No. Losing control through and to drugs can be pleasurable: *toxicity* is inherent in *intoxication*, and desire for poison is not uncomplicated, but drugs can also offer welcome opportunities for play and transformation (Pollock 2016).

In a time in which scholars across the humanities and the humanistic social sciences are increasingly interested in materiality, it is not surprising to find a fluorescence of interest in drugs. Paying attention to the physiological mechanisms by which drugs operate can have value for feminist theory (E. Wilson 2006). At the intersection of cultural anthropology and science and technology studies, analysts attend to "the movement and flow of pharmaceutical materials through research and development, regulatory regimes, advertising, and care practices" to illuminate "the always-emergent nature of pharmaceutical action" (Hardon and Sanabria 2017, 126).

For the health humanities, the drug in its medical sense is an inevitable topic for analysis that offers a route into deeper engagement with materiality and social worlds. The clinical encounter is arguably the foundational scene for the medical humanities, and the drug is archetypally central to the clinical encounter. As anthropologists of medicine have argued, in biomedicine as in other medical traditions, the "thinginess" of drugs "provides patients and healers with a means to deal with the problem at hand," to "transform the state of dysphoria into something concrete" (van der Geest, White, and Hardon 1996, 154). That is why a drug is often the *end* of the clinical encounter in at least two senses: it is both the goal and the chronological conclusion. A drug is what the patient comes for, and it is the physician's "benediction" (Pellegrino 1976, 155): "Go in peace." Yet the drug has layered histories prior to the clinical encounter, and the drug also travels beyond that encounter as it infuses the patient's body and the broader social world with both poison and salve. As health humanities scholars increasingly focus attention beyond clinical settings to scales of social and material environments, "drug" will likely become an even more vital site of inquiry.

20

Emotion
Kathleen Woodward

The word *emotion* belongs to a constellation of overlapping terms under the general category of feeling, including affect, mood, sensation, and the passions as well as emotion. *Emotion* is psychological and social, emphasizing the subjectivity associated with inner life (examples include love and hate, shame and guilt, and hope and despair), while *affect* is a precognitive capacity emerging in large part from sensory experience and the effect that bodies have in relation to one another (a philosophical term, *affect* was articulated by philosophers Baruch Spinoza and Gilles Deleuze and has recently been elaborated by Brian Massumi). Seldom invoked today, *passion* was used before the mid-eighteenth century to describe the strong emotions—wonder and anger among them. While *emotion* is the term commonly accepted today by the general public, *affect* is most in favor in scholarly circles where many understand it to carry the potential for social change.

In what follows, I suggest connections among these terms, tracing subjectivity in relation to sickness through the lens of emotion across three intertwining scales of the human—the individual, the community or population, and the species, with a corresponding movement from the psychological and social emotions of anger and grief to knots of feeling of being at risk. This trajectory roughly parallels the expansion of the medical humanities to health humanities, or, better, the global public health humanities. My conviction is that a rich emotional life—at the level of the individual, the community or population, and the human species—is a crucial dimension of health.

First, consider emotion in terms of the inner life of the individual. In 1988, psychiatrist and medical anthropologist Arthur Kleinman introduced the important concept of the "illness narrative," distinguishing between the clinical object (the biomedical entity) that is the *disease* and the personal experience of *illness*. The latter includes the distress of symptoms, cultural connotations of the affliction, one's own lifeworld, and the moral meanings attached to the experience, all of which may entail "emotional turmoil" (44). Crucial to healing, Kleinman insists, is the "empathetic witnessing of the existential experience of suffering" (10). With physician Rita Charon, the pedagogy of narrative medicine gained traction in US medical schools. In her words, the competence of physicians includes the "narrative skills of recognizing, absorbing, interpreting, and being moved by stories of illness" (2006, 4) (see "Narrative"). Key is the cultivation of empathy for those who are suffering; not a specific emotion, empathy is the capacity to understand another (some go further and define it as the capacity to actually experience the feelings of another; see "Empathy"). As with Kleinman, the physician is depicted as an empathetic witness, with compassion for others an important quality of their care. Significantly, in medical institutions, it is typically not the doctor but the nurse who is called upon to provide emotional labor (Hochschild 1983).

Narrative, as this work suggests, can be a crucial site not only for offering better care to individuals but also for advocating change. And in fact, in the illness memoirs that exploded in the 1980s, individuals voiced their anger at the broken system of health care in the US, positioning the reader as an empathetic witness. Audre Lorde began her 1980 memoir *The Cancer Journals* with an account of its fierce emotional work: "I do not wish

my anger and pain and fear about cancer to fossilize into yet another silence," she writes. "Our feelings need voice in order to be recognized, respected, and of use" (9). The decade closed with "Mourning and Militancy," Douglas Crimp's 1989 compelling essay about HIV/AIDS in which he insists that grief—not only an individual emotion but intensified as a collective emotion—could animate protest, comingling with anger if not rage to produce outrage, a political emotion. In narratives such as these, written by those who are marginalized, the emotions—anger in particular—have an epistemological power, a cognitive edge; these "outlaw emotions," to borrow philosopher Alison Jaggar's (1989, 160) formulation, provide insight into what is morally wrong. The many illness narratives available to us are valuable in no small part because they preserve historically significant emotions, constituting, in Ann Cvetkovich's (2003) wonderful phrase, "an archive of feelings."

Emotions are at the core of the experience of disease. They have also been medicalized. Anxiety and fear, for example, are often conjured in relation to mental illness. Where to draw the line between what is normal and what is pathological is a cultural decision that must be carefully examined for bias; the five editions of the US *Diagnostic and Statistical Manual of Mental Disorders* offer a living archive of these decisions (Horwitz and Wakefield 2012). Numerous diseases, disorders, and conditions—such as bipolar disorder, autism, and forms of self-harm—are related to purported dysregulation of emotions. Others are associated with the very evacuation and absence of emotion. French philosopher Catherine Malabou, for example, explores disaffection (and its cognates: indifference, coolness, and apathy), suffering entailed by brain diseases that diminish and even destroy emotion. Consider also structurally produced emotions, such as the despair leading to deaths by suicide among the US white working class, linked to the lethal failure of neoliberal capitalism (Deaton and Case 2020).

Second, as such deaths of despair suggest, emotions are not only psychological and individual but also social. They are experienced by groups and communities, populations and nations. During the 1980s AIDS crisis, grief and anger were collective emotions, expressions of social suffering. The devastation of the disease was magnified by the stigma attached to the gay community and thus to AIDS itself, both in material terms (the disease was long ignored by the US government) and in affective terms, including the weaponization of shame directed at those suffering from it (I use *affective* because *emotional* continues to carry a negative association, linked with women). The concept of social suffering captures the affective dimension of what today is often referred to as the social determinants of health disparities; among them are poverty, pollution, and state violence and neglect as well as racism, sexism, ageism, and other forms of prejudice (Jenkins 1991; Kleinman, Das, and Lock 1997). How might social suffering, with a focus on structural suffering, be studied in different communities and populations via the emotions? More specifically, what can we learn from ethnographic studies of disease and illness in societies of the Global South that might provide important cross-cultural perspectives to the Global North? Viewing a different society through scenes of medical care will show us not only what we can learn through the lens of the emotions but also the limits of this approach. Emotions rarely come in singular states; they combine with other emotions and mix with other feeling states, including moods and sensations.

A prime example of medical care in the Global South is Julie Livingston's 2012 remarkable ethnography—*Improvising Medicine*—of a small communal cancer ward in Botswana where, notwithstanding severe poverty, the ethos of the country's system of health care

underwrites treatment and palliative care: it is a public good. Here suffering is social. But instead of social suffering, we find social solidarity, a scene of care that is enlivening, not emotionally sterile or toxic. Even pain itself is understood as deeply social rather than, as in the West, isolating and noncommunicable. The space of healing is infused with a rich mixture of emotions, moods, and sensations, including anger and grief, faith, boredom, hilarity, and agony, many of them potentially shared by the members of this community. Especially intriguing is Livingston's discussion of trust, a quality characterizing a relationship that has an affective dimension. What is the source of this trust? In great part, trust at the level of the local derives from the foundational value of a trust that is public and national—a public trust, public health as a public good. This fundamental level of trust in the care of our health we sorely lack in the US. Instead, distrust is one of its defining features.

Third, the emotions constitute a powerful biopolitical discourse, affecting our experience and our future as a species. This dimension of the emotions (and of feelings more generally), as they emerge through political power over populations, both characterizes and creates our experience of health and disease. Today the discourse of risk and fear, security and safety anchors the poles of an omnipresent structure of feeling at the global and local levels; these feelings of risk—of anxiety, fear, dread, and terror—are testimony to the threat presented by multiple sources of disease and to our experience of concomitant emerging forms of social organization (R. Williams 1977; see "Risk"). Countless people around the world, for example, have suffered the devastating effects of toxic environments, with exposure to nuclear radiation resulting in lethal disease a horrifying case in point. For decades people living and working at such sites infected by radioactivity have had to learn how to adjust themselves to the differing levels of risk, finding ways of lowering the feeling of risk to a tolerable level as if it were their blood pressure, seeking the emergence of a feeling of safety they can balance against the risk (Cram 2016). My term for this psychological process is *self-mitigating risk*.

Inarguably, the rampant global circulation of the infectious disease COVID-19 beginning in 2019 offers the most salient illustration of the structure of feeling of risk and security in relation to health and illness. With this wildly contagious coronavirus, four of the five major categories of feeling—emotion, mood, affect, and sensation—combined together in different proportions depending on the situation. More specifically, statistical panic, as I call it, the sense of being at risk derived from large sets of numbers, was a major strain of the dominant structure of feeling (Woodward 2009; see "Panic"). As Melinda Cooper has described it, the state of being at risk is "a state of fear without foreseeable end" (2008, 97). Unlike the cancer ward in Botswana where Livingston finds a rich mixture of emotions and other feelings, a sense of communal vitality in the face of destructive disease, with COVID-19 the dominant structure of feeling contracted—as did feelings themselves—to avoiding risk and seeking safety, signaling the impoverishment of our individual and collective emotional lives and possibly a long-term weakening of the emotional resilience of the human species.

In conclusion, as we look to future research in the health humanities, two areas seem particularly fruitful. First, a comparative history of humanitarian crises in different countries focusing on rhetorics of the emotions deployed in the media to drive people and institutions to provide help. I would like to see studies of pity, benevolence, and mercy, emotional stances largely out of favor in the West. Second, an exploration of the relationships between sickness and emotion in the worlds of nonhuman animals, in terms of both self-care and care of others.

21

Empathy

Jane F. Thrailkill

Empathy is broadly understood as an attunement to the suffering, needs, or experience of another. In health humanities, many see empathic responsiveness as a core value of the field (Johanna Shapiro et al. 2009; Campo 2005; Charon 2001). And yet when it comes to twenty-first-century health care, empathy seems to be that which is too often lacking. This paradox positions us to ask, What exactly *is* this unique sensibility, and how did it become so entwined—problematically so—with the work of clinicians in our current high-tech medical world?

Spliced together from the Greek roots *-em* and *-path* to form *in-feeling*, empathy names the capacity of human beings to feel their way into that which is not them. Despite sounding vaguely Aristotelian, empathy's far shorter genealogy begins with nineteenth-century philosophy. Einfühlung (the German word for "in-feeling") involved a dissolving of the felt distinction between self and object that might arise when, for example, viewing a painting or landscape. In 1909, the British-American psychologist Edward Titchener coined *empathy* to describe a similar experience of spontaneous attunement—not with an inert object but with another *person*.

Titchener describes how this "in-feeling" happens: "Not only do I see gravity and modesty and pride," he writes, "but I feel or act them in the mind's muscles. This is, I suppose, a simple case of empathy, if we may coin that term as a rendering of *Einfühlung*" (1909, 21).

Akin to laparoscopy, empathy involves experiencing another person *as if from the inside*. With empathy, Titchener translates a concept drawn from German aesthetics into Greek for American medicine, endowing a word freshly minted in the twentieth century with the flavor of ancient origins.

Before *empathy*, *sympathy* was the word that described this kind of "in-feeling." Eighteenth-century philosophers Adam Smith and David Hume conceived of sympathy as the capacity, through imagination, to be attuned to the joys and sorrows of another, although Smith thought sympathy involved active reflection and perspective taking (thereby maintaining the self-other distinction), while Hume thought the attunement was instinctive and immediate (dissolving the self-other distinction). That Hume's *sympathy* sounds like Titchener's *empathy* is not a surprise: the nineteenth-century German popularizer of Einfuhlung was a Hume scholar.

Nevertheless, twenty-first century definitions distinguish *empathy* from *sympathy*. With empathy, generally speaking, one feels *with*, putting oneself in another's shoes and suspending the self-other distinction. With sympathy (as with its synonym *pity*) one feels *for*, witnessing and lauding another's joy or bemoaning their sorrows. The self-other distinction is preserved. Empathy provides something different: a responsiveness that is direct, embodied, and mimetic, involving what Rebecca Garden calls "emotional self-attunement and imagining" (2007, 557). The popular inspirational speaker Brené Brown puts it this way: "Empathy fuels connection. Sympathy *drives* disconnection" (2016).

The term *empathy* was coined just as medicine in the US became a "sovereign profession" (Starr 1982; R. Porter 1999). With the founding of the Johns Hopkins Medical School in 1893, essential physician expertise shifted away from feelings and intuition (formerly valued as "bedside manner" and "folk wisdom") toward science-based knowledge and the associated value of detached observation. The 1910 Flexner Report established national requirements for physician education and licensure, mandating systematic training in laboratory sciences. Medical technology expanded to include stethoscopes, X-rays, and microscopes, placing the emphasis on visualizing the body rather than listening to a patient. Competent care, in other words, was increasingly divorced from feeling and tethered to scientific "objectivity."

What was needed, paradoxically, was for the physician to develop a supersensibility to accompany—and to compensate for—their newly penetrative insight into the workings of the body's systems. *Empathy* offered a technical-sounding term that fit nicely into the modern physician's toolbox. Coupled with the knowledge provided by new fields like microbiology, bacteriology, and neurology, empathy provided a way for clinicians to "tune in" to gain a deeper understanding—without being too "touchy-feely" (to use our parlance today).

Empathy was keyed to the impersonal conditions of modern health care. As medicine shifted from home to hospital, twentieth-century clinicians were taxed with what Charles Rosenberg (1987) has called "the care of strangers." Such strangers in the early twentieth-century US included vast numbers of immigrants for whom English was a second language. Cultural differences were compounded in fast-growing northern cities, as Black Americans migrated to escape racist terror in the South. Empathy, at least as an ideal, promised to overcome differences of language, culture, racial affiliation, and national belonging and put the clinician in touch with the patient's needs.

Starting in the 1990s, neuroscientists began to offer a physiological basis for empathy: "Mirror neurons are a specific type of visuomotor neuron that discharge both when a monkey executes a motor act and when it observes a similar motor act performed by another individual" (Rizzolatti and Fogassi 2014, 1). Charismatic popularizer of mirror neurons, the neuroscientist V. S. Ramachandran repeats and aggrandizes the earlier claims of Titchener and Hume, calling them "Gandhi neurons" that succeed in "dissolving the barrier between you and me" (Colapinto 2009).

Now, in the twenty-first century, *empathy* has become a byword. What we might call the applied-empathy book industry has been booming for a decade: starting with Jodi Halpern's (2011) *From Detached Concern to Empathy: Humanizing Medical Practice*, other titles such as *Empathy: Why It Matters and How to Get It* (Krznaric 2014) and *The Empathy Effect: Seven Neuroscience-Based Keys for Transforming the Way We Live, Love, Work, and Connect across Differences* (Riess and Neporent 2018) have touted empathy as a cure-all for social ills and a stimulant for professional success. First-wave health humanities researchers have counted empathy as one of the field's core "Es," along with ethics, education, and experience (Whitehead and Woods 2018).

What's not to like about empathy, insofar as it names the wish to enter into, appreciate, and effectively remediate the distress of others?

For second-wave health humanities scholars, empathy's simple-seeming metaphor of stepping into another's shoes has been diabolically hard to pin down in its ethical entailments and its practical application. Some dismiss empathy as "an unexamined emotional response to the experience of others, a form of false identification and flawed knowledge that disregards distance and difference" (Jurecic 2011, 17). Psychologist Paul Bloom's (2016) *Against Empathy: The Case for Rational Compassion* argues that empathy is biased, shortsighted, unreliable, innumerate (focusing on one over many), and potentially coercive. Empathy centers clinician feeling and can be used as a tool to gain patient compliance and secure customer satisfaction within a competitive, billion-dollar health-care industry. It is notable, in this vein, that top-ranked hospital group the Cleveland Clinic paid dearly for a multipage advertisement in the *Washington Post* announcing they practiced "Empathy by Design," "building empathy into the DNA of their operations" (Cleveland Clinic 2017).

The bureaucratic structures within which modern medicine takes place make the primal scene of empathy, the clinician-patient encounter, seem quaint or indeed a distraction from population-level needs, such as poor, uninsured people's desperate need for Medicaid expansion or the scarcity of abortion clinics in the United States (Cross-Call and Broadus 2020; Ellman 2020). Moreover, faced with acute suffering, complex patients, exhausting hours, and tangles of red tape alongside a demand for empathy, clinicians today are plagued by burnout (Patel et al. 2018).

Perceiving empathy in market terms, as a rare resource in need of replenishment, produces a brutal paradox: the demand appears to make the desired entity evaporate. In my own teaching, I find medical students are acutely aware of the dangers of depersonalization and emotional numbness—the so-called empathy deficit. They take their emotional temperatures, agonize about encroaching negativity, and seek an impossible balance between maintaining calm professionalism and revealing their own feelings, doubts, and vulnerabilities. So, from top to bottom, the question of empathy is both fraught and meaningful in health care today.

Might the term itself be part of the problem? Or put another way, Are we, in the context of health humanities, asking too much of a single, slippery word?

In health care and beyond, we ask empathy to do many things that we believe thinking, colloquy, and theorizing alone cannot accomplish. In aesthetics, to explain human beings' sensory experience of beauty in the object world. In psychology, to answer the question of how we can discern what another thinks and feels. In ethics, to affirm the altruistic impulse to wish another well. In literary study, to center the activities of perspective taking and mind reading. In law, to provide a basis for judicial wisdom. And in health care, to anchor the impulse to care. As one psychologist has noted, "One reason it is difficult to get a good handle on empathy is that it *has so many handles*" (M. Davis 2018, ix).

In the broad field of health care, however, it would seem we have many likely alternatives for our Greek-rooted neologism: these include not only sympathy but also compassion, sensitivity, tact, and concern—or simply the gerund *caring*. The discourse of empathy has tended to eclipse these "softer" terms in discussions about the need to humanize contemporary biomedicine. Perhaps now is a time to consider returning to basics.

Literary scholar Anne Whitehead offers a promising phrase: *care work* (2017, 190). This term describes "something that we *do*" rather than "something that we *have*" (189). It also implies a particular form of (often feminized) labor and brings us back to something essential: while twenty-first-century biomedicine may be de facto an immense economic engine for generating profits, it is de jure a system for providing care (see "Care"). Building from the clinical encounter, care work may also involve instituting operating-room checklists to reduce surgical error (Gawande 2011) or instigating political action to force state legislatures to extend Medicaid benefits even to the "undeserving poor"—disproportionally people of color—who fall outside (primarily) southern lawmakers' sympathies (L. Snowden and Graaf 2019).

Substituting *care work* for *empathy* would emphasize that human concern, at its imaginative best, is fundamentally active, social, and material—applicable across scales, implementable in policy, and not a matter of externalizing and instrumentalizing the inmost regions of the self. Such a shift of terms could be as powerful as trading out the term *prostitution* for *sex work*. Care work would embrace both household and clinic labor while also describing a basic building block of a well-functioning society. Viewed thus, care work is as descriptive as it is aspirational and extends well beyond medicine. "Only by multiplying our circles of care," urge the authors of *The Care Manifesto*, "will we achieve the psychic infrastructures necessary to build a caring society that has universal care as its ideal" (Chatzidakis et al. 2020, 33).

22

Environment

David N. Pellow

The term *environment* emerged with some visibility and circulation during the nineteenth century and is a concept that is as layered and nearly as complicated as the term *nature*, which Raymond Williams once wrote "is perhaps the most complex word in the language" (1976, 219). Vermonja Alston notes that *environment* has been defined in various ways over the centuries but that an enduring understanding is focused on "'surroundings' rather than complex interlinked ecological systems" (2016, 96). For example, my Random House dictionary from 1984 defines *environment* variously as "the aggregate of surrounding things, conditions, or influences"; as "the act of environing"; or as "the state of being environed." Relatedly, the term *environ* is listed in that same source as a verb meaning "to form a circle or ring round; surround; envelop" (Stein 1984, 442). Alston argues that these definitions reflect a colonial logic that supports the kinds of practices involving enclosures of "bodies of land, water, people, plants, and nonhuman animals . . . to exploit and appropriate biodiversity and indigenous knowledge" (2016, 94), as well as the destruction of commons. The myriad ways in which our environments reflect enclosures are sites where the health of our ecosystems and humankind is in considerable jeopardy and where social inequities are amplified. The ubiquitous presence of both environmental harms and social inequality around the globe is indeed a challenge in and of itself, but their frequent and consistent intersections at multiple scales is a major concern for environmental justice scholars and advocates. That is, populations facing virtually any kind of social, economic, political, or cultural marginalization are much more likely to experience greater risks and threats associated with environmental pollution and climate change. That means people of color, Indigenous Peoples, immigrants, working-class populations, women, disabled people, and LGBTQ communities are facing greater health risks than the rest of us (Bullard and Wright 2012). These threats have been the focus of grassroots environmental justice movements for decades, which have sought to confront and repair the harms associated with enclosures in order to ensure improved health for humans, ecosystems, and nonhuman species. And they do so by mobilizing their bodies in protest and their ideas into counternarratives and stories that challenge environmental racism and envision justice.

If one of the primary aims of the health humanities is to "debate and develop the role of the humanities in health as a whole rather than solely in medicine" (Crawford et al. 2010, 8; see also T. Jones, Wear, and Friedman 2014), then the environment and environmental justice are central to this project. First, as numerous scholars have documented, the health of our environment and its constituent ecosystems and habitats is intimately related to public/human health, which requires us to extend our analyses well beyond both the medical system (as a site of health delivery) and a restrictive notion of health that is humancentric (Celermajer et al. 2020; Schlosberg 2007). Second, when social inequalities produce health disparities across racial, income, and gender groups, we find that those same inequalities are associated with environmental disparities, generally referred to as environmental injustices and/or environmental racism. Furthermore, environmental injustices contribute enormously to the health disparities we find across societies (Brulle and Pellow 2006). Third, thinking about the environmental factors shaping health facilitates our capacity to address health concerns on both local and global scales and to focus on the structural forces impacting our health. Fourth, the myriad linkages between human health and environmental health routinely reveal that improving both requires the mobilization of ordinary people in grassroots social movements.

Storytelling is a key tool for work on the environmental justice dimensions of the health humanities (Bleakley, Wilson, and Allard 2020; Sze 2020). What frequently motivates and sustains people's involvements in such social movements are the power and resonance of stories—stories that narrate the injustices that must be confronted and stories that paint a vision of a more desirable and ecologically healthy future. Environmental justice activists and scholars often narrate stories that detail the struggles of marginalized individuals and communities facing terrifying public health threats that directly impact the well-being of their family members and friends who are exposed to exceedingly high levels of pollution in their food, water, air, land, and/or homes. In these stories, the immediate sources of those exposures to disproportionate environmental threats are usually government agencies or corporations (and often both), while the broader causes are associated with racial capitalism, settler colonialism, and white supremacy. Thus, in these stories, activists and community members must mobilize their bodies and their own narratives to engender support (often as much from national and global stakeholders as local ones) to remedy these injustices. A number of scholars—in and beyond the health humanities—have argued that while the hegemonic production of social difference engenders discrimination and oppression, the spaces that difference makes are also sites and opportunities for

realizing and fomenting social justice and counterhegemonic cultural practices (Gutierrez and DasGupta 2016). The environmental justice movement is one such effort: individuals and communities living with health-impairing environmental injustices associated with racial, class, or anti-Indigenous discrimination are also making spaces for using that experience of oppression to critique and transform the arrangements that created that differential value system in the first place. And storytelling is one mode of creating those critical spaces.

The act and art of storytelling can assist communities in thinking deeply about their state of health and their relationship to the environment and in developing ideas and language that have the potential to unsettle dominant narratives through critique and other forms of resistance (B. Rose et al. 2012). These approaches can offer scholars and advocates tools for developing global public and environmental health narratives that step outside of the confines of traditional clinical narratives regarding individual health and medicine. As Hutchings (2014, 214) writes, "Effort must increasingly be made [toward] mobilizing (radical) change 'on the ground,' be it in the form of actively spreading counternarratives or (re)building healthy communities and places." Stefania Barca (2014) and Donna Houston (2013) have both proposed a framework that links the health humanities to environmental justice politics and narrative work. They argue that communities facing industrial contamination have been exposed to a form of "narrative injustice" and "narrative violence" in that their experiences with the negative health impacts of environmental injustice have largely been made invisible and silenced by dominant institutions and ways of knowing. This erasure and silencing carries a triple price: (1) it suppresses the voices of those communities directly affected by environmental injustice, (2) it makes it that much more difficult for these communities to access the health-protective resources they need to address the physiological and psychological effects of environmental injustice, and (3) it serves to produce and amplify ignorance of such struggles in other communities that could also be impacted by industrial toxins and/or where allies and accomplices might be found. Barca (2014) contends that a productive response to this violence is "telling the right story" by uncovering and/or coproducing environmentally just narratives that reflect the experiences and desires of impacted communities. Armiero et al. (2019) build on that idea and argue that storytelling with and by environmental justice community activists is a method and practice that involves both collecting and communicating stories as well as building community. These are methods, tactics, and strategies that can effectively narrate pathways toward racial and environmental justice by mobilizing people around the value of protecting their health, the health of their loved ones, and the health of the land they depend on.

One of the larger lessons of the struggle against environmental injustice and health disparities is not just that people of color and other marginalized communities are facing disproportionate harm but also that the systems of racial domination that produce these inequities also harm the majority's ability to access healthy environments and to secure their own well-being (Metzl 2019). In other words, environmental racism, environmental injustice, and health discrimination result in negative impacts for nearly everyone, not just vulnerable populations. Thus, the enclosures that segregate, dispossess, and target oppressed groups in ways that jeopardize their health and well-being also have much broader socioecological consequences that reveal a global ecology of interdependence and accountability. That is a story in need of telling—repeatedly.

23

Epidemic
Christos Lynteris

The term *epidemic* (from the Greek *epi-*, for "upon," and *-demos*, for a populace as a political unit) is used in modern medicine to refer to outbreaks of infectious and noncommunicable diseases affecting human communities rather than just an individual or her and his immediate social environment. Epidemics have attracted analyses and commentaries concerning their social, political, and economic impact for millennia. Indeed, the emergence of history in classical Greece as a method for examining the past coincides with such approaches to epidemics, with Thucydides's account of the "plague of Athens" being the first historical account of an epidemic and the first work to frame a disease outbreak in sociological and anthropological terms (Orwin 1988). In both medical and nonmedical narratives articulated in Europe since the initial iteration of the term in the Hippocratic Corpus, ideas around the "epidemic" became entangled with shifting aetiological and epistemological frameworks and with associated political, cosmological, and moral configurations of "plague" and "pestilence" (Gardner 2019; Slack 1992; F. Snowden 2020). At the same time, whether through exchange and translation or through conquest and colonization, European ideas about epidemics impacted and were in turn shaped by non-European frameworks of diseases affecting human communities, such as *Wabā* (Arabic) and *wenyi* (Chinese) (Hanson 2011; Stearns 2011; Varlik 2015). At the end of the nineteenth century, bacteriology provided a new ontological framework for diseases that fostered an integration of medical approaches to epidemics in Western medicine and the propagation of the latter's framing of epidemics across the globe within the context of colonialism (Latour 1988; Worboys 2000; Chakrabarti 2012).

From the early nineteenth century onward, epidemics came to be framed anew within the sphere of the humanities. Key to this approach to epidemics and its popular appeal was the development of the idea of the Black Death. As Faye Marie Getz (1991) has shown, the notion of the Black Death, used to describe the devastating plague epidemics of the fourteenth century, became fully expressed in the homonymous work of J. F. C. Hecker (1833), from which it became a concept of lasting impact to our days. The transformation of the 1346–53 plague outbreaks into the Black Death involved what Getz has described as a process of gothification that rendered plague into a manifestation of the forces of nature facing humanity and, at the same time, into a world-historical agent imbued with catastrophic properties. Historical reworkings of this thesis up until the midst of the twentieth century maintained various degrees of catastrophism (Coulton 1929; Creighton 1891; Gasquet 1893; Lipson 1929) or focused on presenting modern science's triumph over infectious diseases (F. Hirst 1953; Zinsser 1935). The focus on discontinuity or the ability of epidemics to usher in radically new social, political, and economic realities was challenged by social, environmental, economic, and cultural histories of epidemics and epidemic control from the 1970s onward (e.g., Carmichael 1986; Brandt 1985; Crosby 1976; R. Evans 1987; Delaporte 1986; Charles Rosenberg 1989b). This led to more nuanced and increasingly theoretically engaged approaches to epidemics by historians as well as to systematic analyses of the ways in which diseases have led to or were impacted by global integration (e.g., Ladurie 1973; Hays 1998; McNeill [1976]

2010; Echenberg 2007). Emerging for the first time in the 1980s from the application of subaltern studies to the history of epidemics and their management in British India (Arnold 1993; Catanach 1988), postcolonial approaches have led to understandings of epidemics as a field for the development and imposition of colonial power as well as for indigenous resistance and innovation (e.g., W. Anderson 2006; Bhattacharya, Harrison, and Worboys 2005; Cueto 2001; Harrison 1999; Kelton 2015; Leung and Liang 2009; Lyons 1992; Mavhunga 2018; Packard 1989; Peckham 2016; Vaughan 1991).

Today the broad field of the medical humanities is informed by nuanced approaches to epidemics that integrate social, postcolonial, comparative, global, and micro- and biohistorical perspectives with anthropological, sociological, geographical, and cultural studies analyses of the social life of epidemics, as both events and ideas, across different sociocultural contexts. Critical medical anthropologists, sociologists, and political scientists, through their interest in the political economy and structural violence, have fostered nondeterministic understandings of the social drivers of epidemics (e.g., Chigudu 2020; Dingwall, Hoffman, and Staniland 2013; Inhorn and Brown 1990; Nguyen and Peschard 2003), most notably through the notion of the syndemic (M. Singer 2009b). At the same time, anthropologists have been active in the study of the way in which the management of epidemics, through prevention and containment, contributes to social inequalities and stigmatization (e.g., C. Briggs and Mantini-Briggs 2016; Farmer 1999a; A. Kelly, Keck, and Lynteris 2019) as well as in developing multispecies approaches to epidemics, especially as regards zoonotic and vector-borne diseases, in dialogue and in critique of emerging One Health perspectives in global health (Bardosh 2016; H. Brown and Nading 2019; Keck and Lynteris 2018). Geographers have in turn contributed nuanced analyses of the spatial aspects of epidemics, with an emphasis on architecture, planning, and the materialities of infection (Hinchliffe et al. 2016; Herring and Swedlund 2010). In the realm of cultural studies, epidemics have been approached both in and as culture. With what started as a focus on diseases as metaphors (Sontag 1989) and enriched by feminist studies, queer studies, and activist approaches to the AIDS/HIV pandemic (Crimp 1988, 2002; Haraway 1991; Martin 1995), cultural studies have focused on the representation of epidemics in novels, films, plays, and video games but also noncorporate cultural practices (e.g., Finkelstein 2020; Hernández 2019; Ostherr 2005; Schweitzer 2018) as well as epidemiology as cultural practice. Understood as based on and in turn promoting the actualization of "outbreak narratives" (Wald 2008), which are derived from synergies between science and the culture industry, epidemiology as cultural practice has been shown to establish contagion not simply as a metaphor but as a central model for understanding social relations and human interactions with the non-human world.

Multi- and interdisciplinary approaches to epidemics and epidemiology both within the humanities and the social sciences and in collaboration with the life sciences have led to analyses of both historical and actual epidemics that allow us to understand these as integrated biological and social phenomena but also develop new conceptual frameworks (Bourgeois 2002; Inhorn 1995; Packard and Epstein 1991; Trostle 2005). Nowhere has interdisciplinarity been more crucial than in the examination of pandemics. The notion of the pandemic, like that of the epidemic, emerged in the Hippocratic Corpus but, by contrast to the latter, was not extensively or systematically used before the end of the nineteenth century. Mark Harrison (2017) has argued that the concept was first systematically

employed to describe the 1889–91 "Russian flu" pandemic. What, however, gave symbolic and epistemic coherence to the term and put it in common use across the globe was the coverage of the chain of outbreaks of bubonic plague between 1894 and 1959 known as the third plague pandemic. Narratives and visualizations of the outbreaks of plague in the late nineteenth century mobilized the notion of the Black Death in forging for the first time a lay experience of "the pandemic." Representing even the slightest outbreak as a herald of a world-catastrophic event, they created what until today remains the interlaced temporality of pandemics: events that refer to a present phenomenon insofar as they describe a chain of global infection like COVID-19 but also one that is rendered meaningful and actionable only to the extent that it is seen in relation and comparison to icons of past pandemics (the Black Death, the "Spanish flu" of 1918–19) and their supposed world-historical, catastrophic potential.

As Carlo Caduff (2015) has argued, this means that, at least since the establishment of the emerging infectious diseases framework in the early 1990s (N. King 2004), the idea of the pandemic is always already linked to that of the "next pandemic," the always deferred epidemiological event that will supposedly face humanity with a crisis of existential risk. Anthropologists have examined in detail how the notion of the "next pandemic" has brought into place biosecurity practices and regimes that have shifted attention away from prevention and toward preparedness (Lakoff 2017; Caduff 2015; Keck 2020; Samimian-Darash 2009). Involving a technoscientific array ranging from sentinels, syndromic surveillance, stockpiling, and culling, preparedness has also come to be seen as a doctrine that frames specific animal species as epidemic "rogues" or "villains" while also framing multispecies interactions (bush meat and wet markets in particular) as the ground zeros of pandemic risk (Bonwitt et al. 2018; Fairhead 2018; Fearnley 2020; Lynteris 2019a; Lynteris 2019b; Narat et al. 2017; N. Porter 2019; Zhan 2005).

The response from the medical humanities to the outbreak of COVID-19 and its management is nested within critical approaches of epidemiology, global health, and epidemic response and is crucially informed by engagements in recent epidemics, such as Ebola and Zika, where a range of scholars became involved both in providing expertise from a distance and in on-the-ground interventions, which have greatly contributed to the development of community-led approaches to epidemic control (P. Richards 2016). Moving away from previous practices of simply "translating culture," emerging collaborative and interdisciplinary practices have sought to proceed through a critique of conceptual frameworks dominating epidemiology and global health as well as the structural inequalities in collaboration and the latter's requirements of toning down conceptual and epistemological disparities, including the very definition of collaboration, in the context of epidemic emergencies (H. Brown and Kelly 2014; Elliot and Thomas 2017; Leach 2019; M. Singer 2009a).

24

Evidence
Pamela K. Gilbert

Evidence, originally meaning "something clearly visible or obvious," has only relatively recently become an important term in science, after a long history of use in religion and law. The term began to be used as we use it now in science—to mean empirical data, gathered in accord with scientific method and used to test a hypothesis—in the late nineteenth century, soon after science research began to be sufficiently specialized that people of broad culture began to find it difficult to understand. By 1959, in a lecture at Cambridge that subsequently became an important book, the novelist and physical chemist C. P. Snow famously identified the sciences and humanities as having become "two cultures," with different vocabularies, assumptions, and interests, and decried the loss of scientists' interest in the humanities (1959, 1).

Medicine has long been considered to be poised between the arts and sciences, and medical practice is often defined as an art based on scientific knowledge. Toward the end of the twentieth century, however, a new term gained traction in medical education and practice: *evidence-based medicine* (EBM). This approach emphasized practical application of the findings of the best available current research in the field and de-emphasized a reliance on the physician's intuition or experience. This also meant an increasing reliance on quantitative data, thought to militate against confirmation bias: the tendency to be more swayed by information that confirms beliefs the practitioner already holds.

Many humanists (and recently educated doctors) are surprised to find that this approach is new. It was in the 1960s that cultural changes and the rise of social science critiques led to attempts to demythologize the authority of doctors (Hanemaayer 2016, 451–52). Responding to this, doctors sought to locate medical authority less in the mystique of individual expertise and more clearly in science. David M. Eddy, an American doctor and mathematical and policy expert, began in the 1980s to critique the lack of scientific evidence in much clinical decision-making. He published the term *evidence-based* in March 1990 in *JAMA*, identifying guidelines for clinicians' use of scientific data. After introducing "evidence-based medicine" into medical education at his own university, Canadian doctor Gordon Guyatt and colleagues wrote in a 1992 *JAMA* article, "A NEW paradigm for medical practice is emerging. Evidence-based medicine de-emphasizes intuition, unsystematic clinical experience, and pathophysiologic rationale as sufficient grounds for clinical decision making and stresses the examination of evidence from clinical research. Evidence-based medicine requires new skills of the physician, including efficient literature searching and the application of formal rules of evidence evaluating the clinical literature" (2420). EBM was heavily influenced by epidemiology and tended to favor quantitative models. It quickly became enormously influential.

Among critics of EBM, there are roughly two subdivisions: one that considers EBM to have a damaging overemphasis on population data with questionable value for the individual patient and one that more actively questions the value and reliability of such quantitative data in the first place (see Marini 2016 for discussion; see also J. Saunders 2001; Greenhalgh 2001). The first questions whether statistical data alone helps the clinician facing a particular patient with complex issues, impacting the patient's ability or desire to follow medical advice: if Mary doesn't speak a doctor's language well, she may not understand her clinician; if she doesn't understand her clinician, she may not communicate a contraindication for this treatment; if Mary isn't insured, she may not be able to afford her medicine; if Mary doesn't trust her clinician, she may withhold important information; if Mary is abused at home, she may not be able to comply with her treatment. And even then, Mary is not simply a human body detached from context—she is enmeshed in a world that includes her environment (she should drink more water, but her drinking water may be polluted) and her human clinician, who has unconscious biases. For example, even with EBM, black women are much less likely to be prescribed pain control in acute care (Hoffman et al. 2016). A recommendation derived from large data sets representing people in vastly different circumstances will not be clinically helpful to all people equally.

If the first set of critiques asks about the individual applicability of data derived from large populations, the second asks about its quality. If, as is often the case, data is drawn from populations from which a certain "messiness" has been eliminated (study participants eliminated for a preexisting condition, comorbidity, or additional prescription), then how useful is that in making a recommendation for people in the real world? What if Mary has cancer, diabetes, and hypertension but is also taking herbs prescribed by her acupuncturist and training for a 5K? Moreover, publication bias, funding bias, and the academic disincentives against publishing negative results mean that the information from quantitative studies is not simply a factual, value-free description of the world (Marini 2016). Moreover, not all clinicians are equally able to evaluate the statistical reliability or individual suitability of quantitative evidence, yet they are bombarded with it, often by adroit pharmaceutical marketers with monetary incentives.

Health humanities has developed over recent decades in part as a supplement to the kinds of scientific knowledge and training promoted in part by EBM, a corrective that would allow physicians to get at issues around the individual nature of patients as well as broader issues such as ethics. In the humanities, "evidence" is more often qualitative. It includes narratives, art, movement, and history, and explicit awareness of the explanatory framework is part of an argument's evidence (what is persuasive within a psychoanalytic framework may not be within a cultural-historical one). It is attentive to questions of affect, the lifeworld, and complex human elements of selfhood and its relation to the environment, both human and nonhuman. It attends to beliefs and values. It is often focused on individuals, although it may also analyze larger populations, as in histories of epidemics or national policies. For example, a health humanities study of an epidemic might use quantitative data (mortality rates), fictional and nonfictional narratives (patient stories, novels), and other historical information to understand not only how people lived and died but how social and cultural attitudes about race, gender, sexuality, class, or ability affect medical and lay responses to minority populations caught in the same epidemic.

There are roughly three approaches at present to the "two cultures" of evidence in medical practice and in the humanities. As we have seen, one questions the integrity and usefulness of the evidence on which EBM depends. Another seeks to balance the overreliance on scientific and quantitative evidence with other kinds of knowledge. In a review essay, "Medicine: Science or Art?," S. C. Panda (2006) determines, "Medicine . . . is not an exact science. It is an applied science, and its practice is an art. . . . In effective medicine, the power imbued in the caregiver is based on trust. . . . Trust blossoms not only out of competency or skill; it involves sensitivity to another world-view. . . . That Medicine is a science is the popular belief, and this has been reinforced by the advent of 'evidence-based medicine.' However, the view of science implied is a narrow one, foreign both to pure scientists and to artists and the art of medicine is devalued by this approach." Rita Charon, a founder of narrative medicine (see her entry in this volume), believes that both kinds of knowledge are necessary and complementary. However, Charon argues, "A scientifically competent medicine alone cannot help a patient grapple with the loss of health and find meaning in illness and dying" (2001, 28). To this end, she advises cultivating the kind of narrative competence that literary scholars use.

So far, we have mostly discussed the critique of evidence related to the first wave of medical humanities that tended to be focused on patient care and the clinical encounter. Some critics on the medical side have faulted the humanities' standards of evidence for being insufficiently rigorous because they tend to be qualitative. In turn, medical humanities advocates often sought to justify their discipline in terms of quantitative evidence of improvements in outcomes for patient health and satisfaction and for medical education. Others, as we have seen, have critiqued that hierarchy of evidence within medicine itself. More recently, especially in the turn to health humanities, the field has questioned the early positioning of the discipline as a kind of supplement to or handmaiden of medicine, making claims for its status as valuable in itself. This is particularly germane to, for example, the history of medicine; the resolute presentism and utilitarianism of clinical medicine make very little space for claims of the importance of historical evidence. However, the tendency to view scientific progress teleologically—as progressing toward greater truth and perfection—also misses the messy human and economic dimensions of scientific research. For example, W. B. Coley discovered in the late nineteenth century that infections could trigger the body to rid itself of cancers—specifically, that erysipelas infection could be beneficial to patients suffering from sarcoma. But radiation was then a shiny new object that didn't seem "dirty" like infections, and so cancer research stopped pursuing Coley's findings and lost decades of potential progress in immunotherapy.

Beyond this utilitarian defense of historical medical humanities, however, lies a larger point. Illness, death, disability, and all permutations of health are human experiences that affect every aspect of our lives—individual and collective—and intersect with every area of study. These disciplines and the forms of evidence that inform them are valuable in themselves. A truly critical health humanities, Des Fitzgerald and Felicity Callard (2016) argue, would take on the subject of medicine not only in its practice but in its epistemological stakes. It would be informed by posthumanist understandings of humans' place in the natural world and in history as well as population- and individual-level biological and sociological issues. Health humanities are "deeply and irretrievably *entangled* in the vital, corporeal and physiological commitments of biomedicine," they argue (35–36). Conversely, as Julia Kristeva et al. (2018) argue, an interdisciplinary health humanities asks us to look beyond the nature-culture divide to realize that the subject matter of the humanities "proper" has never just been culture but also nature, including its medical implications. A successful health humanities must respect the differences between the forms and uses of evidence while embracing the messy creativity of human experience.

25

Experiment
Helen Tilley

In August 2021, twenty-nine-year-old Edrick Floreal-Wooten was treated for COVID-19 with oral medications at an Arkansas prison: "I didn't figure Washington County was going to make me an experiment and use drugs the CDC didn't recommend," he protested. "I'm not livestock. I'm a human being." Despite the availability of state-of-the-art vaccines, Arkansas's prisoners did not receive them. Instead, they were offered a "handful of pills . . . [and] told . . . it was steroids, antibiotics and vitamins." Floreal-Wooten and others incarcerated there later learned one of the medications they were given was ivermectin, an antiparasitic developed for roundworm diseases and used for humans and farm animals. The FDA and CDC explicitly cautioned against its use. Still, the prison doctor, Robert Karas, publicly defended his choices, claiming he had dispensed ivermectin since late 2020 and "not one single patient of the five hundred plus who have followed our plan of care has been hospitalized, intubated or died." He insisted he was not "conducting [his] own clinical trial or study." To his patients and critics, though—including the American Civil Liberties Union, which brought a lawsuit against Karas and the prison—that was exactly what he seemed to be doing (Sissom 2021; Crafts 2021).

The COVID-19 pandemic offers a poignant entrée into the history and politics of the concept *experiment*. Medical professionals and the scholars who study them will recognize what makes the Arkansas case salient:

prison personnel withheld crucial information about treatment and neither sought nor received patients' consent. They abused prisoners' trust, took advantage of their incarcerated status, stripped them of rights, and openly rejected FDA and NIH treatment protocols. Yet the case also highlights a truism in medical history: when a disease is still unfamiliar, much about its control and treatment becomes an experiment of sorts, and murky areas can multiply. Karas may not have undertaken formal drug research, but his decision to eschew vaccines, even as more infectious strains of COVID-19 circulated, guaranteed he had a steady stream of people in the prison on whom to try ivermectin. In many respects, US prisons became a de facto if not de jure experiment for studying the spread, lethality, and treatment of COVID.

The word *experiment*, much like *hygiene*, has cognates in multiple languages, a feature of cross-cultural influences that deserves more attention within global studies of health (Rogaski 2004). In Romance and Germanic languages, it derives from the French word *expérience* (arising from a Latin root), which has the dual meaning of "experience" and "experiment." The Spanish word *experimentar* is similarly dualistic. If we go back far enough, Francophone and Anglophone etymologies of *experiment* reveal it once conveyed ideas about enchantment and sorcery, capturing the uncertainty about who (or what) could control and change reality. Historians have located important struggles to fix *experiment*'s meaning in the seventeenth century, when European scholars debated how best to arrive at true claims—or proof—about how the world worked. Those who sought to privilege experiential or empirical knowledge over claims derived from reasoning alone ultimately triumphed (Shapin and Schaffer 1985). Even so, ambiguities in the concept and its cognates remain, as early modern histories of experiential and experimental

knowledge among people of African descent in colonial Latin America and the Caribbean underscore (Gómez 2017; Schiebinger 2017).

Just what are the roots of experimental logics, and how did experts come to construct arenas of healing and knowing as separate spheres within biomedical traditions? One of the more compelling (if geographically incomplete) origin stories about experimental medicine focuses on western Europe and the United States between 1790 and 1850, when hospitals in urban centers became more numerous and novel pandemics, such as cholera, had acute effects on mortality rates in many parts of the world (R. Porter 1999; Charles Rosenberg 1962). The volume and concentration of patients in these settings allowed doctors to refine diagnostic methods and test new treatments. Along the way, they also began to standardize disease classifications, improve instruments, and practice their empirical skills on both the living and the dead. These changes, in turn, affected how medicine was taught. Dissections had long been part of medical training, but urban doctors working in hospitals now started to perform autopsies more routinely, often taking advantage of indigent patients (whose bodies were never collected) to determine causes of death with greater precision. Doctors and pharmacists also expanded their pharmacopeia and tested different medical compounds more systematically (Weiner and Sauter 2003).

As clinical expertise accumulated, medical professionals began to call for increasingly exact "scientific" studies of bodily states and therapeutic effects. They recognized that hospitals were less than ideal spaces to explore the underlying causes of disease and that there were limits to what could be learned from unwell patients. More controlled conditions were needed in which aspects specific to living organisms could be manipulated. Although laboratories had played an important role in chemical and mechanical studies for decades, in the middle of the nineteenth century, they became central to professional definitions of medical research (Cunningham and Williams 1992). Parisian doctor and physiologist Claude Bernard, alert to the ethical and religious issues involved in testing medical theories and treatments on humans, recognized that modern moral precepts needed to determine what constituted acceptable practice. His 1865 textbook on experimental medicine considered whether physicians had "a right to perform experiments and vivisection on man" (Bernard [1865] 1927, 101). Answering with a qualified yes, he explained he could no longer recommend certain tests, including on prisoners, and concluded, "Among the experiments that may be tried on man, those that can only harm are forbidden, those that are innocent are permissible, and those that may do good are obligatory" (101–2; Coleman 1985).

Bernard and his Euro-American compatriots often failed to appreciate, however, how difficult it was for professions to monitor the borders between trials that harmed and those that helped. They also ignored the entangled political and economic structures that turned so many regions of the world and the people in them into de facto laboratories. Indeed, prisons were just one historical site among many where both *formal* and *informal* medical research on human subjects had taken place and where experimenters compromised people's sovereignty and flouted questions of consent. Colonies, factories, plantations, orphanages, schools, asylums, quarantine zones, battlefields, military bases, indigenous reserves, and concentration camps have all played crucial roles in producing experimental knowledge (Rabinbach 1990; Arnold 1993; Palmer 2009; Tilley 2011; Graboyes 2014). The architects of all these settings distributed political rights in a hierarchical fashion. Few medical doctors needed Claude Bernard to tell them

what they already understood intuitively: some people were more easily studied and experimented upon than others, and some places were sufficiently isolated to avoid institutional or state oversight. These dynamics have been at the heart of both egregious and quotidian medical experiments in the US and its empire (Lederer 1998; L. Briggs 2002; W. Anderson 2006; Reverby 2009; Lanzarotta 2020).

Paradoxically, industrial warfare over the course of the twentieth century served as a further catalyst for both *voluntary* and *involuntary* medical experiments on a massive scale. Soldiers in the First World War, including many from Africa and South Asia, were enlisted by the thousands to serve as research subjects to examine theories about human psychology and intelligence (via standardized tests) and the role of immunity (via new vaccines and drug treatments). Inadvertently, they also became fodder for studies of neurophysiology and mental trauma as a result of poison gases, exploding shells, and their roles in killing (Cooter, Harrison, and Sturdy 1998; Bourke 2000). By the Second World War, military personnel again were used to study penicillin's efficacy and to experiment with insecticides to control diseases. But it was the involuntary research on Jewish subjects in Nazi Germany's concentration camps that led to the infamous Nuremberg trial of doctors (Proctor 1988). Nazi ideologies, as scholars of genocide have pointed out, built upon ideas developed in the violent conquests among Nama and Herero peoples in present-day Namibia and British and American precedents with eugenics (Naimark 2016).

The Nuremberg Code of 1947 codified the idea that a person's "legal capacity to give consent" to a medical experiment meant they were free from "constraint or coercion"; being "informed" meant they were told "the nature, duration, and purpose of the experiment" and were given a clear picture of the "inconveniences . . .

hazards . . . and effects upon [their] health" ("Nuremberg Code" 1996). By 1964, the World Medical Association attempted to extend the geographical reach of these edicts with its Helsinki Declaration, hoping it would serve as "a guide to doctors all over the world" whether they undertook therapeutic research in which patients were also subjects or they designed experiments to be "purely scientific and without therapeutic value to the person subjected to the research" (World Medical Association 1964). As nontherapeutic trials grew in popularity, from the interwar period onward, they dovetailed with new statistical methods of random and blind controls in which testers and research subjects were kept in the dark about who received which treatment (Clifford Rosenberg 2012). Though randomized controlled trials are now a gold standard for medical research globally, it took nearly fifty years for them to become the building blocks for so-called evidence-based and rule-bound medical practice. From the 1980s onward, as people in wealthier parts of the world became overmedicated and overtreated, such trials shifted "offshore" where "treatment-naive" and/or disease-laden subjects could still be found in large numbers (Petryna 2009). The history of ivermectin was caught up in this shift: between 1980 and 1987, Merck Pharmaceutical's research laboratories facilitated clinical trials to study ivermectin's efficacy—for human diseases such as river blindness (onchocerciasis)—in twelve countries in West Africa (Rae et al. 2010).

Experiments, past and present, are an important topic of study in medical humanities because health infrastructures the world over have been built upon them. Such techniques not only validate some definitions of well-being while invalidating others, but they also tend to conceal deep-seated inequalities. The discrepancies help explain why experimental methods have had so many unintended effects, clouding people's understanding of what works, what does not, and why (Adams 2002). These contradictions persist for several reasons. First, existing laws and institutional norms make it difficult to censure those who appear to transgress the rules, precisely because practices alleged to be illicit (in an experiment) can be defended as permissible within regular modes of care. Arkansas's Dr. Karas and the many US physicians experimenting with ivermectin (and denigrating vaccines) during the COVID pandemic serve as a case in point. Second, formal clinical trials still rely on social hierarchies that compromise subjects' autonomy, often preventing participants from being fully informed about the effects of an experiment. Consent itself is something of a legal mirage given how much about medical knowledge and funding are black boxed. Third, powerful actors, including pharmaceutical companies, depend on the ease with which the rules governing experimental protocols can be gamed. Different abuses include ghostwritten articles, cherry-picked evidence, and oversimplified or misleading biological arguments (D. Healy 2012). Geographically and socially inclusive approaches remind us that experiments have long been transnational and transspecies and intersect with biomedical collecting practices of all kinds (Radin 2014; Jain 2020). Studies of medical experiments—formal and informal, voluntary and involuntary—need to take all these dynamics into account.

26

Gender

Gwen D'Arcangelis

Gender is a socially produced category that derives from the essentialization of bodily difference located in chromosomes, hormones, and genitals. These "sex differences," while not completely dimorphic, are often treated as such—in science, law, and public realms. Gender binaries function within many communities, nations, and cultures to govern individual expression and comportment, roles, and life trajectory. An individual assigned the sex "male" at birth is presumed not only to claim the gender identity of "man" but to also be masculine in expression and presentation; the same is true of "female," "woman," and femininity.

Scholars in gender, queer, and trans studies have critiqued the role Western biomedicine has played in reinforcing sex and gender structures and pathologizing the gender identities of nonbinary and trans communities. Medical doctors categorize infants according to genital size (used as the basis for assigning sex at birth) and routinely surgically alter infants who do not fall neatly into the binary (Dreger 2000; Fausto-Sterling 2000). US clinicians and researchers have used the American Psychiatric Association's *Diagnostic and Statistical Manual of Mental Disorders* (through its five iterations) to render trans people as suffering from "gender identity disorder" (fourth edition) and, in the fifth edition, the somewhat less stigmatizing "gender dysphoria." These diagnoses have made medical treatment related to gender transition as well as access to trans-specific medical care dependent on trans people fitting into prescribed narratives of,

for example, being in the wrong body or desiring the "opposite sex." This decenters the self-determination of trans people over their own identities as well as diminishes their medical access (Fink 2019; S. Hsu 2019).

The field of health humanities brings critical insights to issues of gender in medicine and health, questioning medical categories and centering the experiences of marginalized genders as they navigate the medical field. Marty Fink (2019) analyzes the trans coming-of-age novel *Choir Boy* (2005) by Charlie Anders and highlights how the main character in the novel, at the cusp of puberty and facing vocal changes, rejects both "male" and "female" in favor of "choirboy." The main character continues to challenge the medicalization of trans identity when he refuses to perform the "wrong body" narrative to his psychologist to obtain hormones, opting to sing instead. Fink argues that the fictional narrative models the aims of queer and feminist disability theory—by positing that patients' relationship to medical care should be one of self-definition and self-advocacy and, moreover, that reliance on medical providers need not come with acceptance of the hegemonic framing of trans bodies as something to be fixed or cured.

Health humanities scholars also expose how hegemonic Western medical systems regulate women's bodies. The social subordination of women and femmes (feminine-presenting individuals) in Western culture has shaped the post-Enlightenment dominance of biomedicine, which conceptualized reproductive organs associated with womanhood, such as the uterus, as abnormal and categorized processes like menstruation and pregnancy as illnesses. Cultural myths about the predisposition of white, upper-class women to domesticity and frailty in nineteenth-century Europe and the United States led to outlandish biomedical diagnoses: women who complained of a range of symptoms from headache to indigestion as well as a variety of mental states (such as high libido) were diagnosed with the imagined condition known as "hysteria," which at its worst subjected them to unnecessary hysterectomies as purported treatments (Ehrenreich and English [1973] 2011; Lupton 2012; Wertz and Wertz 1981). Rosemarie Garland-Thomson (2005, 1564) has described the medical construction of femaleness as a natural form of physical and mental deficiency as both the "disabling of gender" and the "gendering of disability."

Marginalized women have in particular been pathologized by cultural ideas about fertility, desire, mothering, and ability. Modern gynecology was founded on the famed Dr. J. Marion Sims's experimentation on enslaved Black women in the United States, which he rationalized with the notion of their inability to feel pain, among other cultural myths rendering Black bodies vulnerable (Holloway 2011; Snorton 2017; Washington 2006). Dorothy Roberts (1999) discusses how, in contrast to the chastity attributed to white women, Black women have been negatively constructed: historically, as sexually promiscuous and hyperfertile Jezebels or asexual and maternal mammies devoted to nurturing their white masters' children in lieu of caring about their own children and, in the mid- to late twentieth century, as domineering Black mothers and lazy welfare queens. Roberts describes how this devaluing of Black mothers has served as a technology of social control subsequent to the abolition of slavery: the US medical establishment curtailed Black women's reproduction and policed their sexuality through birth control measures—in its worst form ending in compulsory sterilization. Native, Latina, and Asian American women as well as women who are poor, are queer, and live with disabilities have also been the targets of sterilization abuse—buttressed by eugenic beliefs of their purported unfitness (Garland-Thomson 2005; Tajima-Peña 2015; Stern 2005). In the twenty-first century, women continue to face

limitations on their sexual and reproductive health and autonomy.

Patient narratives receive considerable focus in health humanities scholarship as a means to challenge oppressive cultural norms and reconfigure the relationship of socially marginalized groups to medicine and health care. Noted poet Audre Lorde (1980) mobilized biography, poetry, and analysis to center her experience navigating breast cancer and mastectomy in *The Cancer Journals*. She shared her experience of the isolation of bearing the illness and the physical pain of amputation and also the strength of women-loving support. She also spoke back to the patriarchal and medical gaze, underscoring the pressure on postmastectomy patients to get breast prosthesis in order to maintain norms of femininity. Lorde described her encounter with proponents of breast implants: their investment in implants to secure male companionship and maintain a normalcy of appearance for the comfort of others. Lorde juxtaposed her focus—as a Black lesbian—on survival and productivity to these heteronormative, Eurocentric pressures and also pointed out the lucrative political economy of breast prosthetics. Lorde's far-reaching influence can be seen in, for example, literary theorist Diane Price Herndl's (2002) narrative of her own personal history navigating breast cancer and feminized illness by embracing a posthuman perspective and, consequently, implants.

Health humanities scholars also use patient narratives to interrogate the highly gendered doctor-patient dynamic—where the doctor presumedly embodies an authoritative source and the patient is expected to be compliant and obey the doctor's orders without question. In both *The Cancer Journals* and *A Burst of Light*, Lorde (1980, 1988) describes how doctors were affronted by her asserting her say and control over her body and medical decisions. Scholars have documented extensively the way medical systems in Europe and the US attained the male professional mode of today—most notably, male obstetric physicians usurped midwives' authority over pregnancy and birth in the early twentieth century (Ehrenreich 1972; Wajcman 1991; Wertz and Wertz 1981). In "Three Generations of Native American Women's Birth Experience," poet, musician, and teacher Joy Harjo-Sapulpa (2008) highlights the way US hospitals create an alienating experience for individuals giving birth—their cold, unfeeling sterility and the detrimental effects of the medicalization of birth that results in, for example, immediate postbirth isolation of babies from their parent(s). Physician and essayist Rafael Campo (2014) offers a critical doctor's perspective in "I Am Gula, Hear Me Roar: On Gender and Medicine," critiquing the omission of women's contributions to the profession in medical textbooks as well as the stoic, authoritative air of manliness associated with the doctor profession. Lorde's, Harjo-Sapulpa's, and Campo's narratives, much like the radical achievements of feminist health movements (the 1971 publication of *Our Bodies, Ourselves* and the 1997 founding of SisterSong Women of Color Reproductive Justice Collective are but two manifestations), carve out space for the voices and contributions of women, queer people, and trans people.

Scholars have also transformed established medicine by intervening in education. Like its sister field of medical humanities, health humanities has focused on mining the expressive and reflective strengths of arts and humanities approaches—that is, theater, poetry, music—to improve existing biomedical education and practice, albeit with health humanities' greater focus on unsettling biomedical expertise (rather than bettering health-care providers' communication skills with the tools of the humanities). Health humanities approaches aim to reframe how doctors view patients and their authority as well as the role—and limitations—of

medicine in patients' lives. Susan M. Squier (2020) argues for the utility of comics and graphic narratives in medical education—that their spatial aspect proffers "a zone where one can play with ideas not yet accessible to linear thinking, draw together concepts, communities, and practices conventionally kept separate, and enjoy the fireworks that result" (60). Elsewhere Squier (2014) emphasizes comics as a medium for sex education—that they decenter medical expertise and center embodied experience by encouraging "a broader, more accepting, and distinctly non-normative understand of human sexuality" (228).

Attempts to transform medicine from within have also prioritized incorporating interdisciplinary humanities texts informed by critical theories of power and difference. Gutierrez and DasGupta's (2016) "The Space That Difference Makes: On Marginality, Social Justice and the Future of the Health Humanities" argues for engaging health-care providers in robust methodologies such as feminist philosophy, queer of color studies, postcolonial theory, critical theory, and cultural studies. Drawing on these fields to overhaul health humanities education and textbooks, they argue, pushes the health humanities curricular canon beyond traditional foci on illness, death, and health and toward exploration of social justice praxis outside of the classroom-to-clinic model (e.g., in community spaces or legislative actions). We might query, for example, what future psychiatrists would learn from Stephanie Hsu's (2019) reading—through trans of color critique—of Fanon's footnote on transgender performance in his revolutionary anti-colonial, anti-racist treatise on interracial desire in *Black Skin, White Masks*. These paradigm-shifting frameworks engage future health-care providers in reevaluating existing medical practices and dominant views of health care.

Indisputably, gender forms a site where medical intervention and regulation frequently result in the abuse and loss of autonomy for women, femmes, trans people, and nonbinary people. The field of health humanities, as it continues to center feminist and critical approaches to gender, offers indispensable tools for rethinking notions of illness and health, uplifting patient narratives and expertise, transforming medical education, and ultimately, achieving a reality where people are free from medical abuse and can maintain autonomy over their bodies and self-determine their healthcare access.

27

Genetic
Sandra Soo-Jin Lee

To be "genetic" is to draw a connection. *Genetic* comes from the Greek *genetikos*, meaning "origin" or "resulting from a common origin," as used by Charles Darwin (2002). Based on the *gene*—a heuristic from the Greek *genea*, or "generation," used by Danish botanist Wilhelm Johannsen to refer to a conception of heredity (Johannsen 1911, 130). *Genetics*, or the study of patterns of genes, is used to trace differentiation between individuals and social units—families, patients, communities, and nation-states—through the history of global migration and the "mixing and mating" that result in shared genes. Mapping the frequency of genes across individuals and groups and their association with disease and conditions has become a focus of genetic research. By identifying the presence and absence of genes from one generation to the next, genetic influence becomes a measurable characteristic subjected to statistical analysis used to explain human experience and identity. As such, genetic connection has become a focus of scholarly debate on what it reveals about the past and how genetic explanations can powerfully suggest the future.

The relative contributions of genetics compared to environmental, behavioral, sociocultural, and other forces have fueled interdisciplinary debate and epistemological contention over the power of genetic science to explain life itself. *Genetic* refers to a correlation between observed phenomena and genes; however, correlation should not be conflated with genetic *causation*.

Merely identifying a genetic association can fail to explain why certain people become sick or have a specific trait. A much-cited example of the fallacy of rushing to a genetic explanation is the scientist who is interested in understanding the relationship between genetics and using chopsticks. To answer this question, she might compare the genes of individuals who do and do not use chopsticks and find that there are genetic differences between the two groups. However, upon closer scrutiny, she may also recognize that the two groups differ in other important, more enlightening ways—individuals in group one live in a society where chopsticks are the norm, whereas chopsticks are rare for group two. In this case, cultural practice rather than genes is more likely the "cause" of the difference. This example form of *genetic determinism*, or the belief that genes primarily impact outcomes, can lead to the geneticization of the human condition even when causal mechanisms are elusive. The allure of specificity of the gene belies the inherent uncertainty and ambiguity of genetic connections and their meaning (Dupré 2004; Moss 2004).

Genetics as a focal point in the health sciences has led to the ubiquity of genetic information. Massive public investment in the health sciences has produced an era that has been described as a "genetic revolution" made possible by national initiatives like the Human Genome Project in the late twentieth century that catapulted the study of genes to the forefront of biomedical research. The search for genetic connections is powerfully conveyed through metaphors of promise and peril that describe this emerging "frontier" of medicine and bioengineering (Rapp 1988; Ceccarelli 2013). Geneticists, referred to as "code breakers," are characterized as uncovering the "building blocks" of humanity or as architects, revealing the genetic "blueprint" that contains the hidden "recipe" to the "secrets of life" itself

(Nerlich, Dingwall, and Clarke 2002; Condit 1999). At the same time, cautions against the use of genetic techniques warn of a "biological holocaust" and the specter of human annihilation in the form of a molecular Frankenstein or rogue science that leads to the escape of a genetically manipulated lethal virus outside of the lab. While some scientists expressed concern over the safety of genetic research, the implications of genetic knowledge for explaining and intervening in the human condition have been the focus of humanists and social scientists.

History demonstrates the dangerous use of genetics to distinguish humans into hierarchical groups in furthering racist, sexist, and ableist ideologies. *Eugenics*—a word traced to British scientist Francis Galton in 1883 and derived from the Greek *eugenes*, meaning "wellborn"—refers to reproductive practice to increase the probability of desirable traits (Stepan 1996). In the US, individuals deemed "feebleminded" or prone to criminality or sexual deviance, among other undesirable traits, were considered "enemies to the State" and used as rationale for the application of eugenic policies (Paul and Moore 2010, 36). Local governments in the US activated civic organizations such as the Fitter Families for Future Firesides to sponsor "fitter families contests" in state fairs in the early twentieth century. Backed by the American Eugenics Society's Committee on Popular Education, competitors were required to submit an "abridged record of family traits," and a team of medical doctors performed psychological and physical exams on family members. Families earning the highest grades for "eugenic health" were awarded medals bearing the inscription, "Yea, I have a goodly heritage" (Nelkin 2001; Selden 2005). Scholars have analyzed these normative interventions in the context of the rise of nationalism and conceptions of the "good citizen" that link genetic lineage and notions of biological purity.

Eugenic theories extended to racial and ethnic groups similarly deemed as "the enemy within," leading to state-sanctioned programs of racial hygiene and the use of genetic explanatory models in racist policies on immigration. In the US, statistical research on foreign-born persons in jails, prisons, and reformatories was used to argue that the rising tide of "intellectually and morally defective immigrants—primarily from eastern and southern Europe" was polluting the "American gene pool" (Lombardo 2017, 176). Congressional testimony on population-based genetic research linked the problem of immigrating "social inadequates" to "cost to taxpayers" (Lombardo 2002). These claims supported the passage of the Immigration Restriction Act of 1924, the first bill to establish national quotas that limited what eugenicists described as "dysgenic" Italians and eastern European Jews from entering the country (Ludmerer 1972). The historical conflation of genetics with biological conceptions of race reveals that conceptions of *genetic* are informed by and reproduce categories of difference toward achieving sociopolitical goals.

The gene remains a powerful icon in the public imagination. Rapid commercialization of genetic sequencing technologies has led to an explosion of genetic products, including "recreational" genetic services such as genetic ancestry that connect individuals to geographic locations. The proliferation of genetic tests, once under the purview of the health-care system, has given way to the "genetic marketplace," in which consumers are sold individualized genetic risk profiles for disease and health (Nozick 1974). In the shift from patient to consumer, neoliberal governance of genetic products renders decisions as a matter of individual calculus of risks and benefits. Reframing health in terms of genetic risk, market capitalism fuels expectations that individuals should act on individual genetic information in self-care as responsible, rational, and self-actualizing citizens (Ong 2005). Availability of genetic information on a broadening array of social characteristics, including income, sexual behavior, educational attainment, and cognitive ability, reflects the further entrenchment of the gene to explain variation in the human condition. As anthropologist Mike Fortun described, visions of an ever-expanding genomic utopia stem from public intoxication with the potential for self-discovery and a re-creation (M. Fortun 2008).

The study of genetic connection is fertile terrain for interpretation of what it means to be human and the construction of social relations. As the basis for models aimed at explaining life, health, and disease, individuals increasingly frame and understand themselves and their relationships in genetic terms (Heath, Rapp, and Taussig 2004). Fundamentally a science of comparison, identifying genetic connections relies on the biospecimens and data collected from people across the globe. Genetic connections are inextricable from the sociopolitical histories of groups and their willingness to participate in genetic research. As social knowledge, genetics is informed by and deployed to exercise values and political aims.

28

Global Health

Robert Peckham

From the balcony of our apartment in Hong Kong overlooking the main shipping lane into Victoria Harbour, one of the busiest ports in the world, we watched the megaships pass, among them those of the Evergreen line heading for the Kwai Tsing Container Terminals. For two weeks in the summer of 2020, during the early months of the COVID-19 pandemic, when we'd been tagged with electronic wristbands and quarantined at home, this busy oceangoing and riverine traffic intensified our sense of confinement. Clearly, the draconian lockdowns imposed in Mainland China hadn't stopped all exports; rather, after an initial decline, the pandemic had provided an opportunity for ramping up global trade, at least in certain sectors.

This memory came to mind in March 2021, when the *Ever Given*, a four-hundred-meter-long container ship, ran aground in the Suez Canal, blocking traffic through one of the world's busiest waterways linking the Mediterranean Sea, the Red Sea, and the Indian Ocean. Satellite images showed the logjam stretching far into the Gulf of Suez. The economic impact was immediate: oil prices climbed, and the stranded ship caused an estimated $9.6 billion daily loss in trade. Delayed goods resulted in supply shortages, with knock-on effects to industry—including the health-care industry—compounding markets already reeling from the COVID-19 pandemic (K. Ramos et al. 2021).

Both events—the canal blockage and the imposition of public health measures to disrupt the spread of disease—cohere under the sign of the global. The wedged superfreighter, sailing to Rotterdam from the Yantian International Container Terminal in Shenzhen, China, with its Indian crew, was registered in Panama, owned by a Japanese family, leased to a Taiwanese conglomerate, and managed by the German Bernhard Schulte Shipmanagement company. The cargo on board included IKEA products, Nike sneakers, and Lenovo laptops. The complex financial, legal, and logistical arrangements that made the *Ever Given* and its cargo possible were aspects of an intensifying global interdependence. But images of the stranded ship were also graphic reminders that "globalization" doesn't just connote the accelerated cross-border flow of goods, services, investment, and people. The concurrent lockdowns triggered by the coronavirus and the Suez jam were more than aberrations or system malfunctions; instead, they instantiate a system in operation, disclosing an inherent capacity for deceleration and disconnection. The "global" may signify spatial expansion, but it also connotes violent constriction.

Like the former British colony of Hong Kong, the Suez Canal is a good place from which to reflect on the imperial history of global health and the durable afterlife of that history in the present (Stoler 2016; Packard 2016). While global health may have evolved out of public health and international health in the post–World War II period, its deeper origins lie in nineteenth-century tropical medicine and sanitary science, which developed in tandem with ambitious colonial modernizing initiatives, including the construction of roads, railways, dams, and canals.

The Suez Canal, which opened in 1869, was financed and operated by a British and French concessionary company until Egyptian president Gamal Abdel Nasser nationalized it in 1956. Serving as a crucial connector, the canal also regulated imperial traffic, particularly against the backdrop of increasing scientific awareness of the dangers of infectious diseases (Huber 2013). Cholera pandemics and the third plague pandemic in the late 1890s demonstrated the speed of infections traveling via steamships along global trade routes. The tension between the promotion of "free" trade and anxieties about quickening mobilities found expression in the British Empire's often contradictory approaches to quarantine (Harrison 2013).

Fast-forward to the late twentieth century, when the term *global health* (*salud global*, *santé globale*) began to eclipse *international health*, and globalization connoted both an opportunity and a threat (Yach and Bettcher 1998, 742–44). Global interdependence was beneficial in that it facilitated the diffusion of knowledge, technology, and capital, which could be mobilized to address global health disparities. But it was also harmful, since the uneven spread of investments reinforced embedded inequalities. Meanwhile, global connectivity produced novel pathways for infectious diseases to circulate, necessitating a new infrastructure of global surveillance (Bettcher and Lee 2002).

Given the contemporary promotion of global health by those with vastly different interests and agendas, it's hardly surprising that the term eludes easy definition. Public health specialists, pharmaceuticals, tech companies, aid and media agencies, governments and NGOs, the World Health Organization (WHO) and the World Bank, civil rights activists, academic researchers, and many others all invoke "global health" to describe and valorize their activities. *Global health* may refer to a technical and institutional capacity embodied in the WHO, the United Nations Children's Fund (UNICEF), the UN Population Fund (UNFPA), and the Joint United Nations Programme on HIV/AIDS (UNAIDS), with antecedents in the League of Nations Health Organization formally established in 1924 ("International Health Organization" 1924). It may also pertain to a radical politics of universal rights, articulated in revolutionary claims to health citizenship at the end of the eighteenth century. In this context, rather than used descriptively, it designates an ideal of health equity. In recent years, researchers and practitioners have pointed to global health's colonial roots, arguing that an exclusory and coercive colonial prehistory perpetuates biases and continues to shape global health institutions and practices today, including new epidemiological surveillance methods based on the digital harvesting of big data (Richardson 2020; Peckham and Sinha 2017). As some have argued, however, this reckoning with an oppressive past may produce blind spots, veiling new configurations of cultural, political, economic, and military power (Horton 2021).

Since the HIV/AIDS epidemic in the 1980s and the growing recognition of the threat to human health posed by new and reemergent infectious diseases, global health has also been promoted by state and intergovernmental agencies as a facet of global security (Heymann and Rodier 1998; Elbe 2010). Humanitarian interventions that seek to prevent disease, alleviate poverty, and build capacity in "unstable" postcolonial regions of the world are construed as ways of protecting the West from emerging threats. Viewed from this perspective, global health isn't just tied to expanding capitalism in the form of Big Pharma; it's also enmeshed with Western humanitarian and peace interventionism that ultimately provides a form of covert neocolonial governance over the people of other countries. Instead of diminishing the gap between development and underdevelopment, global health could be said to legitimate structural asymmetries (Duffield 2007). It thereby represents a form of "cruel optimism" by holding out the promise of a better future while impeding the realization of that future (Berlant 2011).

Those who teach global health find themselves confronting these contradictions. For the most part, it is taught in privileged Western universities and disseminated via policies and funding that emanate from the West to the rest. At the same time, global health tends to be understood by researchers and practitioners within a uniquely Western and largely Euro-American framework, even by those intent on problematizing it. The role of other nations, including the People's Republic of China (PRC), is often downplayed or relegated altogether. While Mao's "barefoot doctors"—a network of community-based medical workers in China's rural areas—provided an inspiration for the WHO's espousal of primary care and "health for all" enshrined in the Declaration of Alma-Ata in 1978, the PRC has more recently been at the forefront of a new global health drive. Even as President Trump's administration announced plans to cut funds to the WHO in 2020, China pledged millions of dollars to the organization.

The global health humanities seek to elucidate this entanglement of health with economic, social, and cultural processes by drawing on cross-disciplinary insights from the social sciences and humanities, including history, philosophy, and literature. In a China context, engaging with works of fiction, such as Yan Lianke's 2006 novel *Dream of Ding Village*, can provide fresh perspectives on the HIV/AIDS blood contamination scandal in Henan Province in the 1990s (Peckham 2016). Poverty, avaricious "blood kingpins," and a booming plasma economy that serviced a nascent Chinese biotech sector in a market-liberalizing one-party state were factors driving infection (Anagnost 2006). Similarly, engaging with the writer Fang Fang's diary, written in the form of daily online postings during the government-imposed lockdown of Wuhan in 2020, not only yields insights into the psychological impact of enforced isolation but furnishes an important

counternarrative to epidemiological analyses and the official Chinese COVID-19 story (Fang 2020). Expanding the remit of global health to include the study of this creative archive is important because it can further our understanding of how global forces intermesh with individual, community, and state relations and how behaviors are shaped by entrenched power relations and economic systems that perpetuate injustices (Stewart and Swain 2016).

Meanwhile, this essay was written in the United Arab Emirates (UAE), where I was stranded during the COVID-19 pandemic in September 2021, unable to rejoin my family in the United States after the imposition of visa restrictions. While vaccinated US citizens were able to move freely across the world, citizens of many other countries were unable to travel even when they had been fully vaccinated. In Dubai, a Pakistani taxi driver from Peshawar told me that the evacuation of US troops from Afghanistan and the Taliban takeover of the country in late August 2021 had created a refugee crisis along the Pakistani border. In his homeland, he said, the health challenges from this exodus far outweighed those of the pandemic. Later, a young woman from Cameroon working in a hotel in Jumeirah complained about the disparities in access to COVID vaccines. While UAE citizens received the Pfizer-BioNTech vaccine, foreign workers, she claimed, were given the Chinese Sinopharm and Russian Sputnik V vaccines, which she worried were less safe and efficacious.

Today, "global health" seems tautologous. How can health *not* be global when many challenges to human health, such as those posed by infectious diseases, are manifestly cross-border? The voices of these migrants, who account for well over 80 percent of the UAE's population, however, are reminders that while the business of health may be global, even planetary, health is always local, grounded in social worlds and lived experience. All the while, like the *Ever Given* in the Suez Canal, the conduits that enable global health cooperation too often fall prey to blockages that exacerbate inequalities, benefiting the few at the expense of the many.

29

Harm
Tod S. Chambers

As a keyword in health care, *harm* possesses the characteristics of what the rhetorician Richard Weaver (1953) refers to as a *devil term*. A devil term is a rhetorical absolute in a particular culture that when expressed causes almost universal revulsion. While there are a number of devil terms in medicine and the health humanities—such as *suffering, objectification*, and *dehumanization*—*harm* is a particular type of devil term: an *ultimate* one, or "prime repellent" (Weaver 1953, 222). Harm is also the foundation of several other key concepts in medicine, such as nonmaleficence (the duty not to cause harm), risk (the potential harm that might be caused directly or indirectly by a medical intervention), and even beneficence (which includes the positive moral duty to prevent harm). Finally, the often-quoted Latin dictum *primum non nocere*, commonly translated as "first, do no harm," demonstrates that harm is not simply something that should be avoided but something the avoidance of which should in most cases take priority in medical practice. This status can be discerned in the manner physicians' writings assume that evoking *primum non nocere* will end any further debate on a topic. So one can find *primum non nocere* used by physicians to argue against capitation (Thomison 1987), for routine digital rectal exams (J. A. Moran 1992), against physician-assisted suicide (Lema 1993), and for psychiatrists' involvement in the state-sanctioned torture of prisoners (Kottow 2006).

The immense moral weight given to harm can be traced, according to Virginia Sharpe and Alan Faden, to the nineteenth century's focus on natural healing as opposed to the concept of medicine as entailing heroic interventions (2001, 42). As Western medicine, especially American medicine, became more interventionist, evaluating what forms of harm would be acceptable became a key part of medical practice. In his discussion of the history of the injunction against harm in medicine, Albert Jonsen notes that among its different meanings, one can distinguish between the "risk-benefit ratio" and the "benefit-detriment equation" (1978, 829–30). The risk-benefit ratio is the recognition that any procedure almost always entails only a probability of benefit as well as a probability of possible harm. In the benefit-detriment equation, the treatment will concurrently occasion a detriment; Jonsen's example is an amputation to remove a diseased part of the body.

The phrase *primum non nocere* is not without its contemporary detractors, of course. Some, like Raanan Gillon (1985), find that the priority given to this dictum—that is, the priority given to avoiding harm over doing good—is philosophically suspect. Determining what constitutes harm cannot be done without reference to wider cultural values. In his discussion of measuring harm in pharmaceuticals, Jacob Stegenga illustrates this by noting that the drug methylphenidate (Ritalin) is used to treat attention deficit disorder—yet the drug's success can be "considered a benefit or a harm depending on one's broader normative commitments and sociocultural position" toward a particular notion of the behavior of a "normal" child (2017, 343). Furthermore, medical interventions rarely present themselves as a simple option with only a single possible harm. Instead, each presents an entire range of possible harms, and because of this, decisions must be made through some form of ranking. In her entry on harm in the *Encyclopedia of Bioethics*, Bettina Schöne-Seifert (2014) observes that debates over the term are divided between those who argue there can be objective criteria for ranking harms and those who believe that there are only a plurality of subjective definitions and rankings.

The use of the term *harm* in medicine—aside from those harms caused by the disease process itself—is almost always understood as the result of actions taken by health-care professionals, most often physicians, in the course of caring for patients. Many of the key fictional texts used in the health humanities have this form of harm as their key theme; these include William Carlos Williams's (1984) "The Use of Force" and Richard Selzer's (1982) "Brute" as well as Samuel Shem's (1978) *The House of God*. The first two are, as Anne Hudson Jones remarks, both told from the physician's point of view and "offer insight into why a presumably good doctor with beneficent intentions none the less ends up harming his patient in an abuse of power" (1999, 254). These examples and many others prompt Leslie Fiedler to observe that the history of representations of physicians gives rise to a "doctor with many names but only a single face—the face of evil with good intentions" (1996, 120).

In developing moral principles to guide medical practice in the twentieth century, it was deemed necessary to distinguish different obligations concerning harm. In *The Principles of Biomedical Ethics*, Tom Beauchamp and James Childress (1979, 97–98) argue that one should not, as was proposed by William Frankena, view beneficence and nonmaleficence as part of a single principle. They contend that beneficence should be considered a positive duty to promote the welfare of the patient as well as a duty to prevent harm from occurring to the patient: nonmaleficence is a negative duty to refrain from causing harm or imposing risks of harm. Yet in contemporary medical ethics, the principle

HARM TOD S. CHAMBERS

of autonomy can be regarded as having superseded the principle of beneficence; once the risks of a medical intervention have been identified, the patient has in large part replaced the physician as the one evaluating those risks and deciding whether the intervention is appropriate. This has shifted the expectations for physicians in terms of assessing and explaining the risks of harm.

Cases in which autonomy carries less moral weight than beneficence and nonmaleficence often turn on the question of potential harm. So, for example, as an expression of respect for patient autonomy, physicians have an obligation to tell the truth to patients—but under the notion of "therapeutic privilege," information can be withheld if it is thought that the disclosure would harm the patient (Berg and Appelbaum 2001). Similarly, physicians have an obligation to keep patient information confidential—unless revealing that information could prevent serious harm. Psychiatric patients, too, cannot be involuntarily hospitalized—unless there is also a likelihood they will do harm to themselves or others. Each of these instances illustrates the manner in which the ethics of health care has been profoundly influenced by the "harm principle" first set forth by John Stuart Mill in "On Liberty": civil liberties can only be curtailed when there is potential harm.

Since the twentieth century, the way harm is understood has been challenged in a number of debates. In 1982 in the United States, capital punishment entered directly into the sphere of medical practice with the advent of lethal injection. While for some the notion that having physicians use medical procedures to cause death seemed an obvious violation of the profession's moral code, others framed the issue of physician involvement as something that could minimize harm by ensuring a painless death (Emanuel and Bienen 2001). In the 1990s, a similar debate emerged when physician-assisted dying took center stage following a number of highly publicized cases. Medicine's traditional stance against being the agent of death was displaced by a discussion as to "whether physicians should have any role in facilitating one harmful event (a patient's self-destruction) in order to help the patient avoid other harms . . . that the patient regards as worse" (Weir 1992, 124).

During this same period, public concern over harm in medicine zeroed in on medical error. In 1999, apprehension over iatrogenic harm was epitomized by the Institute of Medicine's report *To Err Is Human*, which suggested that in United States hospitals, medical errors were potentially responsible for ninety-eight thousand deaths per year (Donaldson, Corrigan, and Kohn 2000). This increased apprehension over medical intervention as itself the cause of harm, David Armstrong argues, is in line with a cultural perspective greatly altered from that of the nineteenth century. Over the course of the twentieth century, he explains, public health began to concern itself with the hazards of the environment to health, for "just as the New Public Health was discovering dangers everywhere, so clinical medicine found that everyone was 'at risk'" (2006, 875). Advances in genetics in health care forced a new discussion of harm in terms of the subjunctive mood. Harm became reconceived as the potential injury that would occur if a person decided to have children with the knowledge that the future child was likely to have a "harming condition" (Feinberg 1986; Steinbock 1986; D. Brock 1995; D. Davis 2010); in this formulation, however, it is not the health-care professional who is the agent of harm but rather the prospective parents (Steinbock and McClamrock 1994).

Perhaps the most radical change in the notion of harm in medicine is how medical interventions that were traditionally viewed as "successful" are increasingly conceived as forms of oppressive normalization.

Cochlear implants developed as a "cure" for deafness were radically critiqued by the deaf community as posing harm to the individual child as well as to the community itself. As Alicia Ouellette argues, even if one concludes that it is morally defensible to allow the parents of the child to decide the matter, it "does not justify indifference to the potential physical, psychological, and social harms carried with implantation" (2010, 1267). Similarly, in calling for a ban on the medical management of intersex children through early genital surgery, hormone treatment, and secrecy, the intersex community claimed that a "misplaced focus on gender distorts the perspective of clinicians in many ways that are harmful to patients" (Chase 2003, 240). Implied in these critiques is that medical interventions based on social norms cause harm. Indeed, some interventions once considered treatments are now seen instead as enhancements, a shift revealing what Margaret Olivia Little refers to as medicine's "complicity with harmful concepts of normality" (Parens 1998, S9). A more complex example perhaps is that of individuals who may identify as "transabled"; these people argue that they are being harmed when physicians refuse to modify their bodies in order for them to acquire desired physical disabilities (M. Gilbert 2003; Reynolds 2016).

Technological advances can also have profound impact on larger social injustices, as, for example, Dorothy Roberts observes in the racial disparities in the use of IVF, so that "harm occurs at the ideological level—the message it sends about the relative value of Blacks and whites in America" (1999, 283). Even the promotion of health, it has been argued, should be considered a form of "iatric disease" for the "moral and physical harm that is done to the public by particular nostrums of public health" (Klein 2010, 17). In each of these examples, social prejudices toward particular bodies and desires, the "tyranny of the normal" (Fiedler 1996, 154),

lead medicine to act (or not act) in ways that can be interpreted as forms of harm. In the end, medicine must come to recognize that it is the social mores outside the profession that determine what harm is, that so central a keyword as *harm* lacks an objective definition and shifts with changes in social mores.

30

History
David S. Jones

The idea of "history" conveys many meanings. It can be chronology, the "aggregate of past events; the course of human affairs." It can be scholarship, the "branch of knowledge that deals with past events." And it can be craft, a "narration" or "representation" (*OED Online* 2020, "history").

In the context of health, history can also claim an intimate relationship with healing. Clinicians in many healing traditions diagnose patients through histories, often with formal methods. When a patient presents with a chief complaint, the physician conducts a diagnostic interview that traces the patient's history of present illness, the past medical history, the family history, and the social history. The goal is to construct a narrative of the patient's experience, identify what has changed over time, consider possible causes (i.e., the differential diagnosis), and make an argument about the best explanation. What historians do for societies, doctors do for individuals.

Historians long ago realized that the act of history is not a simple task of assembling chronological narratives and deciphering their unambiguous meanings. Historians understand that different histories can be written of any specific event. This subjectivity is both a problem and an opportunity. William Cronon captured these postmodern anxieties in his analysis of progressivist and declensionist narratives of the Dust Bowl: historians risked becoming "rudderless in an endless sea of stories" (1992, 1371). Historians also worry about who

has a right to write histories. All historical scholarship appropriates someone else's past.

Physicians also grapple with these anxieties. Medical students meet the problems of subjectivity and selectivity right away, tasked as they are with conducting the most thorough histories of their patients. They are then asked to distill these complex tapestries into brief vignettes that will motivate the clinical team to act. Appropriation, meanwhile, is explicitly what doctors do: they "take" a history. As Katharine van Schaik describes, "Patient information is, to an extent, appropriated, then processed, reorganized, and interpreted. It is this process of appropriation—of 'taking'—that permits the transformation of patient information into a form physicians find useful" (2010, 1159). She asks physicians to reconsider this presumption, perhaps "recording and interpreting a history, rather than taking it," or even asking patients how they would want their own histories to be written (1160).

Medicine has a special relationship with history in another way as well. Until the nineteenth century, European physicians studied history to learn medicine. Galen wrote extensive commentaries about his predecessor's ideas (Nutton 2020). His medical knowledge informed medical practice for millennia. Thomas Sydenham's 1676 *Observationes Medicae* earned him the title the "English Hippocrates," one meant clearly as an honorific. René Laennec, celebrated for introducing the stethoscope (and diagnostic technology more broadly) into medicine, had written his 1804 medical school thesis about the continuing relevance of Hippocratic theory (Duffin 1998). Thomas Jefferson hired his own physician to teach medicine and its history at the University of Virginia, believing that "the student should learn something of the earlier progress of the science and the art" (Dunglison 1872, iii). As late as the mid-nineteenth century, even as French and

German physicians broke with the past and sought new knowledge in clinical and laboratory science, they continued to celebrate Hippocrates as an icon of rationality, empiricism, and professional virtue (J. Warner 2003, 169–77).

However, the new medical sciences did soon transform the relationship between history and medicine. Biomedicine, a modernist endeavor, celebrated rupture over continuity, new knowledge over ancient wisdom. It idealized laboratory discoveries. The history of medicine no longer seemed relevant (Huisman and Warner 2004; D. Jones et al. 2015). But history found new advocates and new rationales. Consider Johns Hopkins University School of Medicine. Modeled on German research universities, Hopkins celebrated the emerging medical sciences. Nonetheless, William Osler and its other founders believed that they could teach history to inculcate professional virtue and to inoculate students against the increasing reductionism and commercialization of medicine. Osler sought to train gentlemanly physicians who were well versed in the liberal arts, especially history (J. Warner 2011).

A different model of medical history had also emerged, beginning in the late eighteenth century. German historians had recognized that they could learn much about a society by studying disease and caregiving (Huisman and Warner 2004). This approach flourished periodically throughout the nineteenth century. It achieved prominence with the rise of social histories of medicine and disease in the 1960s. Charles Rosenberg (1962) demonstrated how social responses to disease—in his case, the cholera epidemics that struck New York City in 1832, 1849, and 1866—offered insights into fundamental questions of urbanization, immigration, race, and governance. William McNeill ([1976] 2010) looked more broadly to demonstrate the impact of disease on the sweep of human history.

Proliferating scholarship in the late twentieth century produced many new visions of what the history of disease, medicine, and health might be. It also demonstrated how deliberately crafted histories could be used to advance various agendas. Historians continued to produce intellectual histories of medical theory and practice (Feudtner 2003; Greene 2007; Aronowitz 2015). Social historians placed disease and health care into their economic and political contexts (R. Evans 1987; Wailoo 2001; Metzl 2009). Cultural historians explored questions of meaning and value (Sontag 1989; Tomes 1998; Linker 2013). Applied histories drew lessons from the past to guide current policy (Brandt 2007; Lakoff 2017; Benjamin 2019a). Historians moved past the traditional focus on elite white men and offered new histories of women in health care, whether midwives, nurses, or physicians (Morantz-Sanchez 1985; Reverby 1987; Ulrich 1990). Others foregrounded the experience of patients (R. Porter 1985; S. Rothman 1994; Nayan Shah 2001). Colonial historians examined the many roles that medicine and public health played in the systems of surveillance and discipline created by European empires (Arnold 1993; Birn 2006; W. Anderson 2008). Scholars now seek decentered and decolonized histories (Amrith 2006; N. Davis 2011; Clapham 2020). Disease and caregiving are fundamental and pervasive features of human life. It should be no surprise that they have been productive of an astonishing diversity of histories. These histories can serve as a basis for advocacy on many fronts.

The new scholarship that has emerged since the 1960s and 1970s has bifurcated histories of health. On one side are academic historians of medicine, disease, and health. Working from roots in history, history of science, science studies, cultural studies, ethnic studies, and other disciplines, they often take a critical stance toward the healing professions and their practices. On the other side are the physicians and historians who instead see historical inquiry as a way to reflect (often favorably) on the calling of medicine and instill professional values.

Both groups have struggled to find a place for their vision in medical education. Osler complained in 1902 that increasingly crowded medical curricula left little time for formal instruction in history (1902, 93). Things have not gotten any easier. Part of the problem, as Lester King argued in 1968, was that advocates for history could not easily argue that knowledge of history made people better doctors (L. King 1968, 28). This has not stopped physicians from continuing to argue that history can be used to instill professional virtue in students (Bryan and Longo 2013). Such celebrations have now met headwinds: medicine's race reckoning has tarnished the reputations of Osler and other past icons (Buckley 2020; Persaud, Butts, and Berger 2020). Some historians have attempted a more ambitious argument for history, arguing that it actually is "an essential component" of medical theory, thinking, and practice. It provides insights into disease and therapeutics, things that physicians must understand to be most effective for their patients (D. Jones et al. 2015, 626).

Even as present-day historians debate among themselves how best to make the case for histories of medicine and disease, they negotiate their relations with like-minded disciplines in the humanities and social sciences. Some historians have allied with medical anthropology and sociology to pursue the theory and practice of social medicine. Others have signed on as part of the medical humanities, first established in the United States at the Pennsylvania State University College of Medicine in 1964. In this vision, the constituent disciplines of the medical humanities—typically philosophy, literature, history, art, and religion—examine "questions of value and meaning within and around medicine." The medical humanities equip students with specific "qualities of mind," including critical reasoning, perspective, empathy, and self-reflection (Barnard 1994, 628). Efforts to create space in curricula for the medical humanities have been stymied, in part, by the emergence of bioethics in the 1960s. Advocates have argued that ethics is the one domain of the health humanities that is indeed essential. This raises an important strategy question for historians (and a parallel one for scholars in each of the health humanities): Does each discipline simply contribute to a shared mission—for instance, fostering empathy or teaching students to tolerate ambiguity? Or should each discipline emphasize its own unique contributions (Greene and Jones 2017)?

Working to make the case for history in 1902, Osler reached back to Thomas Fuller's 1639 *Historie of the Holy Warre*. History could grant the wisdom of age without the attendant debilities: "History maketh a young man to be old, without either wrinkles or grey hairs; privileging him with the experiences of age, without either the infirmities or inconveniences thereof" (Osler 1902, 93). In the original passage, Fuller took this further: "Yea, it not only maketh things past, present; but enableth one to make a rational conjecture of things to come. For this world affordeth no new accidents. . . . Old actions return again, furnished over with some new and different circumstances" (Fuller 1639, A3–A4). This admonition holds up well. Despite some claims to the contrary, scholarship on the histories of health, disease, and medicine remains lively and relevant (Timmermann 2014). Any doubts about history's usefulness were cast aside by the COVID-19 pandemic, during which doctors, policy makers, and the suffering public turned to history for insight into their predicament. Historians appeared regularly in media and scholarly forums, trying to help make sense of it all.

History does indeed have much to offer. As Huisman and Warner argued in 2004, historical insight can help patients, doctors, government leaders, and citizens make difficult decisions as they respond to the challenges of disease. Historians have enumerated many specific contributions. History offers perspective on the social contexts of medicine. It fosters humility in place of overconfidence. It rehumanizes medicine and reminds clinicians that medicine is a social practice of caregiving. It can help socialize students into the profession while warning them against the risks of this socialization (D. Jones et al. 2015). It can suggest valuable avenues for intervention. We cannot understand health, disease, or medicine without history. But we cannot understand these only through history. We need a capacious conception of the health humanities in which history works with other disciplines to illuminate the human experience of suffering and caregiving.

31

Human Rights
Jaymelee Kim

The intersection of health and human rights continues to expand as stakeholders concerned with social vulnerability realize the interrelated nature of all human rights and health outcomes. As health practitioners and scholars engage more deeply with a human rights lens, they are forced to acknowledge the deep-seated social processes and relationships that endanger people's mental health, physical health, and well-being. Using a human rights lens in health humanities provides insight into advocating for social change that addresses the subversive forms of oppression that impact health status, morbidity, and mortality. Such advocacy requires increased collaboration between health entities and other rights-focused organizations. Power, biases, and discriminatory practices ebb and flow not only within the health-care system but throughout all facets of societies. To examine the relationship between health humanities and human rights, there must be a basic knowledge of the trajectory of international human rights law and its applications to health and well-being.

At the close of the Second World War, the United Nations drafted the 1948 Universal Declaration of Human Rights (UDHR), the first document in an ever-growing body of international human rights laws and norms. The document became foundational for framing human rights across cultures. Unlike a covenant that would only apply to signatories, a declaration applies to all nation-states. The UDHR and subsequent human rights treaties seek to clarify protections and freedoms afforded in society regardless of "race, colour, sex, language, religion, political or other opinion, national or social origin, property, birth or other status." Article 25.1 of the UDHR states, "Everyone has the right to a standard of living adequate for the health and well-being of himself and of his family, including food, clothing, housing and medical care and necessary social services, and the right to security in the event of unemployment, sickness, disability, widowhood, old age or other lack of livelihood in circumstances beyond his control" (UN General Assembly 1948). This recognition of health and access to medical care as a human right is further reinforced by the 1976 International Covenant on Economic, Social and Cultural Rights (ICESCR). Article 12 of the ICESCR outlines the "right to the highest attainable standard of physical and mental health" (UN General Assembly 1966). The Siracusa Principles on the Limitation and Derogation Provisions in the ICESCR allow the state to "limit certain rights . . . to allow a State to take measures dealing with a serious threat to the health of a population or individual members of the population" (para 25). The Siracusa Principles align with international human rights law that further considers collective rights as legitimate, which is a concept particularly relevant to health needs. While originating in legalistic terms, the application of human rights law quickly permeates diverse fields—including those of health and medicine. UDHR and international human rights law provide a platform for health-care practitioners and those in health humanities to identify and address health inequity and social vulnerabilities.

Internationally, health as a human right has been levied to address myriad health concerns, including access to reproductive rights, prevention of domestic violence, prevention of female genital mutilation, freedom from environmental violence, access to affordable health care, freedom from torture, freedom from medical intervention without consent, and freedom from medical experimentation. The use of a human rights lens in health humanities also exposes the sociocultural arrangements that impact health. Jonathan Mann (1947–98), MPH, MD, quickly saw the utility of this approach. Shepherding the theory and praxis of a combined health and human rights model (Gostin 2001), Mann argues that "the human rights framework provides a more useful approach for analysing and responding to modern public health challenges than any framework thus far available within the biomedical tradition" (1996, 924). He ardently not only emphasizes health as a human right but goes a step further to frame human rights as a health concern. Because human rights are interdependent, deprivation of rights to shelter, consumable water, and other resources will ultimately impact health status.

Continued research in both the sciences and health humanities has established that health indicators extend beyond personal behaviors and are inextricably tied to social factors, economic status, living and working conditions, and access to medical care (Farmer 1999b; Braveman 2010). This understanding undergirds what has become known as human rights–based approaches in health care. The Office of the High Commissioner for Human Rights (2022) describes human rights approaches as aiming for "better and more sustainable development outcomes by analyzing and addressing the inequalities, discriminatory practices (*de jure* and *de facto*) and unjust power relations." It is no longer adequate for health-care fields to narrowly diagnose pathology without considering power relations that steer human rights and violations. Assessing violations of human rights law, structural inequalities, and sociocultural barriers enables practitioners and health scholars to identify risk factors that influence health status.

Health humanities are well positioned to examine how human rights are bestowed and deprived and to offer improvements for implementation of preventative medicine measures, holistic treatments, representation, and diagnostic capabilities. Denial of the right to adequate health care is often subversively entrenched in implicit biases and learned behaviors that target marginalized social groups. The United States has a long history of violations of human rights through, for example, the exploitation, experimentation, institutionalization, and forced sterilization of racialized minorities. The 1930s Tuskegee Syphilis Study on Black men and the common practice of sterilization of Native American and Hispanic women without their consent through the 1970s exemplify the United States' historic targeting of racialized groups. Similarly, nutritional deprivation research and other medical experiments were conducted on Canadian Indian residential school system children in the 1940s and '50s. While these overt violations of human rights are readily identified, they are also aspects of systemic policies, practices, and beliefs within a society that can take less obvious forms but are prevalent in health humanities discourses.

Scholars of history and human behavior have long recognized that psychological responses to social conditions are likely to be among the most important explanations of the social gradient in health in affluent countries (Braveman 2010). To this end, the International Federation of Gynecology and Obstetrics maintains that women's health requires social and cultural factors experienced by marginalized women to be addressed. An example of an issue underscored by a human rights–based approach is that of maternal mortality rates. For instance, the United States has the highest maternal mortality rate among developed nations. Furthermore, Black, Indigenous, and people of color (BIPOC) in the United States are disproportionately impacted. Since race has no biological foundation to explain the increased risk, health researchers using a human rights lens study sociocultural factors that impact quality of prenatal care, preexisting health status of mothers, and stress levels related to race-based discrimination. The latter includes examination of a range of human rights, such as access to housing, healthy environments, cultural life, and education. Similarly, Yancy (2020) reports the disproportionate impacts of COVID-19 on people of color in the United States resulting from structural factors, including housing density, inability to work remotely, comorbidity with other socially influenced health conditions, and limited access to healthy food.

Just as human rights law provides a common language for those pursuing social change to engage with policy making, it also is vulnerable to being politicized, co-opted, or narrowly defined. The language of human rights law can also be used to create barriers to health. The question of who bears the burden of educating policy makers on the sociocultural variables and discriminatory practices that impact health can also become a point of contention and a space of constant negotiation.

However, because a human rights approach to health is rooted in international law, it provides a common language for health-care practitioners to use with policy makers and reinforces a perspective that encourages the medical field to advocate for change. Nation-states and local governments can be held accountable for contributing to health risk factors, including those that disproportionately impact underrepresented subsets of the population. A human rights approach includes sensitization and capacity building of communities as a component of public health. In combination, capacity building and sensitization on rights to health care and on how to advocate for them also pave the way for sustainable change. Health-care providers, civil societies, community members, and others invested in improving mental and physical health also face the challenge of how to institute change, such as the upheaval of currently inequitable social arrangements that continue to impede access to the highest attainable standard of health. As human rights discourse continues to expand, so too will its implications for the health-care fields. As such, health humanities scholars familiar with human rights frameworks can illuminate violations of human rights and reveal the sociopolitical shaping of human rights rhetoric that negatively impact health and well-being.

32

Humanities

Sari Altschuler

The word *humanities* is at the core of the medical and health humanities. Still, anyone who has walked into a room of health-care practitioners, students, and humanities professors ready to do *medical humanities* or *health humanities* work knows all are eager to improve the practices of health care, but individuals differ—sometimes radically—in their understanding of what that work is. Today's debates over defining the health humanities frequently focus on the differences between *health* and *medicine* (Crawford et al. 2010; T. Jones et al. 2017), but some of the most challenging differences emerge from divergent understandings of the word *humanities*. These differences are not merely inside baseball: they determine what kinds of interventions into the practices of health care are possible.

In medical contexts especially, the term *humanities* names something missing from health care today: a way to cultivate humaneness. These *humanities* offer a sorely needed antidote to the callous dollars-and-cents logic and baroque bureaucracies of today's Western health-care systems. As recently as 2014, the American Academy of Medical Colleges identified training in feeling and therapy for physicians, with an emphasis on empathy, as the core of humanities work in medical schools (Krisberg 2014). This understanding of the *humanities* is best captured by a 2005–6 *JAMA* exchange over the value of medical humanities for medical education. Physician-poet Rafael Campo began by offering a passionate defense of the medical humanities. While the field lacked definition, he recalled a meeting where those who had been debating the field's contours were left "speechless" after an art therapist staged a play for health-care workers and the loved ones of dying patients. Here was "elusive proof" of the medical humanities' work (2005, 1011). Howard Spiro echoed this view: "Instilling a feeling for the human condition," he declared, "is what the humanities are all about" (2006, 997). *JAMA*'s "Humanities" section promotes this sense of the term as a universal human ideal best developed through the arts, publishing "original poems," "personal vignettes," and "essays that demonstrate the relevance of the arts to the science and practice of medicine" ("Instructions for Authors" 2020).

For humanities experts, however, the word means something different: the *humanities* are a set of disciplines organized around the analysis of human culture broadly understood. As Catherine Belling writes, "The humanities are not defined by their impossibly huge set of objects—human activities and its products— but by their method," which "question[s] the epistemology, ethics, and language of both biomedical science and clinical practice" (2017, 23, 20). Inspiring empathy and feeling for others may be a side benefit, but the *humanities* names a set of disciplines that train capacious, creative, and ethical thinking as well as rigorous, precise, and flexible analytical skills that are essential for fields like health care. The category *humanities* (literature, rhetoric, film, history, philosophy, art history, religion, musicology, some anthropology, and certain interdisciplinary fields) in university settings is used to distinguish study and training methods from the *social sciences*, which investigate broad social phenomena using more empirical methods (economics, political science, psychology, sociology), and the *natural sciences*, which analyze the natural world empirically (biology,

chemistry, physics). Here the *humanities* in the *health humanities* cultivates the ability to navigate the complexities of interpersonal interaction and their ethical implications, to relate the individual to the structural, to historicize encounters, to communicate accurately and effectively across a variety of media, and to engage in creative analytical thinking about health care.

The *Oxford English Dictionary* recognizes only this second definition. While derived from the word *humanity*, in the "sense relating to HUMANE," the *humanities* has, for at least half a millennium, referred to "literary learning or scholarship; secular letters as opposed to theology, *esp.* the study of ancient Latin and Greek language, literature, and intellectual culture (as grammar, rhetoric, history, and philosophy)," or, since the nineteenth century, "the branch of learning concerned with human culture; the academic subjects comprising this branch of learning . . . typically distinguished from the social sciences" (*OED Online* 2020, "humanities"). The medical use of the term tracks better with a definition of *humanism*, "sympathetic concern with human needs, interests, and welfare; humaneness" (*OED Online* 2020, "humanism"), or *humanity*, "the quality of being humane" (*OED Online* 2020, "humanity").

The *humanities* (a pedagogical project studying the human rather than the divine) first split from *humanism* ("zealous faith in an ideal") in the sixteenth century (Grafton and Jardine 1986, xvi). Still, this ideal of *humanism* or *humanity* and the *humanities* continued to intersect at times, becoming somewhat more entwined, for example, in the nineteenth-century idea of the *humanities* as a practice of expanding sensitivities to the human (Graff 1987, 3–5).

Both medicine and the humanities were fundamentally restructured in the US at the turn of the twentieth century, when they emerged as modern disciplines through educational reform that valued rigorous training and research programs indebted to the German university model and developed through the modern research university (Veysey 1965; Wellmon 2015; for medicine, see Flexner 1910; Starr 1982). At that time, both medicine and the humanities cultivated more technical language and systematic inquiry, broadening subject matter and methods beyond classical training and emphasizing specialized knowledge (During 2020).

Medicine's transformation opened vital new avenues for research and treatment, but something was lost; William Osler (1919), often described as the founder of modern medicine, called it "the humanities." In fact, the humanities had been lost in both senses. Over the course of the nineteenth century, historical study ceased to be the "meaningful" part of physicians' "intellectual life" it had been for centuries (Charles Rosenberg 1992, 1). And following Abraham Flexner's 1910 report, which revolutionized US medical education, Latin, Greek, and philosophy were replaced by biology, chemistry, and physics as ideal prerequisites for medical school (Altschuler 2018). By 1925, Flexner himself lamented these shifts: "Scientific medicine in America" had become "sadly deficient in cultural and philosophical background" (18). Osler also regretted this loss of training but understood it as a perilous devaluation of a universal human ideal. Osler's view valorized medicine for its modernity, while the humanities were historical and timeless, as the title of his 1919 essay "The Old Humanities and the New Science" announced. Still, Osler knew himself as a humanities "amateur" and deferred to experts (4). Considering the humanities the "greatest single gift in education" and vital for medicine, Osler's vision for reintegration began from what experts in humanities and medicine could offer one another (26).

Contemporary humanities scholars have expressed legitimate concerns about definitions of the humanities in the health humanities that romanticize a preprofessional ideal. For example, arguments that emphasize "exposure to the humanities," defined as time spent with "literature, music, theater and visual arts," obscure the need for expertise (e.g., Mangione et al. 2018, 628). Furthermore, humanists worry that a timeless sense of the humanities not only mischaracterizes the work but represents it as unequal to health expertise (soft and feminized but also common sense and universal). It can spread dangerously diminished views of the humanities as disciplines lacking rigor—a damaging misconception already culturally ubiquitous (Altschuler 2018; J. Williams 2019). These fears are grounded in experience: some medical humanities programs make no space for the analytical work of the humanities (Wachtler, Lundin, and Troein 2006). Furthermore, as Sam Dubal warns in the following entry, efforts undertaken "in the name of humanity" necessarily emerge from white, Western ideas of the liberal subject and are thus constitutively "insufficient in truly addressing structural problems" wrought by racism and capitalism (see "Humanity").

But blaming health-care professionals alone for obscuring the humanities' analytical contributions to health care is unfair. Differences between popular and expert ideas about the humanities trace back to the original split between humanism and the humanities half a millennium ago (Grafton and Jardine 1986). And humanists themselves have, not infrequently, obscured these differences to extend the broad cultural authority of their fields and to secure funding, even if they risk devaluing their own expertise.

Tensions stemming from divergent definitions of the humanities, usually buried, exploded in a September 2020 LISTSERV debate over who should teach health humanities. Craig Klugman began: "Having a non-PhD holding MD teaching health humanities is like having a PhD in literature perform surgery. Suggesting that a PhD in humanities is not needed to teach these areas feeds into the hidden curriculum that these areas are not as important and that 'anyone can do it'" (2020). Rita Charon agreed: "Let us raise a chorus on the dangers and ineptness" of "self-canoniz[ed]" clinicians "who trade on their status as doctors to proclaim authority in fields they may be attracted to—literature, history, visual arts—and have no advanced training in" (2020). Douglas Binder countered: "This is tribalism, and nothing more. Instead of welcoming physicians with an interest in the humanities you seem too eager to push them away. . . . There is a great deal of humanistic knowledge to be gained by the actual practice of medicine" (2020). Other MDs defended their ability to teach poetry and ethics in medical settings without formal training. While some responses sought to mend rifts, the exchange surfaced tensions central to the field since its founding.

Given what can seem like an unbridgeable divide, some scholars have turned away from defining the *humanities* toward thinking about the spirit of health humanities endeavors; they describe the field in terms of shared political projects and a social justice mission. Framed positively, this emphasis invites a capacious perspective on health, bringing together like-minded health-care practitioners, humanists, social scientists, and artists toward the common goal of a more just and equitable health care (e.g., T. Jones, Wear, and Friedman 2014). Here health humanists are joined by values, not method (Klugman and Lamb 2019). Nevertheless, as recent contentious debates suggest, setting definitions aside has not resolved the problem of what the humanities are for the health humanities.

Framing the issue differently can move the conversation forward: the *health humanities* is not, as the name might suggest, a kind of humanities but a field that builds from humanities work and draws in the expertise of collaborators interested in making the culture of health care more equitable, just, and humane. Such a reframing preserves the field's inclusiveness without diminishing humanities expertise; *health humanities* remains a capacious term for people joined by a common mission, while *humanities* names an intellectual origin and set of core tools for that work. Significantly, the purpose of the very first US medical school humanities department was "to recruit scholars trained in the methodology and subjects of traditional humanities to bring their unique perspectives to bear on medical education and practice"—a project that began from the promise of collaboration among experts (A. Hawkins, Ballard, and Hufford 2003, 1001).

Obscuring or avoiding divergent understandings of the humanities may seem useful, but underlying tensions hamper the field's progress (e.g., Hurwitz 2013). Instead, we ought to clarify and elaborate on what humanities experts offer the health humanities to sharpen and extend the analytical power of the humanities for health care.

Here *humanities competencies* offers a useful umbrella concept that describes the collection of analytical skills—narrative, historical perspective, observation, ethics, and judgment—the humanities offer health care (Altschuler 2018; "Social Science and Humanities Competencies" 2018; cf. Johanna Shapiro et al. 2009). This concept provides a humanities complement to Metzl and Hansen's (2014) "structural competency," which elaborates social science contributions to health care. Humanities competencies underscore the unique tools the humanities supply for moving between and connecting scales of analysis and care in ways that the social and natural sciences—because they are largely dependent on empirically verifiable data—have difficulty doing. A competency in observation, for example, trains students not only to sharpen their techniques of observation and their attention to individual difference and idiosyncrasy but to understand how individual observations are shaped by broader social, cultural, and historical forms and factors. Likewise, a competency in historical perspective, as historians of medicine have recently argued, "offers essential insights about the causes of disease (e.g., the non-reductionistic mechanisms needed to account for changes in the burden of disease over time), the nature of efficacy (e.g., why doctors think that their treatments work, and how have their assessments changed over time), and the contingency of medical knowledge and practice amid the social, economic, and political contexts of medicine" (D. Jones et al. 2015, 623). "Narrative competence" provides a ready model, highlighting the need for health-care practitioners to be better receivers of stories, as narrative medicine teaches us, but a competence in narrative should, moreover, train students and practitioners in close reading skills (Charon 2006) and to identify the formal features of narrative that shape not only the clinical encounter but community and population health, paths of infection, and treatment protocols (Wald 2008). Using outward-looking, translational language for health educators and professionals who already think in terms of training competencies, *humanistic competencies* nonetheless authorizes humanities experts to define their own contributions, particularly those that connect individual and structural issues. (Some prefer *humility* to *competence*. While useful, I worry this use of *humility* unwittingly deskills the humanities [cf. DasGupta 2008; Tsevat et al. 2015].) The key terms of humanities competencies are not new, but together they more clearly articulate a program to structure interdisciplinary collaboration that foregrounds the analytical contributions humanities disciplines offer the study of health and practices of health care.

33

Humanity
Samuel Dubal

Defining the field of "health humanities" requires careful attention to the fraught concept of humanity itself. As Raymond Williams (1976) points out, the use of "the humanities" to define an academic field inclusive of classics, philosophy, and modern literature arose in the eighteenth century. In this sense, the field of health humanities strives for an inter- or multidisciplinary approach to health inclusive of history, the arts, bioethics, and the social sciences, among countless other forms of thought.

Elsewhere in this volume, Sari Altschuler delves into the complexities of this contested discipline and its history in detail (see "Humanities"). Among the genealogical threads she identifies is how the humanities and modern medicine diverged and came to be seen as antithetical. One narrative in this story is that the health humanities (originally "medical humanities" but rightfully expanded to a broader and less elitist scope) historically arose and grew in medical education as a counterbalance to what was seen as corrosive effects of biological sciences—the decline in empathy of clinicians and the loss of a "human" touch (Bleakley 2014). Put bluntly, the soft arts were to restore sensitivity and humanity to the hard sciences that, under the influences of rationality and capitalism, tended to dehumanize both the sick and their healers by forsaking a certain ethical and insidiously gendered idea of care.

The process of rehumanizing the sick was to take place under several different forms but perhaps most prominently through illness narratives or narrative medicine. The subfield of narrative medicine developed to recenter stories of illness in medical treatments that had become impersonal, overtly technical, and bureaucratic in an effort to reinstate what was seen as a lost genuine engagement with the patient, whose human illness experience had been reduced to a technical disease case (see "Narrative"; Kleinman 1988; Charon 2006; Jurecic 2012). The illness narrative was to refocus attention on the meaning ascribed to disease—a practice common to nonbiomedical healing practices but usually jettisoned in biomedical practice.

The sick have not been the only objects of rehumanization. Increasingly, humanism is also being called upon to rehumanize their healers. Provider "burnout" is a serious concern among many health professions, including physicians, nurses, and pharmacists, as healers suffer from "depersonalization," among other forms of alienating distress including depression, suicidality, and substance abuse. The strains of capitalism, bureaucracy, excessive workloads, and similar structural problems lead them to treat patients "as objects rather than human beings" (West, Dyrbye, and Shanafelt 2018, 516). Some of those attempting to counter burnout suggest that humanities education can help increase tolerance to ambiguity and build emotional resilience in providers (Mangione et al. 2018). Others have called for increasing training in mindfulness, stress management, and other forms of "wellness"—treating healers as though they are deficient and lacking in "resilience" rather than attempting to revolutionize the violent infrastructure of the US health-care system that afflicts the healers and the sick alike. At its worst, this kind of resiliency building naively calls on practices like yoga and meditation to restore the humanity of healers broken by a failing system. Some advocates proclaim these approaches as "revolutionary"—not because they get to the root of

systemic injustice but because they cost less than the financial or welfare benefits that might alternatively be implemented to combat burnout (Cocchiara et al. 2019).

Narrative medicine, humanities education, provider "wellness," and similar humanizing approaches have thus far largely failed to seriously challenge existing discourses and practices of clinical biomedicine, particularly their devotion to technocracy and evidence (see "Evidence"). These discourses are so entrenched that they dictate how such humanization might take place and be evaluated. In order to maintain its precarious seat at the biomedical table, the field of health humanities has often had to justify its legitimacy and value in clinical terms, often by being required to provide scientific evidence that their interventions had impact (Bleakley 2014, 18). Within the subfield of medical anthropology, this legitimization occurred via clinically applied work that sought to functionalize scholarship to improve doctor-patient relationships and measurable clinical outcomes. By providing "cultural sensitivity" and "explanatory models," clinically applied anthropologists were to be negotiators or brokers of the patient-doctor relationship, interpreting illness narratives in ways that would facilitate biomedical care. Anne Fadiman's (1997) *The Spirit Catches You and You Fall Down*, which became a staple in American medical school curricula, embodies this approach. It highlights how a lack of "cultural competence" on the part of medical providers can impair effective care and lead to poor clinical outcomes. Adding a human touch was to be not only ethically imperative but also therapeutically effective by improving clinical outcomes. This practical philosophy has given birth to such grotesque concepts as "compassionomics," which suggests that compassionate care is virtuous not simply in itself but because it reduces health-care costs (Trzeciak and Mazzarelli 2019). In short, within the health humanities, there is a conscious, burdensome, and utilitarian expectation instilled (in particular by clinical training schools) that the humanities will counter dehumanizing tendencies of biological sciences by developing a moral compass in healers—making them more humane and, by perverse extension, more effective carers (T. Jones 2014).

On the surface, all this striving toward humanity may not come across as particularly objectionable, especially in spaces of health in the United States where care becomes robotized through technological, legislative, and corporate restructuring (Pine 2011). Who could seriously object to reforming systems that dehumanize both the afflicted and those who attempt to heal them? The more elusive problem is that these and other turns toward "humanizing" medicine do little to call into question deeper assumptions of biomedicine and in particular its way of creating and reproducing unequal power relations. These "humanizing" turns do not bring into question systematic political, economic, and racial underpinnings of the US health-care system (Fox 2005); they do not fundamentally change the relationship of the bourgeois clinician to the marginalized sick (Scheper-Hughes 1990), nor do they challenge fundamental white Western ideals of what it means to be human, including the presumed duality of mind and body (Gordon 1988). As Jeffrey Bishop (2008) puts it, "Humanism is the add-on that makes the power more palatable" (22).

It is this use of "humanity," in relation to its close cousins "humanism" and "humane," that continues to pose problems in the struggle toward justice in the health humanities. These debates over "humanity" and humanism are not, however, exclusive to the discipline. They have been raised elsewhere—primarily by Black scholars, scholars of color, and their allies—as part of a broader critique of the violence of liberalism. In the largely white academic field, liberal humanism proclaims the equality of individual selves with rights, liberty, and freedom—an equality that does not actually exist but is perpetually postponed (Maldonado-Torres 2020). For people of color and colonized subjects, "humanity" has always been a mirage, a false promise, a "dishonest ideology" (Sartre 1961, lviii). An abstract universality, "humanity" in practice violently made men of Europeans and slaves and savages of others. The exclusionary perversions of European humanism refused (and continue to refuse) the recognition of a Black humanity or the humanity of other subjugated peoples. Part of the problem is that the supposedly universal concept of humanity is usually taken as synonymous with Western-bourgeois Man, a particular code exclusive of the experiences and dreams of nonwhite peoples (David Scott and Wynter 2000). This is a partial, not a full, humanism. To speak of this kind of humanity as a universality is violent insofar as it precludes alternative visions of humanity, new kinds of radical humanisms that decolonize what it means to be human (Weheliye 2014; Dubal 2018; Jobson 2020).

What these critiques of liberalism highlight for the health humanities are the ways in which discourses of humanism are built on the scaffolding of exploitation, providing reformist window dressing in place of revolutionary change. Training more "humane" clinicians who treat their patients as people rather than disease cases will not undo the pathological processes of racism, capitalism, and techno-utopianism, among other ongoing mechanisms of health injustice. Indeed, the danger of humanism lies precisely in its masquerade—it offers universal fulfillment in a supposedly common state of freedom while ignoring the problematic terms and conditions on which that fulfillment is built. In doing so, it reproduces inequity and injustice under the guise of good intentions.

The desire and need for change from the unjust status quo is clear to clinicians, patients, scholars, and activists who have literally grown sick of the structural inequities produced by American biomedicine. The challenge today for the health humanities in particular and for scholars and activists in general is how to enact that change. Many, including those in a long Black humanist tradition, advocate for new emancipatory humanisms that finally recognize the equality of people that has hitherto only been theoretically described. This tradition has found its public voice in the Black Lives Matter movement, an intersectional process that asks for the recognition of humanity that its detractors (among them those who retort that "all lives matter") accept in theory but deny in practice (Pierce 2020). Repudiations of the human as it stands have also thrived in parallel in arenas such as ontological studies, where racial justice is not necessarily at the forefront of disciplinary thinking. As the effects of climate change intensify, posthumanist scholars identify the "human" as a limit that prevents scholarship from seeing and attending to alternative worlds inhabited by plants, cyborgs, spirits, and animals (to name a few) in a movement away from, or at least critically interrogative of, the Anthropocene (Kohn 2013; Kirksey and Helmreich 2010). This kind of departure from the human is increasingly being linked with radical liberation and decolonization, in which violence to nonhuman worlds is recognized as part of and integral to broader projects of elite racial capitalism and settler colonialism (see, e.g., Todd 2016). Despite the important work of Zoe Todd and others challenging the colonial assumptions within the field, there are nonetheless reasons to remain vigilant about the kinds of political visions that these fields more broadly construct through different forms of posthumanism. There is historical precedent for this suspicion—as Richard Pithouse notes, Western poststructuralist and postmodern elites were proclaiming the end of humanism precisely when colonized peoples were vehemently demanding and fighting for their own recognition as human beings (quoted in Pierce 2020, 13).

The question of "humanity" will likely continue to animate the health humanities as a foundational liberal philosophy. Despite its problems, "humanity" will remain for some a rallying cry against certain kinds of "dehumanization" taking place in and through health care and health interventions. Reformers will combat what they see as ongoing losses of "humanism" in medicine, pining for more compassionate systems of care in the face of "antihumanistic" immigration law, autocracy, and nationalism (Thibault 2019). However well intentioned, these efforts "in the name of humanity" are nevertheless insufficient in truly addressing structural problems. Teaching healers to be more compassionate to their patients will not cure the collective diseases of racism and capitalism, among others, that afflict the corporate body. Humanism may bring some comfort to the sick, but it will not bring justice; alone, it continues a tradition of change that is more clinical than critical, more concerned with individual sicknesses than structural or social sicknesses. One wonders how much progress can and will actually take place in the name of "humanity." As adjacent disciplines consider burning down the house by abandoning the universal liberal subject (Jobson 2020), might the fire spread to the health humanities?

34

Immunity

Cristobal Silva

Before the emergence of the global COVID-19 pandemic, *immunity* had become a relatively abstract concept in the industrialized world. For those who had easy access to health care and functioning immune systems, formerly life-threatening diseases like measles, polio, diphtheria, and influenza had been reduced to acronyms associated with vaccine schedules: MMR, IPV, DTaP, and Hib, among others. And yet even as the vaccine era dominated public health responses to infectious diseases, pockets of vaccine resistance persisted, and new diseases began to loom large in the cultural imagination: Zika, West Nile, SARS, Ebola, H1N1, and HIV/AIDS seemed to elude treatment and cure, raising the specter of global apocalypse. By mid-2020, COVID-19 embodied the worst fears and greatest promise of modern public health: a contagious disease that spread rapidly through casual social interactions but for which an effective vaccine could be developed, tested, and deployed in record time. By early 2021, the promise that vaccination would mean a quick return to prepandemic life was shattered: even as tens of millions of people were vaccinated in the United States alone, suspicion of governments and private corporations hardened into persistent anti-vaccine conspiracy theories. As vaccination rates plateaued, so did resistance to the SARS-CoV-2 virus. By mid-2021, new variants continued to evolve as waves of infection put pressure on US health systems, wreaking havoc on economic infrastructures and leading to distressing

levels of mortality. In what follows, we will consider the complex relation of biological, political, historical, and personal factors that make a seemingly simple idea like immunity such a critical and controversial concept in modern society.

How, one might ask, does a society that possesses a clear solution to a public health crisis fail to follow through on it? How does the very idea of immunity expose political and cultural fault lines in a community? To explore these questions, I will set COVID-19 aside for a moment and examine the history and meaning of *immunity* itself. Doing so will not add to the development of practical treatments and medicine, nor will it add to debates about the effectiveness of vaccines. And yet reflections by literary and cultural critics as well as historians working in the medical and health humanities help clarify the core tensions between individual and communal rights that lie at the heart of modern public health debates. Rather than resolving questions about the limits of state power, they underscore how rhetorical and ideological structures determine the historical equity and effectiveness of public health policy. This history begins with an acknowledgment that the word *immunity* (*immunitas*) existed two thousand years prior to its use in medicine. An idea firmly rooted in Roman law, it was used to describe the exemption from tribute and taxation that a sovereign power could grant to an individual or state. In other words, an individual who was granted immunity to a certain tax did not have to pay it. Immunity remains a key concept of civil and criminal law, but it has long since expanded to signify a protection from liability or prosecution. Although *immunity* would not be used in medicine until the modern era, physicians have known that individuals could be susceptible or resistant to certain illnesses for millennia. However, it was only in the age of microbiology—the period that begins roughly with the work of John Snow and Filipo Pacini on cholera and of Louis Pasteur on anthrax and rabies in the late nineteenth century—that medical practitioners began to feel the need for a word that could internalize the idea of resistance to infectious disease (i.e., that immunity comes from within one's own body rather than from an external force like God).

There is no inherent reason that medicine should have settled on *immunity* as its word for resistance to disease, but *immunity*'s early association with law and exemption proved to be important for several reasons. First, because regardless of how accurate or sophisticated the modern understanding of human immune systems is in helping develop new vaccines and medical therapies for rare diseases, the term's prehistory reminds us that medicine's appropriation of it emerged from an analogy to the law. Acknowledging this analogical character should prompt us to resist the essentialism that otherwise lurks at the heart of modern Western medicine—an essentialism made concrete in immune-system models of the human body that define health as a private function of individual persons (my body and my health are my own).

Second, *immunity*'s legal origins tell a story about the role of sovereignty in Western medicine. While the biological concept of immunity has no obvious association with forms of sovereignty that define a state's political and legal powers, the medical profession's appropriation of *immunity* as a controlling metaphor for resistance and susceptibility to infectious disease may in fact be rooted in history. Taking the long view, Western history and literature are filled with examples of writers who portray epidemics and pandemics as punishments meted out by sovereign deities against sinful populations. Consider Apollo's plague at the beginning of the *Iliad* or the plague of Thebes at the start of *Oedipus*. Or the European justification narratives that represent devastating New World epidemics as acts of divine

providence to support their colonial dispossession and appropriation of Indigenous lands. Or even the modern jeremiads that figure contemporary epidemics like HIV/AIDS as divine punishments for national sins.

Modern medicine can of course make sense of such events by pointing to interactions between pathogens, vectors, modes of transmission, and differential susceptibilities, but it would be naive to imagine that the accuracy of those explanations somehow erases the ideological foundations of medical narratives that themselves date back to at least the ancient Greeks. So that if divine sovereignty no longer has purchase over Western medicine, immunity models of susceptibility and resistance may still internalize political sovereignty in the forms of its narratives. Looking back to justification narratives, for example, once divine sovereignty lost its appeal as a model for explaining Indigenous susceptibility to contagious diseases, narratives centered on the apparent immunological and genetic inferiority of Indigenous People (the so-called virgin soils model) became dominant (see Crosby 1976; D. Jones 2004). No less appealing in their simplicity than those earlier narratives, virgin soils models substituted biological determinism (the death of Indigenous People from exposure to European pathogens was inevitable) for divine sovereignty and fed into historical colonialist tropes by flattening the relation between epidemics and complex demographic patterns.

This seemingly narrow debate about the structure of historical epidemiological narratives is critical to struggles over Indigenous sovereignty and reclamations precisely because of the state's ongoing interest in regulating health. More pointedly, where governments determine how to define immunity, public health policy becomes the embodiment of sovereignty and political power. This dynamic becomes clearer to broader public audiences in the wake of COVID-19. During the vaccination phase of the pandemic, vaccine mandates

IMMUNITY   CRISTOBAL SILVA

became avatars of state power. They stood as gateways to employment, to schooling, to travel, and to the enjoyment of public spaces. Even as people resist vaccination for a number of reasons, the state's sovereign interest in mandating vaccines arises because they help moderate the risk of epidemical outbreak via a concept known as herd immunity. In contrast to personal immunity, herd immunity is expressed as the percentage of a given population that is resistant to infection at a specific point in time. For example, when a community has a high level of herd immunity to a disease (say, 90 percent), it has a low risk of epidemical outbreak because contagious individuals have a low likelihood (one in ten) of randomly encountering and passing the pathogen on to susceptible people. On the other hand, communities with low levels of herd immunity (say, 10 percent) are at a high risk of epidemic outbreak for exactly the opposite reason. Though they share a term, an important difference between *individual immunity* and *herd immunity* is that immunity tends to be a relatively static state for individuals, whereas herd immunity changes day by day as people are born, die, migrate, or develop immunities of their own through vaccination and exposure. Herd immunity is an important tool in public health because large swings in the ratio of susceptible to unsusceptible people have dramatic effects on the likelihood that epidemics will erupt or peter out in a population.

An important point to clarify about public health policies during early phases of the COVID-19 pandemic is this: among the various strategies for combatting the outbreak, *herd immunity* was used as loose shorthand for policies that sought to increase rates of resistance to the SARS-CoV-2 virus by allowing it to circulate freely. As people became infected and recovered, they presumably developed their own resistances and contributed to higher levels of herd immunity against the virus. Notwithstanding the fact that as of late 2021, the estimated rate at which herd immunity becomes an effective barrier against COVID-19 (the herd immunity threshold) is believed to be well above 80 percent, the social cost of such policies is that mortality is considerably higher in the short term than it would be with strict mitigation efforts like quarantines, lockdowns, face masks, and social distancing (see Aschwanden 2020). Furthermore, as the virus circulates freely in the world, the risk of new, more infectious, and vaccine-resistant variants evolving also rises. This particular shorthand glosses over the fact that herd immunity is a key component of mitigation strategies that aim to keep infection rates low until effective vaccines can be developed and distributed to the public—at which point they would help raise overall rates of resistance. Though both of these strategies rely on herd immunity, the former proved to be a failure based on total and per capita mortality; its use among critics of quarantines and lockdowns was a euphemism for state-sanctioned policies whose direct effect was more sickness and death.

Pointing out the multiple entanglements of medicine, culture, politics, and law in the term *immunity* is not a criticism of the tremendous advancements that medicine and science have made over the past century. Instead, situating immunity within its larger history as a word and an idea shows how our understanding of resistance and susceptibility to infectious disease reflects larger political and cultural trajectories in the field of medicine and public health. Working with this longer temporal horizon reminds us that before the era of professionalization and specialization in the late nineteenth century, fields like law, theology, medicine, history, philosophy, art, and literature were not nearly so distinct, and words like *immunity* drew promiscuously from them. While *immunity* may conjure the disciplinary expertise of health professionals (like epidemiologists, immunologists, and infectious disease experts) in the twenty-first century, the role of the medical and health humanities in revisiting the histories of such words is to highlight the interdisciplinary entanglements that have always been part of public health and to offer insights into the narratives and forms that modern public health debates share with their predecessors.

35

Indigeneity

Michele Marie Desmarais and
Regina Emily Idoate

We have our own names.

Placing and *Re*placing Terminology

Indigeneity is a word in English that refers to the state of belonging to a Place or a Peoples. The word is linked in origin to the perspectives of colonizers.

Regarding terms such as *Indigeneity* or *Indigenous* that refer to belonging, Distinguished Professor Aileen Moreton-Robinson (Goenpul from Minjerribah, Quandamooka First Nation) explains, "Who belongs, and the degree of that belonging, is inextricably tied to white possession" (2020, 18). And yet despite centuries of colonization, we have our own names and ways of belonging that are unique to each of us.

Across Turtle Island, there are 574 Native American Nations in the areas now known as the United States and more than 630 First Nations, as well as the Métis Nation and the Inuit, in the areas now known as Canada. The United Nations Declaration on the Rights of Indigenous Peoples recognizes more than 370 million people as "Indigenous," but respecting Indigenous Peoples' rights to name themselves, the authors purposely do not define "Indigeneity" or offer any suggested qualifiers to establish what makes a person "Indigenous" (UN General Assembly 2007). We have our own ways of referring to our People that translated into English can mean Original Peoples, Principal Peoples, First Peoples, from the People's origins, the Real People, the People. We have our own words for referring to the Places to whom we belong, Places that English speakers call rivers, waterfalls, lakes, oceans, mountains, prairies, deserts, forests, or sky.

We have our own names for who we are.

The quality or state of being who we are is unique to each of us. The diversity of Peoples, Nations, names, Places, histories, and languages that we find across Turtle Island and beyond is vast. While respectfully listening to and recognizing the distinct ways of knowing, being, and doing among Indigenous Nations and Peoples, some Indigenous scholars also recognize certain commonalities among us that can aid in decolonizing the terms *Indigeneity* and *Indigenous*. We can, for example, understand the meaning of Indigeneity to refer to the quality or state of being Indigenous, which Murri scholar Lorraine Muller describes as "a statement of physical, cultural and spiritual heritage" (2020, 14). Leanne Betasamosake Simpson, Michi Saagiig Nishnaabeg scholar, outlines seven commonalities among Indigenous worldviews as summarized by Michael Anthony Hart, a Kaskitémahikan scholar and citizen of Fisher River Cree Nation: "First, knowledge is holistic, cyclic, and dependent upon relationships and connections to living and non-living beings and entities. Second, there are many truths, and these truths are dependent upon individual experiences. Third, everything is alive. Fourth, all things are equal. Fifth, the land is sacred. Sixth, the relationship between people and the spiritual world is important. Seventh, human beings are least important in the world" (Hart 2010, 3).

We have our own names for what we know.

Thus, the term *Indigenous*—as defined and explained by Indigenous Peoples such as La Donna Harris (Comanche) and Jacqueline Howell Wasilewski (Cherokee)—can therefore elucidate some "common core cultural values shared by most Indigenous Peoples" while simultaneously supporting an understanding of Indigeneity as "the ability to hold our core values even while we entertain and create new ideas" (Harris and Wasilewski 2004, 490–91). Indigenous knowledges are inheritances passed down through place, community, and family that are alive in our diverse ways of knowing, being, and doing. In contrast, non-Indigenous perspectives of Indigeneity too often reveal an explicit or implicit essentialism in their characterizations. Such essentialism most clearly manifests itself in colonial dichotomies such as traditional versus modern, subjective versus objective, authentic versus assimilated, static (read museum pieces) versus living.

Countering colonial dichotomies, Kānaka Maoli scholar Maile Arvin writes that "critical indigenous scholarship can unsettle the ways these categories were formed in colonialism in the first place and imagine indigeneity otherwise" and that such work can "enable both a critique of how indigenous peoples are always seen as vanishing as well as opening up the boundaries of indigenous identity, culture, politics, and futures to new, productive possibilities" (2015, 125–26). Professor Chelsea Watego (Mununjali and South Sea Islander) and co-authors explain that in the health humanities, Indigenous research investigates "the ways in which power is configured to the detriment of Indigenous peoples' health and wellbeing" and that "Indigenous ways of working based on relationality" offer "an alternative vision of scholarship and knowledge production" and "a new way of thinking about health and Indigeneity" (Watego et al. 2021, 9).

Indigeneity embodies resilience; the state or quality of being Indigenous comes from generations of peoples who have survived and thrived, generations of peoples who have, in the face of adversity, demonstrated the ability to adapt to maintain their values or transform to create new ones. Māori scholar Darryn Russell and Stephanie Rotarangi reason that "to be indigenous is to be resilient" (Rotarangi and Russell 2009, 209). Marion Kickett, a Noongar Aboriginal scholar, defines resilience as "the ability to have a connection and belonging to one's land, family and culture: therefore an identity. Resilience allows the pain and suffering caused from adversities to heal. It is having a dreaming, where the past is brought to the present and the present and the past are taken to the future. Resilience is a strong spirit that confronts and conquers racism and oppression strengthening the spirit. It is the ability not just to survive but to thrive in today's dominant culture" (2011, ii).

Our Indigeneity—alive in our ways of being, knowing, and doing—is resilient. Sisseton-Wahpeton Oyate scientist Kim TallBear reiterates this point, noting that global Indigenous movements and narratives in the twenty-first century are about our "will not only to survive but also to thrive" (2013, 516). Indigenous health humanities is a vital part of that movement, a countering or balancing force in medicine and academia that embraces the healing practices of our relatives and communities as a whole.

Indigenous Health Humanities

Indigenous Peoples have practiced, and continue to practice, a range of topics now referred to as health humanities. Ojibwe scholar Megan Bang and colleagues suggest that "Indigenous sciences build knowledge about the world through a distinct set of orienting values, concepts, and questions. These include: What is worthy of attention? What needs explanation? Who is related? How? Why does it matter?" (Bang, Marin, and Medin 2018, 149). Our aim in this section is to briefly highlight how we answer these questions and to share examples of Indigenous health humanities.

We have our own names for what we do.

In his book *Research Is Ceremony: Indigenous Research Methods*, Opaskwayak Cree researcher Shawn Wilson shares a research paradigm grounded in Indigenous ways of knowing, being, and doing. He writes that "if Indigenous ways of knowing have to be narrowed through one particular lens (which it certainly does not), then surely that lens would be relationality. All things are related and therefore relevant" (2008, 58). From there, Wilson illuminates some principles and practices of Indigenous research methods that are widely shared among Indigenous researchers: ethical protocols, ceremony, relationality (including with Places, Ancestors, Peoples, Environments, Cosmos), knowledge of and respect for our distinctive Indigenous ontologies and epistemologies, representation (nothing about us without us), and relational accountability (Chilisa 2012; Kirkness and Barnhardt 1991; Kovach 2009; L. Smith 2013; Cajete 2020). This decolonized and Indigenized approach to research recognizes that Indigenous Peoples have long engaged in knowledge gathering and sharing, in healing practices that recognize the whole person whose well-being is dependent upon community, other-than-human persons, and the health of Water, Air, Earth, and many more Relatives. Our research and our arts carry medicines that are beneficial to our Peoples and Places and not merely to an individual or to academia. As Maxine Noel, a Santee Oglala Sioux visual artist from the Birdtail Sioux Dakhóta Oyáte, writes, "At its simplest, my art is the way I offer healing to the worlds around me" (2015, 57).

Story medicine is another example of how we, as Indigenous Peoples, share medicine and research in accordance with our own cultures and knowledge systems. Michif artist Dylan A. T. Miner succinctly notes, "Storytelling and healing are interconnected, within ourselves and within our respective communities" (2013, 321). A recent expression of this is the report *COVID-19 and Indigenous Health and Wellness: Our Strength Is in Our Stories*. The Indigenous scholars, practitioners, and learners present their findings through stories because "stories emphasize the values embedded in, and purposed through, the practice of our Indigenous Knowledge systems" (Richmond et al. 2020, 10). Furthermore, stories function in this report as "a way to articulate how COVID-19 has shaped the nature of our own relationships—with self, family, community, land, and as self-determining peoples—and how this impacts health and wellness. Together, the stories act as demonstrations of our existence and highlight our efforts to document, share, and mobilize action based on those experiences" (10).

Another recent example of Indigenous art-medicine research is an art exhibit and study that asked a circle of Indigenous women, "*What does it mean to be an Urban Indian Woman who advocates for Native health and wellness in Omaha?*" (Idoate et al. 2020, 36). Each woman responded in her own words, in her own ways, through sculptures, poems, a speech performance, prayer, paintings, dolls, shawls, nests, moccasins, containers, beadwork, and a tapestry. The inquiry process was embodied by these women as they created and analyzed all artworks related to the exhibit. After publicly exhibiting these works in *INDIGENIST* and examining their collective response to the original question, they identified an Indigenist theory of health advocacy: the bundle of seven strands. They found their own words for the essence of being an Indigenist: remember, respect, relate, reconstruct, reflect, reciprocate, and rally. Relating the data to the People, who they belong to, what they know, and what they do enabled them to mutually construct, deconstruct, and reconstruct

meanings to ground stories into this framework (Idoate et al. 2020).

The examples above show how decolonized and Indigenized research can contribute toward promoting the health humanities and addressing the many adverse effects of colonization on the health of Indigenous Peoples. Indigenization and decolonization strengthen the resilience of Indigeneity.

We are here.

In an earlier article we asked, "What happens to all the people, all our relatives, whether clinician, patient, survivor, Indigenous or settler, if silence remains the dominant narrative related to Indigenous Peoples?" (Desmarais and Robbins 2019, 9). Cherokee-Greek writer Thomas King, reflecting on the power of stories, writes, "So you have to be careful with the stories you tell. And you have to watch out for the stories that you are told" (2003, 10). As the field of health humanities grows, we invite you to continuously question dominant culture narratives by asking, "Who is telling this story? Who am I not hearing from and why?" Here we offer a brief example of the breadth and depth of Indigenous knowledges in health humanities and show how research can recognize and respect Indigeneity in its diversity and solidarity. In keeping with the spirit of belonging to a Place or Peoples, we have emphasized positionality and have featured the work of Indigenous scholars, artists, activists, writers, and researchers. We have used direct quotes to respect the integrity of their voices because we have our own names for who we are, what we know, and what we do.

We are here. We have our own names for Indigeneity.

36

Life

Matthew A. Taylor

"Life" isn't easy. Despite being the foundational premise of Western medicine—the precondition of health, the opposite of death—life chronically resists definition (Mayr 1982; Tarizzo 2017). Simultaneously biological (life-forms) and cultural (lifestyles), physical (mere living) and metaphysical (living well), it is a concept with myriad referents but no coherent meaning. This "polysemy of life," to use Donna V. Jones's (2010, 7) phrase, is evident in a quartet of recent *New York Times* articles that ask whether SARS-CoV-2, bioengineered xenobots, planet Earth, and reanimated brain cells from a dead pig, respectively, are alive (Burdick 2020; Sokol 2020; Jabr 2019; Kolata 2019). And to these examples we might add the more prominent, contentious cases of human embryos and persons in persistent comas. Such debates demonstrate not only life's inherent amorphousness—and thus its essentially interpretive or discursive nature—but also and relatedly its supreme significance in contemporary society. As Alain Badiou has argued, "What is life?" is the question of modernity (2007, 13), organizing modern science, religion, economics, politics, ethics, and subjectivity in spite, or perhaps because, of its constitutive imprecision. The answers vary; the question—and its life-or-death stakes—does not.

Although assuming a unique form today, the fact-value conflation attending concepts of biological life is at least as old as Aristotle (Thacker 2010). In his teleological account, a principle of end-directed agency and self-directed activity animates nature as a whole, with the result being that animal life—and, more specifically, self-reflective human life—becomes the highest (because the most organized, actualized, and ensouled) expression of being (Aristotle 1984d, 1:436; Aristotle 1984b, 1:684). Life is both synecdoche and apex of Aristotle's cosmological order, modeling within itself a "continuous scale of ascent" (Aristotle 1984a, 1:922) that elevates the complex over the simple, the active over the passive, the animal over the vegetal, and the male over the female (Aristotle 1984c, 1:1008).

This subordination of "mere life" to "life of high degree" (Aristotle 1984c, 1:1021) would become the template for the medieval Christian Great Chain of Being (Lovejoy 1976), and its indirect influence can be seen much later in the otherwise dissimilar precepts of turn-of-the-nineteenth-century British Romanticism and Anglo-Franco-German evolutionism, both of which rejected prevailing mechanistic, reductionist natural philosophies and histories in favor of organic, holistic ones (Riskin 2016). Aristotelians and Great Chain adherents emphasized an immutable natural hierarchy with static orders of life; however, the Romantics (e.g., Samuel Taylor Coleridge) and early evolutionists (e.g., Erasmus Darwin, Johann Friedrich Blumenbach, Jean-Baptiste Lamarck) broadly imagined a diachronic, transformationist biology in which both individual beings and life itself developed dynamically over time (R. Richards 2002; Gigante 2009; R. Mitchell 2013). Movement and change, that is, became inherent, causal features of the order of things, not simply aspects of epiphenomenal entities; the Great Chain's links became temporalized. Consequently, as outlined by Michel Foucault and others, the taxonomic classification of living beings was supplanted by ontological inquiries into the force, principle, or law of life as such (Foucault [1966] 1994). Whether understood as transcendental or immanent, vitalist or materialist, life itself increasingly was isolated from the living, positioned as the subterranean power inspiriting organic things (and, often, inorganic things too) while also being beyond them. The paradoxical complement to this life-living distinction was an increasing conviction that life was, in some sense, itself alive, with its own desires, directions, proclivities, and imperatives. "Yielding to . . . [this] tremendous push" became, in Henri Bergson's phrase, "the key to life" (1944, 295, 36). Life, in other words, became more vital than the living, became their source, destiny, truth, and sovereign. Here, life isn't what you make of it; it's what makes you of it.

This subjection of the living to life had profound implications, especially as evolutionism began to consolidate disciplinary and cultural authority at the turn of the twentieth century. Despite a concerted effort, for instance, Darwin could not prevent a progressive teleology from entering his—and many other evolutionists'—theories. The notion of evolution as advancement maintained the Aristotelian hierarchy of the living, as life—now simultaneously a positivist scientific concept and a noumenal postulate—assumed the function of a god or an ideal in judging beings' conformity to its dictates (Ruse 2016). Those beings that best embodied life's propulsiveness, adaptability, agency, complexity, and freedom—that is, the most *lifelike* beings—were deemed more evolutionarily advanced, more valuable, more worthy of life. By contrast, those beings regarded as naturally out of step with life's imperatives due to degeneracy, feebleness, primitiveness, or other abnormality were regarded as unworthy of protection, care, or even existence. In the name of life, late nineteenth-century laissez-faire social Darwinism naturalized the elimination of supposedly inferior life-forms through a zero-sum survival of the fittest (Hofstadter 1955; M. Hawkins 1997); in the name of life, early twentieth-century state

eugenics authorized the segregation, sterilization, and murder of those labeled unfit (Degler 1991, 42–50; Kevles 1995). And if, following Foucault, we categorize such endeavors as biopolitical because they exemplify how modern governmentality identifies biological life as the necessary site for the exercise of power, then we must also recognize that they are only the most extreme examples of a general culture of life whose fundamental principle demarcates healthy from unhealthy, normal from abnormal, the rightfully living from the naturally dying (Foucault 2003; E. Cohen 2009)—and thus, in Achille Mbembe's formulation, "who is *disposable* [from] who is not" (2013, 174). In this sense, death is less life's opposite than its catalyst or purifying agent. Life's normativity precipitates its lethality.

Of course, as Mbembe (2013), Donna V. Jones (2010), Ann Laura Stoler (2000), Alexander G. Weheliye (2014), Kyla Schuller (2018a), Stephen Knadler (2019), and many others have noted, the biopolitical cleaving of healthy and unhealthy forms of life always has been adjudicated by race. From the scientific racism used to justify slavery and settler colonialism in the long nineteenth century; to the forced movement of Indigenous Peoples to reservations; to Jim Crow lynching; to the Holocaust of communities identified as Jewish, disabled, gay, or Romani; to the drastically lower life expectancies for people of color—especially LGBTQ+ people of color—in the US both before and during the COVID-19 pandemic, race is the arbiter for internally dividing life, the blueprint for the "creation of *death-worlds*, new and unique forms of social existence in which vast populations are subjected to conditions of life conferring upon them the status of *living dead*" (Mbembe 2013, 186). Communities designated as aberrant relative to the heteronormative White standard, that is, have been and continue to be exposed to death—as well as to what we might call microdeaths—as a matter of both policy and social infrastructure. From this perspective, White lives matter to the exact extent that Black lives do not, and systematic zombification therefore can be seen as the uncanny, inverted mirror of prospective cybernetic or genetic augmentation. Given the racializing operation at the heart of biopolitics, this is inevitable. Life isn't fair, but it is light-complected.

It is also, correlatively, anthropocentric. The same absolutist, exclusionary logic that aims to denominate and deanimate non-White life is also the logic that denigrates nonhuman life through habitat devastation and industrial agriculture alike. This is the shared insight of environmental justice movements, animal studies, certain versions of critical posthumanism, and certain forms of Black feminism (see, for instance, Wynter 2003; Z. Jackson 2020), and the concept of the Plantationocene represents one attempt to name its common root (Haraway 2015, 160n5). The Plantationocene—along with the Anthropocene, the Capitalocene, and so on—also gestures to the fact that the modern articulation of life is not only genocidal and ecocidal but also, finally, suicidal. The self-destructiveness immanent to this conception of life is evident in the patent unsustainability of continuing to live as if evolutionary progress and modern personhood are marked by ever-increasing autonomy from and mastery over the definitionally nonhuman environment—a common tenet across Lebensphilosophie, evolutionary biology, liberalism, and neoliberalism throughout the nineteenth and twentieth centuries (see, for instance, the work of Friedrich Nietzsche, Bergson, F. C. S. Schiller, Lester Frank Ward, Julian Huxley, John Maynard Keynes, Milton Friedman). When White supremacy erases the difference between non-White and nonhuman and when the domination of nature indexes racial vitality, then eugenics and anthropogenic climate change become coeval.

Recently, scholars in a wide range of disparate fields have argued convincingly that there is no necessary relationship between life's essential nature and the regressive political and cultural agendas that long have claimed it. In fact, these scholars contend, biological life's true essence actively counters such conscriptions through its innate horizontality, interconnectivity, open-endedness, diversity, and deconstruction of false binaries (Grosz 2011; Pitts-Taylor 2016; Kirby 2017; Puig de la Bellacasa 2017; Braidotti 2017; Vitale 2018). Life's values, that is, are actually progressive, which means that they can be enlisted in the struggle against racism, sexism, heterosexism, ableism, and speciesism. What's more, much work in this vein also radically expands the newly reconfigured conception of life as freedom to encompass everything, from atoms to planets to the universe as whole; according to the so-called new materialism, anything embodied partakes of the intrinsic vitality, agency, and dynamism of matter, which entails, for humans, new ethical responsibilities and potentially new forms of political recognition and collaboration (Bennett 2010; Coole and Frost 2010). Perhaps the most prominent incarnation of this philosophy is the resurgence of interest in Gaia, the theory that Earth itself is "a kind of living organism" of which conventional lifeforms are constitutive parts or organs (Lovelock 2016, xxi). Such a vision does not question life's primacy, only its artificial, prejudicial limitation; the solution to life's tyrannies, therefore, isn't to abandon life's reign but to universalize it, to reimagine it as democratically omnipresent.

Such optimism, while understandable, is unfounded. In both history and prospect, life is not a reliable ally. It can't be: on the one hand, it is too nebulous to ground any definitive political or ethical commitments, any actually binding investment (the mere recognition that something is alive has never afforded protection from harm); on the other, when life is, in fact, sutured to a fixed ethico-political program, it necessarily involves privileging some beings over others, with life's definition—whatever it may be, "conservative" or "progressive"—serving to naturalize such discriminations. This is the point of invoking life: it ontologizes what otherwise could seem arbitrary, relativistic, merely linguistic; it provides a standard, and for the standard to be functionally useful, it must value certain forms of life while disvaluing or disavowing others. In the abstract, all lives may matter, may be grievable; in practice, politics and ethics require cuts that, by definition, can't be equal to all (Butler 2009; Derrida 2009). Biological phenomena aren't normative in any straightforward sense, but instrumentalizations of them inevitably are, as evidenced in the current convergence of "biological (re)production and capital accumulation" and in the concomitant "rise of markets in biological commodities and services" that perpetuate the structural racisms of global colonialism (M. Cooper 2008, 3; Vora 2015, 2). Repurposing, reengineering, or revitalizing life, therefore, is not a viable solution to its—or our—problems; life will never save the living, and believing that it will risks writing only another chapter in its bloody biography.

But what is medicine in the absence of life? What is health? Living? It's hard to say—which is precisely the point. Freed from the monolith of life, the plurality of living—and of the living—might experiment with other, less deterministic, less mortifying forms of being. This is not, then, to advocate for abandoning life in favor of some other, truly innocent means of securing or naturalizing ways to live; it is to argue that a nonontological approach to ethics and politics is the only way to attend to the diverse existences and needs of the concretely living (Putnam 2004; Geuss 2020). Inspired by disability studies and hospice care, among other practices, such an approach might allow for the health humanities to explore quality-of-*living* issues rather than the vital-dead polarization that follows from valorizing the numinous abstraction of life itself. Living without life will not be easy—it may even prove unimaginable given life's centrality not only to modern thought but also to modern ways of thinking (Foucault, for example, links a vitalist ontology to the surface-depth, symptomatic hermeneutic that informs much contemporary humanities criticism). There is, furthermore, no easy or necessary nonbiological answer to how to adjudicate among the competing needs of living beings. Such solutions will have to be constantly constructed rather than found, divined, or birthed once and for all. In this sense, health justice, equity, diversity, and inclusion can only come at the end of "life."

37

Medicine

Sayantani DasGupta

The Origin of Medical Terms suggests the word *medicine* is originally from the Latin *medicina*, implying the art of healing. The verb *medeor* may have more complex Indo-European roots, meaning "to think" or "to reflect" (Charyn 1951). In modern usage, *medicine* implies something more practical—both the pharmaceutical drugs used to treat disease and the profession of medicine itself. Indeed, this transition from a reflective meaning to an active one might be at the root of mainstream Western medicine's often fraught relationship with the health humanities, a field that asks those whose professional identities are built on agentic "doing" to reflect, analyze, and consider in unfamiliar and often discomfiting ways (Boler 1999).

Although the word *medicine* is often used interchangeably with *health care* as a whole, this conflation erases the particular and unique skills and contributions of nurses, nurse practitioners (NPs), physician's assistants (PAs), social workers, respiratory therapists, occupational therapists, physical therapists, and other health-care professionals. Indeed, the history of the professionalization of medicine, through the formation of medical schools and professional organizations and the certification of trained physicians, is a history of exclusion. Moves to professionalize medicine in the mid-nineteenth century were as much to regulate ill-qualified and ill-trained practitioners from treating the sick as they were to eliminate the economic competition (usually male) physicians faced from midwives

and other types of healers (I. Waddington 1990). The rise of the American Medical Association (AMA) saw the solidification of the identity of "physician" around upper-middle-class white masculinity. When, in the aftermath of the Civil War, the issue arose of admitting women physicians and African American physicians to the professional organization, it was quashed at the national level and deemed a decision to be made by local chapters. Indeed, "the AMA's policy of tolerating racial exclusion was pivotal in creating a two-tier system of medicine in the American South and border states—racially divided, separate and unequal" (Baker 2014). The 1910 Flexner Report, whose aim was to make consistent training across the country's medical schools, was "explicit in its racism" and found that most Black medical schools did not meet its standards, although it suggested that training some Black doctors was necessary so that they might relieve white doctors from treating Black patients, who were, according to Flexner, "a source of infection and contagion" (Flexner 1910, quoted in Steinecke and Terrell 2010, 238).

Approximately this same time period that saw this organization of physician identity around dominant race, class, and gender identities saw shifts in Western societies from feudal to capitalist economies. With that shift came medicine's increased role in commodifying and classifying productive and profit-making bodies from those considered less or nonproductive. Michel Foucault ([1961] 2001) and others have written about medicine and the rise of prisons, asylums, hospitals, and poorhouses at this time to sequester, control, and diagnose nonnormative bodies. Indeed, medicine's history is steeped in histories of oppression toward marginalized groups, from the medicalization of disabled individuals (DasGupta 2015) to racist experimentation upon bodies of color, such as the development of the pelvic speculum by the so-called father of gynecology

Dr. J. Marion Sims through unanesthetized experiments upon enslaved African American women (Washington 2006). Into modern times, these tensions and oppressions continue alongside attempts to address medical violence and oppression through disability activism, anti-racist initiatives, and health humanities training in narrative humility (DasGupta 2008) and structural competency (Metzl and Hansen 2014).

In the meantime, historic tensions between medical and other health-care practitioners continue today. For instance, modern-day physicians in the US are often disgruntled by terms like *health-care providers* that might more fairly encompass the variety of professionals who provide health care, as well as family caregivers, pointing to the term's "demoralization" and "deprofessionalization." These conversations reveal hierarchical tensions within the health-care fields, with physicians arguing that NPs have far less training and are therefore not equivalent to those who have earned MDs. In the words of one family physician, "Calling me a 'provider' lumps my physician colleagues and me with individuals who are frankly less qualified and yet aspire to do the same work we do. Although I believe that physicians respect the work of physician assistants and nurse practitioners, such respect does not justify the use of terms that, although 'politically correct,' diminish us as professionals" (R. Taylor 2001, 2340).

The evolution of the term *health humanities* is very much tied to these tensions, as it emerged in response as alternate terms for the field that often centered medicine and therefore physicians: literature and medicine, arts and medicine, medical humanities, humanities and medicine, narrative medicine, and so on (Charon 2000, 2001; H. Evans and Greaves 2010). Indeed, alongside non-health-care-trained scholars (those trained in English, anthropology, philosophy, bioethics, etc.), these fields were often dominated by physicians and

continue to be so. The centering of not just physicians but biomedical practice is reflected in the fields' early focus on the writings of physicians as well as the focus on illness narratives, memoirs, and other reflections by "patients," a category of person necessarily defined in relation to biomedicine. Centering the hospital, clinic, or medical school rather than the community or broader society as a location of praxis, teaching, and analysis is another way that "medicine" has made its presence felt in the "health humanities." With that presence comes not only histories of medical oppressions and tensions with other professionals but deep-rooted disciplinary perspectives, including what Arthur Frank (1995) has called the "restitution narrative": medicine's belief that all conditions are "treatable" through medical intervention, which then returns the sufferer from a state of sickness to "health." Such a perspective clearly does not make room for chronic illness, disability, or even death, which is, from the perspective of the restitution narrative, always and necessarily a failure of medicine.

In their 2010 call for the term *health humanities*, Crawford et al. argued that it was a "more inclusive, outward-facing and applied" term and would "engage with the contributions of those marginalized from the medical humanities" (2010, 1). Pushback to the terminology of *health humanities* has included those who urge to retain the *medical* in *medical humanities*, arguing, "Critical engagements with 'the medical' which open out and interrogate the multiple ways in which 'the medical,' medicine and health are encountered and experienced are not only important and desirable in their own right . . . but would also facilitate recognition of the breadth and vibrancy of medical humanities research without the need to draw disciplinary lines" (Atkinson et al. 2015, 73). Yet as health humanities scholar Daniel Goldberg has asserted, "Part of the rationale [for the health humanities] . . . reflects the critical importance of distinguishing between delivery of medical care and the pursuit of health. . . . Overwhelming evidence suggests that health and its distribution in human populations is mostly not the result of medical care. . . . I believe our primary goal should be directed to health and human flourishing rather than to the delivery of medical care" (as quoted in T. Jones, Wear, and Friedman 2014, 7).

This is not to suggest that "health" as a term is somehow free from entanglements with "medicine." As Jonathan M. Metzl and Anna Kirkland have argued, "'Health' is a term replete with value judgments, hierarchies, and . . . assumptions that speak as much about power and privilege as they do about well-being. Health is a desired state, but it is also a prescribed state and an ideological position" (2010, 1–2). "Health" becomes a way to morally legitimize and mandate certain configurations of behavior, appearance, weight, and so on. Additionally, the enforcement of these frameworks of "health" lies most often with medicine itself, from obesity and plastic surgery clinics to pharmaceuticals, including weight loss and anti-smoking products.

Despite all its problems, there is room for medicine as a profession to shift and change. At this historical moment, as medicine is facing the challenges of both the COVID-19 pandemic and our country's epidemic of racist and institutionalized violence, the profession is experiencing seismic shifts. While traditional organizations like the AMA have provided what has been described as mere "lip service" (M. Ramos, Lanzarotta, and Chandler 2020) to issues of structural racism and the Black Lives Matter movements, activist groups led by younger physicians of color such as White Coats for Black Lives (WC4BL; Charles et al. 2016) organize die-ins and marches, calling attention to the public health emergency of racist state violence. There are movements for physicians to organize against gun violence and for

better working conditions, including adequate personal protective equipment (PPE) and other safety measures (M. Ramos, Lanzarotta, and Chandler 2020; Topol 2019). Calls for medical professionals to participate in conversations about police abolition and anti-racism appear in major medical journals (Iwai, Khan, and DasGupta 2020), envisioning an abolition medicine akin to what W. E. B Dubois (1998) termed *abolition democracy*. Speculative visions abound about such a future incarnation of the profession, a medicine invested in freedom and justice rather than oppressive and exclusionary formulations of health, professionalism, and power.

38

Memory
James Chappel

Perhaps no single word has as many different meanings and valences as *memory*. While this is not true of all languages, in English, at least, it has a vast scope, encompassing the faculties by which I recall the location of my keys, the sound of my mother's voice, and my nation's responsibility for the slave trade. Endel Tulving (2007), one of the pioneers in the psychological study of memory, made the tongue-in-cheek suggestion, complete with a list, that there were 256 kinds of memory. As such, a vast array of scholarship, from every conceivable discipline, has barnacled around the study of memory. The so-called memory boom has infiltrated our popular culture too. As responsible citizens, we are urged to remember our nation's sins and atone for them; as medical subjects, we are enjoined to pursue various kinds of memory training to stave off dementia.

My modest goal here is not so much to summarize the interdisciplinary research into memory, which would take up a great deal of space and has been adequately done already (for collective memory, see W. Hirst, Yamashiro, and Coman 2018; for individual memory, see D'Esposito and Postle 2015). My goal, instead, is to provide a few of the key findings that are most relevant to the medical humanities.

Most of us, in our daily lives, presume what scholars call the "container" or "archive" theory of memory. The idea is that our brains are like large buckets or hard drives, containing pieces of information that we search for and find or fail to. This conception of the mind is not at all universal. For one thing, it is a relatively recent view, even in the West. As Ian Hacking (1995) has shown, this particular conception of memory and selfhood has been encoded into Western science and common sense since the nineteenth century. It certainly extended into the twentieth century as well. Alison Winter (2012) has shown how it was central to American visions of mind and memory, especially during the Cold War, when Americans flocked to *The Manchurian Candidate* and indulged a strange obsession with forensic hypnosis.

Simply because an idea is new does not, of course, mean that it is false. And yet in this case it seems to be, as scientists from multiple disciplines have shown for decades now. The work of Daniel Schacter—a student of Tulving, in fact—is exemplary here. As he explains, the container view presumed "a single or unitary faculty of mind," while researchers now see "a variety of distinct and dissociable processes and systems," each involving "different neural structures, each of which plays a highly specialized role within the system" (2008, 5).

Schacter is alive to the ways in which cognitive psychology and neuroscience, after working separately for years, have arrived at complementary views about memory. And as Jens Brockmeier (2015) has pointed out, there is yet another convergence between this scientific perspective and the memory research carried out in the humanities.

Humanists have been concerned, in their own ways, with rejecting the container theory of memory: less by looking at how we behave in clinical settings than by how we behave in social reality. From this perspective, it is not simply that our brains are inaccurate storehouses for memory but that our brains are not the only sites in which memory exists. Language, architecture, ritual, and religion—all these cultural formations, and many more, can profitably be viewed as forms of memory existing outside of our individual consciousness.

Jay Winter (1995), for instance, has influentially traced the emergence of a continent-wide culture of memory and trauma in the wake of the First World War. Much of this work has centered on trauma and specifically on the Holocaust. Holocaust memory, this work teaches, is a historical creation and one that will not and should not remain static (for one classic example, see J. Young 1993).

In recent years, humanistic studies of memory have, like humanities research more broadly, moved in more inclusive directions. Memory is global; memory has a gender, and memory has a race. Rothberg (2009), another professor of English, globalizes the study of Holocaust memory, showing how decolonization affected the memory of the Holocaust and how the Holocaust in turn paved the way for other narratives of genocide and trauma to be articulated and received. Hershatter (2011), in her study of modern China, shows how memory is "gendered": how, in other words, men and women might experience the passage of historical time differently, singling out different events as significant and creating distinct sorts of periodization. Lastly, the sociologist Ron Eyerman (2002) has influentially reconstructed the place of slavery in the memory of African Americans. Using theories of cultural trauma and collective memory, he shows how the place of slavery, like that of the Holocaust, has changed over time and created different sorts of communities and subjectivities in different historical contexts. In certain times and places, the memory of slavery, as a vanquished evil, endorses a triumphant account of American nationhood; in others, the same memory, reframed instead as a trauma with a long afterlife, endorses a more tragic account.

The imperative to remember has, in recent years, led to something of a backlash, as scholars and intellectuals have begun to ponder the virtues of forgetting. There are, of course, many studies of "forgetting," but the point has normally been that this erasure was problematic and in need of redress through memory. A different vein of scholarship has studied forgetting in its own right as a necessary component of individual and social life. This, too, has a venerable history: Plato, Nietzsche, and Freud, to take three obvious examples, were all obsessed with the virtues of forgetting. In recent years, these musings have taken more rigorous forms. Fawcett and Hulbert (2020) argue for the virtue of forgetfulness for individuals. To remember everything, they suggest, would stand in the way of coherent self-formation and rational action in the world. They include a discussion of Jill Price, a remarkable woman who has been diagnosed with highly superior autobiographical memory (HSAM): essentially, she is unable to forget what has happened to her, which has been, in her telling, more of a curse than a blessing. The psychologists William Hirst and Alin Coman (2018) have pursued empirical studies of collective forgetting and its relation to collective memory. Likewise, the public intellectual David Rieff (2016), drawing on his experiences in Kosovo and elsewhere, has made a normative case for collective forgetting as, in some cases, a necessary predecessor to intergroup harmony.

Most of the work on memory, including the work just cited, does not belong in the category of health humanities. It is striking how bifurcated the work has been. On the one hand, clinicians and scientists study the memory of individual people, mainly in lab settings; on the other, humanists of many stripes study collective memory as it persists in culture, architecture, and politics. This is not a recent phenomenon. These two sorts of studies have different genealogies. The medical-scientific study of memory traces back to Ebbinghaus ([1885] 1913), while the more humanistic study of collective memory begins with Halbwachs ([1941] 1992). The former was a German psychologist fascinated by individual feats of memorization; the latter was a French sociologist fascinated by how class differences led to different interpretations of social life.

Given the salience of memory culture, in our doctors' offices and in the public square alike, it is to be hoped that genuine health humanities research on memory will grow in the future. The site at which this field is most developed is the interdisciplinary study of aging, which has begun to organize around the rubric of "aging studies." For it is here, in the minds and bodies of the elderly, that the contemporary and medicalized concern with memory is most apparent.

Old people have not always been defined, either culturally or scientifically, by their impaired cognitive functions or impaired memory. If anything, the elderly have tended to be linked more with successful memory: with tradition, oral storytelling, and so on (Fischer 1977). This was true into the early twentieth century in the United States and the pioneering works of gerontology. Cowdry's (1939) *Problems of Ageing: Biological and Medical Aspects,* for instance, without a doubt one of the pioneering works of American gerontology, spares little space for brains, memory, or cognitive processes at all: the approach was variously physiological and psychological, concerned with reflexes and sensory perception. At the same time, Alzheimer's disease did exist as a diagnosis, but it was not used to think about old age: indeed, the whole point of the disease for most of the twentieth century was to give a name to "presenile dementia," appearing in the young.

Between the 1960s and the 1980s, this changed (compare Cowdry 1939, for instance, with Chown and Riegel 1968). Ballenger (2006) chronicles this process, which had multiple components. It involved, on the one hand, attitudes toward health and aging broadly construed. In the era of "active aging," it was no longer assumed that the decline of faculties was an inevitable component of aging but rather that these were pathologies to be warded off through therapeutic intervention. This happened just as "the brain" assumed immense significance in cultural and medical accounts of well-being and health. Together, these trends coincided to turn Alzheimer's and the fear of dementia more generally into major components of the aging experience.

This particular field of health humanities is taking some of the same innovative turns that I sketched above. As for a diversification of sources and voices, some recent work has begun to think about the expansion of memory cultures into the Global South (L. Cohen 1998 was a pioneer here). This particular field, too, is well placed to take advantage of the turn toward "forgetting" as an axis of research. Scholars from a number of fields have been probing the cultural and medical meanings of dementia, hoping to dislodge the persistent attempts to equate memory with meaningful selfhood (Harper 2020).

Aging studies, and specifically dementia research, is one possible growth area for health humanities scholarship on memory. It is certainly not the only one. The "memory boom" has swept the world since the end of the Cold War: the meaning of memory, as an individual faculty and as a social construct, is being contested every day and is one of the main sites on which social reality is being reconstructed. But what is memory, and where does it reside, and why are we willing to fight and die for something we understand so dimly? These are questions that ought to interest all of us and that merit an answer if we hope to create a world worth remembering.

39

Microbe

Kym Weed

Microbe is the shortened form of *microorganism* that describes any organism that is too small to be seen without magnification. Unlike the word *germ*, which names "the causative agent or source of a disease, esp. an infectious disease" (*OED Online* 2020, "germ"), *microbe* refers to a broader range of microorganisms like bacteria, fungi, and viruses, whether or not they cause disease. In the scientific, medical, and popular lexicon, *microbe* can describe anything from the "helpful" microbes living in the human digestive tract to the viruses that cause influenza or the common cold.

Although early microscopists like Robert Hooke and Antonie van Leeuwenhoek observed microscopic forms of life in the seventeenth century, the term *microbe* did not appear in English until the 1880s (*OED Online* 2020, "microbe"), when bacteriology emerged as a new scientific discipline after the germ theory of disease, which posited that a specific microorganism causes a specific disease, gained traction in scientific and medical discourse. Despite the existence of earlier theories of contagion (see "Contagion"), it was not until scientists like Louis Pasteur and Robert Koch established laboratory procedures to isolate and identify microorganisms that they could generate a consistent theory through a series of experimental proofs. Bacteriological findings related to fermentation, disease etiology, and decomposition demonstrated the diverse role that microorganisms play in health, disease, and ecology. Meanwhile, improved microscopy techniques made possible dramatic visualizations of everyday objects teeming with microorganisms that the popular press circulated with a dual sense of wonder and terror (e.g., "Through the Magic Glass" 1880, "Germ-ane" 1884). By the 1880s, bacteriology had made a considerable scientific and cultural impact, shaping understandings of infectious disease and perceptions of microorganisms as both an invading threat to personal and national health and an essential partner in human and planetary health.

This dual understanding of microbes is most apparent during two formative periods that have shaped cultural and medical thinking about microbes: the advent of bacteriology (the study of bacteria) in the nineteenth century and the launch of the Human Microbiome Project (the genomic study of microbes living in the human body) in the twenty-first century. The rapid identification of the microorganisms that cause anthrax, rabies, tuberculosis, and cholera in the 1880s launched a period of fervent "microbe hunting" as bacteriologists traveled the globe in search of the next pathogenic microbe. While authors like Paul deKruif hailed these microbe hunters as heroes of humanity now at war with germs, their enterprise was both scientific and colonial in nature, as it promised to eventually conquer microbial life alongside ever-expanding colonial territories (Otis 1999). In addition to these projects of conquest, bacteriologists were also invested in establishing the importance of their field of study by promoting the work of nonpathogenic microbes in everything from fermentation industries to planetary conservation (Weed 2019).

In the past decade, scientific and popular representations of microorganisms have shifted, as anthropologists Heather Paxson and Stefan Helmreich put it, from "an idiom of peril to one of promise" (2014, 165). Representations of the human microbiome often explicitly link microbiome health to individual health, thereby recasting microbes as partners in rather than a threat to human health and shifting health practices to involve the cultivation of microorganisms rather than the avoidance of them. And yet as Paxson and Helmreich point out, this shift in perception of microorganisms from one of "peril" to "promise" is possible only because most epidemic diseases have been eradicated or controlled in the Global North. As the SARS-Cov-2 pandemic has made abundantly clear, we are further from the post–infectious disease world than previously imagined. Instead, we are living with a paradoxical view of microorganisms: we are simultaneously aware of their power to both cause catastrophic disease and support human health.

Health humanities scholarship attends to the ways microbes shape public health practices. According to historian Nancy Tomes, the "gospel of germs," or "the belief that microbes cause disease and can be avoided by certain protective behaviors," transformed American habits at the turn of the twentieth century (1998, 2). The germ theory of disease marked a shift in disease etiology from bad air and filthy spaces to isolated microorganisms that was accompanied by a shift in public health responses to infectious disease. Rather than focus on cleaning up environments as hygienists advocated, preventative measures became more focused on people, making it an individual responsibility to maintain cleanliness and therefore health. As Tomes explains, this period established a set of behaviors like handwashing and covering a sneeze as well as a set of assumptions about who is responsible for protecting individual and collective health that continue to shape contemporary health discourse and practice. The urgent public health messaging to "flatten the curve" during the early months of the COVID-19 pandemic, for example, demonstrates the continued emphasis on individual health behaviors in response to a global public health crisis.

Microbial science has also shaped social relationships and narrative form (Belling 2003; Choi 2015; K. Nixon 2020). For example, while germ theory rhetoric emphasized isolation and sanitation as a response to risk, Kari Nixon shows how Victorian fiction writers advocated for the benefits of contact, even infectious contact. In their reinterpretation of germ theory, these writers figured germ-free spaces as antithetical to life itself and "risk encounters" as necessary for meaningful, intimate relationships. Tina Young Choi furthers that the germ theory of disease created new representational possibilities in the form of "germ narratives" (2015, 130). Microbes, she suggests, reveal "the existence of another narrative, with its own spatial and temporal coordinates" that helped generate new narrative conventions (148). According to Catherine Belling, narratives written from a microscopic perspective require readers to "imagine themselves in relation to nonhuman spatial and temporal scales," thereby challenging anthropocentrism (2003, 85).

Nevertheless, scientific and literary representations of germs tend to restore the primacy of humanity by casting microbes primarily as enemies of humankind. This characterization of microbes is perhaps best demonstrated by the "military metaphor" that Susan Sontag argues "came into wide use in the 1880s with the identification of bacteria as agents of disease" (1978, 65–66). The metaphor of a body battling an anthropomorphized microbe, which as she demonstrates circulates in representations of illnesses from cancer to HIV/AIDS, not only shapes the stories that can be told about illness but also becomes a metaphor itself for other social phenomena from immigration to crime. Understanding the disease process as a "battle" operates on the individual level, pitting person against disease, and on the population level, pitting bacteriologist against microbe. More recently, in his study of the origins and implications of what he calls the "martial metaphor" in medicine, Lorenzo Servitje extends Sontag's analysis beyond individual illness experience to examine the "broader cultural work performed by the specific metaphor of war as it developed historically" (2021, 3). He argues Victorian literature played a crucial role in naturalizing the martial metaphor that continues to have material consequences that range from antibiotic overuse to social determinants of health.

One of these consequences is the association of disease microbes with individuals and groups of people (Kraut 1994; Wald 2008). For example, Mary Mallon, an Irish immigrant who was incarcerated for decades after being identified as a "healthy carrier" of typhoid fever, became "Typhoid Mary" (Wald 2008; also see "Carrier"). In her analysis of George Soper's epidemiological storytelling, Priscilla Wald suggests that the close association between Mallon and the typhoid fever microbe "called attention to the bodily interconnectedness of people" that required new forms of social relationships—namely, individual responsibility in preserving one's health and the health of a community (2008, 70). While Mallon is an example of how this plays out on the individual level, entire groups of immigrants have been associated with contagious disease as a justification for their exclusion in the name of protecting national health, a process that Allan Kraut calls "medicalized nativism" (1994, 3). These ties between populations and microbes, from "Asiatic cholera" in the 1830s and "Spanish flu" in 1918 to the "Wuhan virus" in 2020, stigmatize and dehumanize entire groups of people, making them scapegoats and perpetuating myths about the impermeability of national boundaries.

Scholars identify these contested boundaries of the self from the nineteenth century onward. In her study of the coconstruction of cell theory and the politics of imperialism, Laura Otis identifies bodily boundaries, especially those threatened by microbial incursion, as essential to the concept of the individual that emerged in the nineteenth century. She argues that "fears of infiltration"—of the individual body or national borders—produced a concept of selfhood based on exclusion that she calls the "membrane model" (1999, 6–7). For Otis, this bounded model of selfhood is at best a myth and at worst a tool of imperialism that obscures global interconnectedness. In the past decade, Kyla Schuller argues, a new model of selfhood, "the microbial self," has emerged to account for "interspecies entanglement" (2018b, 54). This shift from the bounded individual to the microbial self is important especially because scientific and popular interest in the human microbiome has renewed questions surrounding the boundaries of the self. As scientists document the vast number and variety of microorganisms living on or within the human body, the myth of the bounded individual becomes difficult to maintain. The human microbiome, then, is an occasion to rethink the value of individuality and independence that has dominated neoliberal thought in favor of interdependence, which opens new possibilities to understand human health as communal.

While the human microbiome has the potential to undo the centrality of the individual in our social, political, and medical systems, the language of microbiome optimization in health practices like probiotic consumption and fecal transplants tends to reify individual responsibility over collective health practices. Moreover, the urgency of the Sars-CoV-2 pandemic has refocused our collective attention on microbial threats and reintroduced the myth that with the right precautions, we can seal off an individual body, home, or even nation from microbial incursion. As Sarah Atkinson et al. suggest, health humanities scholarship ought to move "beyond a neoliberal, humanist notion of the individual body-subject and associated conceptualization of responsibility, rights, and risk management to really explore alternative 'collective' and 'relational' approaches to 'flourishing'" (2015, 77). Acknowledging that human health neither begins nor ends in an individual body may offer a model for health humanities scholarship to imagine collective health programs and promote health justice.

In this intersection of pandemic reality and microbiome possibility, health humanities scholars can examine the competing priorities of microbial protection and cultivation. Especially in times of multiple global crises, thinking in terms of interconnectedness—across individuals, communities, and species—can facilitate previously unimaginable solutions. As we navigate the pandemic and study its impact, health humanities scholarship can and should continue to examine the assumptions that shape representations of microbes, whether pathogenic or not, and the thinking that these representations both make possible and, perhaps more importantly, foreclose.

40

Narrative
Rita Charon

The word *narrative* seems omnipresent in our contemporary world, having escaped from an obscure corner of literary studies to accrue power in social sciences, in popular culture, in politics, and throughout the humanities. One early definition of the word is Barbara Herrnstein Smith's: narrative is "someone telling someone else that something happened" (B. Smith 1981, 228). *Narrative* has become a health humanities keyword because central events of health care occur when a person or group gives an account of ill or good health to another person or group, whether in a private conversation in a clinical encounter or a virally spreading social media story of trauma or illness. Such health-care fields as narrative medicine and reflective practice propose that the telling of a patient's or community's situation begins not only the factual report of a health matter but the discovery of the matter itself (Charon et al. 2017).

Such narrative acts as close reading, radical/critical listening, and advocacy allow the health humanities to approach many of its commitments: to improve clinician-patient relationships, to critique assumptions of bioscience, to unite with patient communities in activism, and to interrogate the power/economic/ethical dynamics of structural health care (Gilligan 2015). Dimensions of power and privilege along race, class, gender, and ideology positions are enacted in scenes of telling and listening, placing narrative at the core of efforts toward bias-free health-care justice.

Beginning at least forty-four thousand years ago with Neanderthal cave paintings, the story of narrative winds through origin tales of Gilgamesh and Homer and through Plato's and Aristotle's studies of poetics and rhetoric. Much of the sentinel works of modern literary criticism, from Henry James's *The Art of Fiction* to James Baldwin's *Collected Essays*, shows how narrative accounts bridge the gulf between emitter and receiver, in effect asking, "How do stories work?" The field of narratology (i.e., the study of narrative) itself emerged in the late nineteenth century, when Russian literary scholars Vladimir Propp and Viktor Shklovsky studied the structures of Russian folktales to catalog the functions of the tales' characters and plots and to distinguish between the *fabula*, the events being represented, and the *syuzjet*, the narrative account produced (Propp [1928] 1968; Shklovsky [1917] 1965). The early twentieth-century rise of the fields of linguistics and semiotics added to narrative theory's conceptual foundations. Later twentieth-century literary theorists furthered the intellectual paradigms of narrative with close attention to time, space, poetics, metaphor, and voice (Genette 1980; Todorov 1977; Ricoeur 1984–88; de Certeau 1984). Among his many contributions, Gerard Genette introduced a third dimension to the story/narrative dyad—*narrating*—to complete the impersonal and abstract process of *fabula/syuzjet* with the flesh-and-blood action of the teller: "The narrative can only be such to the extent that it tells a story . . . and to the extent that it is uttered by someone" (Genette 1980, 29).

By the early 1980s, narrative escaped the sectors of literary study and linguistics to show up in far-flung disciplines—history, phenomenology, cinema studies, psychoanalysis, sociology, psychology, and law (Kreiswirth 1992). Those who were early drawn to narrative in these fields overturned the conventions of their own disciplines to uncover the paradoxes, biased perspectives, storied uncertainties, and untestable grounds upon which many of the convictions of their fields were based.

Whether one examines Toni Morrison's *Beloved*, a Bach fugue, or the transactions of a death-row exoneration trial, the receiving listener/viewer/reader enters a contract with the teller, inheriting ethical duties toward the one whose messages are communicated (Miller 1987). Although one can recuse oneself from the contract by choosing not to read the book, leaving the concert hall, or ignoring public wrongdoing, the demands placed upon the receiver by the presence of the Other—that is, a person other than oneself—cannot be negated (Butler 2005; Levinas 1979).

Among the scholars and artists early attracted to narrative ways of knowing were clinicians and bioscientists who recognized the salience of narrative in health care. I remember sitting in narrative theory graduate seminars in Columbia's English Department realizing that what I learned about narrative process was fundamentally changing how I practiced my internal medicine. Shocking realizations about my science and about my patients' situations emerged from the shadows cast by professional training. How complex were these accounts I heard and witnessed from my patients and their families once I could hear/see with my newfound narrative skills. Many of us in the early days of literature and medicine—Joanne Trautmann Banks, Kathryn Montgomery Hunter, Anne Hudson Jones—discovered how *actionable* were the connections between literary studies and clinical practice. The more recent works of Lisa Diedrich, Catherine Belling, Ann Jurecic, and Rebecca Garden, among many others, expand health humanities' commitment to narrative into areas of critical health studies, disability studies, illness autobiographies, and activism.

Narrative skill allows health humanities practitioners not only to examine their own clinical work in health care but also to powerfully read the records of the past to recognize how current injustices got baked into what has been passed down as knowledge and practice (Metzl 2009; Matthew 2015). Using the affordances of narrative ethics and qualitative and archival research methods, clinicians and humanities professionals trained in narrative can elicit or exhume persons' accounts of their own health situations. These accounts spell out individual lived experiences of embodied and socioeconomic conditions, producing convincing evidence of otherwise unseen forces that influence health (Charon et al. 2021). Narrative skills equip clinicians to challenge the hierarchies of the health professions and to equalize power across members of a health-care team. Advocacy efforts join health humanities practitioners with community groups for shared efforts toward health-care justice—identifying local social determinants of health, revealing underlying mechanisms of a community's health disparities, and exerting collective force to alter them.

The complexity of stories requires attention to the hazards as well as the dividends of using them. Corporate name branding, polarizing and misleading political utterances, and public access story slams oversimplify or exploit the complex phenomena of narrative. Some narrative scholars warn that casual sharing of private stories with an unknown public may endanger tellers and listeners with invasion of privacy, commitment of voyeurism, psychic dangers of unlicensed psychotherapy, and being lied to (Mäkelä et al. 2021). If the human processes of narrative require not just attention to words but attention to the relationships that cull meaning from those words, then narrative acts themselves unite us story-using creatures and require ethical attention to networks of power and domination.

Taking into account both its risks and its benefits, a narrativized medicine contributes demonstrably to health-care quality, humanistic clinical education, and social justice in health (Remein et al. 2020). Beyond clinical settings, expanding intellectual foundations of narrative studies now address such conceptual and practical health humanities concerns as posthumanism, ecocriticism, digital storytelling, cognitive literary studies, rhetorical narratology, and the vast media transformations of how we see ourselves, represent ourselves, and place ourselves in the widening cosmos (Lanser and Rimmon-Kenan 2019; M. Ryan 2017; Zunshine 2020; Phelan 2010). I can already see—both at Columbia and beyond—the forward contributions of a narrative medicine to health humanities in increasingly rigorous methods of assessing the consequences of humanities interventions in health care, tested pedagogic methods to deepen self-awareness and collaborative practice among clinicians, partnerships with community-based organizations in facing health disparities, and literary/visual scholarship exposing means of comprehending one another's perspectives.

All these narrative concepts and practices further display why narrative has become both an increasingly complex and an increasingly necessary concept in health and health care. As a bonus, the concept of narrative has constructed bridges among otherwise seemingly unrelated endeavors, intimating that there may be some possibility of uniting our fractured human experiences. Together, perhaps, literary scholars, anthropologists, clinicians, philosophers, rhetoricians, historians, archeologists, painters, and players of Bach can overlay our varied concepts of narrative to emerge with a transcending mosaiclike understanding of human lived experience while, at the same time, the *local* uses of narrative concepts are practical tools for each field.

Roland Barthes wrote in 1966, "International, transhistorical, transcultural, narrative is *there*, like life" (1988, 95). Maybe he was right.

41

Natural

Corinna Treitel

Natural is a term so protean, its field of meanings so large, that it almost defies disciplining as a keyword. In the original *Keywords*, Raymond Williams makes much the same point about *nature*, calling it "perhaps the most complex word in the language." Williams identifies three areas of meaning: an essential quality of something; a force that inheres and directs people and/or the world; and the material world, including the people within it. *Natural* has a similarly broad range of meanings, and as with *nature*, many of these meanings still resonate today. Within the health humanities, at least four senses are discernible: natural as signifying an essential quality, relating to the material world, identifiable with human reason, and unsullied by human intervention.

Natural has, in the first place, been a key term in Western approaches to health, illness, and the body from Greek antiquity onward. According to the Hippocratic tradition, health is a state of dynamic equilibrium in the body, while disease is a general state of imbalance. Since disease is nature's way of trying to restore equilibrium, healers should seek to imitate this "natural medicinal action" (*vis medicatrix naturae*) to restore health. In this task, healers have recourse to the six nonnaturals (*res non naturales*): air, food/drink, movement/rest, sleep/wakefulness, evacuation/retention, and the passions. These factors are *non*natural in the sense that they are not part of a person's constitution (nature). Manipulating them through carefully constructed dietetic regimens is the best way to restore the body's own

equilibrium, as in *The Natural Method of Cureing the Diseases of the Body, and the Disorders of the Mind Depending on the Body* by Scottish physician George Cheyne (1742).

Since the Scientific Revolution, *natural* has also referred to a rational understanding of the human body as belonging to the material world of nature and being subject to its laws. In the nineteenth century, this view was popularized in a flood of hygienic texts on right living that sought to teach laypeople how to take "natural care" of their own bodies. "Natural care" involved two actions: first, gaining a rational understanding of the laws governing the human body through the study of basic anatomy and physiology, and second, applying these laws to the care of one's own body. The message was simple: individuals who observed these laws would be rewarded with a long and healthy life followed by a quick and painless death; those who broke them, in contrast, would soon find themselves on the road to illness and an early, painful death.

In his best-selling *Book about Healthy and Sick People*, for instance, German physician Carl Bock (1855) sought to furnish his readers with a "rational viewpoint about the natural care of the human body in health and sickness." Here, natural served as a warning: govern your body according to natural laws or face the consequences. Bock even discussed natural death as the reward of right living. A natural death involved no particular illness, disability, or pain but simply a gentle running down of the body's material structures and functions. Typical of a secular worldview in which ultimate authority rested with nature rather than God, *natural* in this sense enshrined physicians as nature's lawyers. Without necessarily naming them, these legalistic approaches to the body also recycled the six nonnaturals for popular audiences.

Since the eighteenth century, *natural* has become a keyword in critiques of professional medicine. These critiques have important intellectual roots in the thought of French philosopher Jean-Jacques Rousseau about civilization and "natural man." Civilization, Rousseau believed, "denatures" human beings. As he wrote in his best-selling novel *Émile*, "God makes all things good; man meddles with them and they become evil. He forces one soil to yield the products of another, one tree to bear another's fruit. He confuses and confounds time, place, and natural conditions. He mutilates his dog, his horse, and his slave. He destroys and defaces all things; he loves all that is deformed and monstrous; he will have nothing as nature made it, not even man himself, who must learn his paces like a saddle-horse, and be shaped to his master's taste like the trees in his garden" (Rousseau [1763] 1993, 5). At birth, we are in our natural state: strong, healthy, and free. Through false education, however, civilization corrupts, sickens, and enslaves us. The solution is to educate children according to nature from birth. In *Émile*, the eponymous protagonist is brought up to be a natural man. He is breastfed, left unswaddled, bathed only in cold water, fed a vegetarian diet, put to sleep without coverings on a hard bed, and sent out to learn from nature in his bare feet. He has no fear of pain, suffering, or death, which are in any case natural to life. Émile is a natural man, educated to be free of the "artificial" pathologies induced by civilization, and the postmonarchical future of republican citizens belongs to him.

Rousseau's opposition of "natural" and "artificial" in his critique of European civilization has had wide resonance across many fields of human activity, including medicine and wellness. Many of the physicians who popularized hygiene in the nineteenth century feared the health-damaging consequences of industrialization and found inspiration in Rousseau's writings about natural man. But by the end of the century, as physicians sought to leverage the clinic and the laboratory to gain professional power, *natural* became a keyword used by laypeople in battles with medical experts over how best to promote health. This is most visible among adherents of naturopathy. From the 1880s onward, naturopaths criticized physicians for doing violence to the body's natural equilibrium through excessive drugging, a tendency to cut (perform surgery), and an insistence on vaccination (which introduced artificial poisons into the body). Better, naturopaths claimed, to maintain the body's own natural state of health by embracing the natural lifestyle. Among other things, this meant fresh-air exercise, a mostly vegetarian diet, bathing in air/sunlight/water (preferably in a natural state of nudity), sleeping on mattresses and wearing fabrics that "breathed" naturally, and so on. At this point, the six nonnaturals were reframed as "natural factors."

More than one professional physician has embraced this vision of the natural. A good example is Max Bircher-Benner, the Swiss physician-turned-naturopath who invented muesli and cured his patients with a raw plant-food diet. His invocation of the first law of thermodynamics to justify this diet—raw plant foods cure because they deliver solar energy to the body in its least thermodynamically transformed state—suggests the ability of natural lifestyles to hybridize with more scientific forms of medicine. Conversely, in some cases laypeople have co-opted techniques pioneered by physicians and repackaged them as "natural" to signal their liberation from medical expertise. This happened in the 1970s, when American second-wave feminists adopted a breathing technique invented to manage obstetric pain from F. A. Nikolaev and Fernand Lamaze (physicians in the Soviet Union and France, respectively), renamed it "natural childbirth," and used it to exclude physicians from the birthing room.

This sense of natural as a term of opprobrium toward professional physicians and scientific medicine is still with us today, as numerous studies in prestigious medical journals bemoaning the popularity of alternative medicine testify. Given the ongoing attraction of "natural" herbs, remedies, and lifestyle choices to millions of consumers, it is perhaps worth closing this entry by calling on health humanists to cultivate a wide-ranging ethnographic curiosity about the role of *natural* in health-seeking behaviors that have little to nothing to do with professional medicine.

42

Neurodiversity

Ralph James Savarese

Almost a decade ago, general internist and health services researcher Christina Nicolaidis published an essay titled "What Can Physicians Learn from the Neurodiversity Movement?" (2012). The mother of a child with autism, she was deeply invested in providing better health care to people on the spectrum. She argued that doctors had to become much less pitying and alienating if they wanted to more effectively treat some of autism's less salubrious aspects—anxiety, for example. She called on doctors to do two things: (1) learn from autistics about autism and (2) abandon what self-advocates and others call the "deficit model." "Such a model, which focuses almost exclusively on impairments and limitations, leads us," she wrote, "to see autistic individuals as broken people who are ill" (503). The neurodiversity model, in contrast, moves beyond illness—without sacrificing treatment—to difference.

The concept of neurodiversity stipulates "infinite variation in neurocognitive functioning within our species" (Walker 2014). Such variation includes, but is in no way limited to, ADHD, bipolar disorder, Parkinson's disease, dyslexia, schizophrenia, and autism. It views neurodivergent people as "possessing a complex combination of cognitive strengths and challenges" (Nicolaidis 2012, 503) just like so-called neurotypicals. That it's harder to spot the latter's challenges only confirms what the field of disability studies teaches: environment, broadly construed, plays a significant role in producing disability. The world, to put it simply, has been set up to let neurotypicals thrive.

The piece by Nicolaidis was big news in 2012. The medical community wasn't accustomed to conceiving of a physiological or cognitive problem as diversity, let alone as a potential boon. If doctors were familiar with the term, they had likely encountered a caricature (autism is nothing but sweetness and light) or produced that caricature themselves, so at sea were they in this new framework. In her article, Nicolaidis was careful to insist that "neurodiversity, support, services, and therapies are not mutually exclusive" (506). As Ari Ne'eman, founder of the Autistic Self-Advocacy Network, wrote in 2010, "None of this is meant to deny . . . that autism is a disability. It is only to point out that disability is as much a social as a medical phenomenon and that the 'cure' approach is not the best way forward for securing people's quality of life."

Thinking contradictory things at once—difference *and* disability, gift *and* impairment—has proved difficult for many doctors, scientists, clinicians, and parents, especially in cases of so-called severe autism, bipolar disorder, and schizophrenia. Every time a self-advocate has promoted an affirming view of neurodivergence, the charge of whitewashing "suffering" has attached itself like Velcro. Cleanth Brooks famously described paradox as the "language appropriate and inevitable to poetry" (1947, 3). The art form strives, he said, for a "balance or reconciliation of opposite or discordant qualities" (18). A poetic or paradoxical understanding of neurodiversity would dispense with reductive binaries, resulting in both a better understanding of neurological differences and more humane care. It would also yield a startling insight: those most in need of the concept are those most affected by their conditions.

While 1998 marks the first appearance of the term *neurodiversity* in print (in an article by Harvey Blume—the term itself is attributed to Judy Singer), the concept emerged earlier. In 1992, Jim Sinclair co-founded Autism Network International (ANI) with Kathy Grant and Donna Williams. Sinclair's movement-founding piece from 1993, "Do Not Mourn for Us," set the agenda for neurodivergent people: self-affirmation and self-advocacy. During this period, Williams published two important memoirs, *Nobody Nowhere* (1992) and *Somebody Somewhere* (1994). These books tracked her emergence less from autism, PTSD, and dissociative identity disorder than from the pernicious ideas that people had about these conditions. In 1998, someone named Muskie created a satirical website, "Institute for the Study of the Neurologically Typical." "Neurotypical syndrome," it explained, "is . . . characterized by preoccupation with social concerns, delusions of superiority, and obsession with conformity." Like many self-advocates, Muskie was dismayed by how experts talked about autism: "This site is an expression of autistic *outrage*. . . . I am in awe of the mind that I have."

The internet played a crucial role in the development and dissemination of the concept of neurodiversity. Larry Arnold and Laura Tisoncik were both quite active on the web in the late 1990s; the latter started Autistics .org in 1999, a project that Mel Baggs joined shortly thereafter. In 2002, Valerie Paradiz published a parent's memoir of Asperger syndrome, *Elijah's Cup*, which celebrated autistic culture. In 2003, Kevin Leitch inaugurated his blog *Left Brain / Right Brain* (Leitch 2020), and Kathleen Seidel started the website Neurodiversity.com. The year 2004 saw the publication of Dawn Prince's memoir *Songs from a Gorilla Nation*, which spoke of autistic beauty and, unlike the work of Temple Grandin, categorically denounced the killing of animals. That same year, psychology researcher Morton Gernsbacher published an opinion piece, "Autistics Need Acceptance, Not Cure," and *New York Times* reporter Amy Harmon wrote a story, "Neurodiversity Forever: The Disability Movement Turns to Brains."

In 2005, Susanne Antonetta's *A Mind Apart: Travels in a Neurodiverse World* came out; this book linked autism and bipolar disorder under a pride banner. Some important blogs appeared as well, including Éstee Klar's *The Joy of Autism* and Mel Baggs's (2005) *Ballastexistenz*. The latter's YouTube *In My Language* would garner more than a million views (Baggs 2007). The next year, Ne'eman founded the Autistic Self Advocacy Network, which is entirely led by people with autism. And the year after that, Ralph James Savarese (2007) published a memoir of autism and adoption, *Reasonable People: On the Meaning of Family and the Politics of Neurological Difference*. CNN aired a segment about Baggs called "Finding Amanda" in 2008; the program examined the concept of neurodiversity and explicitly deployed the terms *neurotypical* and *neuroatypical*. In one segment, Baggs and fourteen-year-old nonspeaking autist DJ Savarese discussed the importance of activism and self-definition. When the host, Dr. Sanjay Gupta, asked if autism should be treated, DJ typed on his text-to-voice synthesizer, "Yes, treated with respect" (*Anderson Cooper 360* 2008). ("The Superior Part of Speaking" [Savarese and Savarese 2010] gives a more exhaustive treatment of the early development of the neurodiversity concept.)

This brief history takes us roughly to 2007, the moment when neurodiversity had penetrated the culture at large, a backlash was well underway, and scholars were vigorously writing about the topic. The next thirteen years would see an intensification—and, indeed, a normalization—of all three phenomena. Neurodiversity would not only find its way onto additional TV and movie screens but also become big business as employers, having been tutored in neurodivergent strengths, sought a competitive edge. More and more young people with ADHD, bipolar disorder, depression, autism, and schizophrenia would be leading inclusive lives. Health-care professionals would begin to take seriously the needs of atypical patients. Yet despite the obvious gains of the neurodiversity movement, opposition to the concept would remain strong.

For every proneurodiversity blog that sprung up in the first decade of the twenty-first century, an antineurodiversity one followed. The vitriol spewing out from these sites was striking. One called *Hating Autism* spoke of "expos[ing] the lies of a collection of scoundrels who oppose curing autism" (Best 2006). These parent bloggers regularly depicted their "severely" autistic children as swimming in shit, rubbing it on the walls and furniture—the rhetoric of poo and pee, as I call it, quickly became a kind of dog whistle. They contended that the movement refused to recognize autism as a disability, willfully ignoring its debilitating challenges. For them, neurodiversity was a luxury that only those with milder forms of autism could afford.

This line of attack continues today. A parent reviewer recently criticized a new book about reading literature with autistic people. "Although [these readers] vary in abilities and difficulties," he wrote, "all can read and write, interpret texts, and analyze their own responses, which in itself places them among the more fortunate of autists" (Osteen 2019). For this reviewer, the issue of diversity in autism can be reduced to something like the Calvinist notion of the elect and the reprobate (see Savarese 2020). Any attempt to celebrate autistic possibility suggests a betrayal of the most impaired—even as much of the old science on autism is being overturned and even as we're still discovering the scope of that possibility *across the spectrum*. The "severely" autistic, or at least some portion of this group, may not be what we declared them to be. My son, for example, graduated Phi Beta Kappa from Oberlin College in 2017.

When one reads the work of neurodiversity's critics, one soon discovers their discomfort with the social model of disability and the identity politics to which it gives rise. "The need to cling to autism as a marker of identity," writes the aforementioned reviewer, "has resulted in reifying the condition such that certain self-appointed spokespersons presume to speak for all autists and reject any contribution from neurotypicals. This approach risks minimizing impairments, potentially withering supports for those most in need of them" (Osteen 2019). Presented without evidence, this latter worry works, like the poo-and-pee trope, to create fear.

A recent piece by a prominent neurobiologist, "Against Neurodiversity" (Costandi 2019), follows the same recipe, spicing it up with the chili powder of condescension and the unsupported beliefs of extremist parent groups. He calls most neurodiversity advocates "well-intentioned" but argues that they trivialize the suffering of the "severely" autistic and those who care for them. More "militant" and "authoritarian" self-advocates, he contends, have bullied those who don't agree with their view, shutting down free speech and directing research dollars away from finding autism's cause and treating the most impaired. Of course, what is suffering to an able outsider may be something else entirely to a disabled insider.

Into the fray recently stepped Simon Baron-Cohen, whose own changing views of autism—he's famous for saying, without qualification, that autistics lack empathy—reflect the salutary influence of the neurodiversity movement (2019). Unlike the neurobiologist above, he sees the advantage of the social model of disability but only selectively and when the level of impairment is modest. Some things in autism, such as the attention to detail, he labels as difference; some, such as limited social cognition, he calls disabilities. "In sum," writes Baron-Cohen, "there is a case for all of the terms 'disorder,' 'disability,' 'difference' and 'disease' being applicable to different forms of autism or to the co-occurring conditions. . . . By taking a fine-grained look at [autistic] heterogeneity . . . we can see how sometimes the neurodiversity model fits . . . and . . . sometimes the disorder/medical model is a better explanation" (2019).

Baron-Cohen ends up closer to the position adopted by self-advocates, though they refuse such reductive parsing. Context changes not only how the features of neurodivergence are viewed but also what they are. Their meaning, in other words, isn't fixed. For instance, a recent study showed that social interaction difficulties diminish when autistic people interact with other autistic people and increase for both groups when they interact across neurotypes (see K. Morrison et al. 2019).

As important, the social model of disability reminds us of the deleterious effects of stigma, which arises in part from our commitment to norms. It also reminds us of eugenics, which found a vast and receptive audience in the US. Tying the concept of neurodiversity to the severity of autism is like offering passengers on a perfectly functioning ship, as opposed to those struggling in the water, a life preserver. It reveals how superficial our commitment to difference really is. Only some shall be offered the appellation *human*. A "balance . . . of opposite or discordant qualities" helps preserve the fullness of neurological difference (Brooks 1947, 18); it also protects against demeaning simplification. From the beginning, proponents of neurodiversity have argued that we can treat and respect, alleviate and affirm.

43

Normal

Peter Cryle and Elizabeth Stephens

Normal regularly functions as an approximate synonym for "healthy." The word emerged in writing about medicine and health at the start of the nineteenth century and has played a prominent role there ever since. But even as the term continues to hold a central place in the field, its precise meaning can appear vague and elusive. A useful way to bring this ambiguity under control is to identify the series of meanings, some of them inconsistent to the point of contradiction, that the word has taken on in the two centuries or so since it first appeared.

Normal came into use as a term in the medical sciences around 1820 in France, when Étienne Geoffroy-Saint-Hilaire, a leading comparative anatomist, used it to characterize organs whose function presented a high degree of integration with the organs around them. Normal organs were by this definition neither dominant nor subordinate: they simply played their structural role. But while Geoffroy-Saint-Hilaire came later to be regarded by many as a pioneer of evolutionary anatomy, his classificatory innovation proved to be less consequential in the nineteenth century than the slightly later use of some physiologist colleagues. Around 1830, French physiologists began to use the concept of the normal to redefine health itself. Until that time, medical thinkers had tended to speak, following Aristotle, of "perfect health" as the full integration of form and matter and thus the optimum natural tendency in humans. Materialist medical thinkers like

François-Joseph-Victor Broussais broke with that tradition, turning away from any teleological account of health. Broussais sought to characterize the general condition of patients by locating them within a range that extended from a minimal degree of irritation, associated with debility, to an excessive degree of it, associated with disruptive vigor. It could no longer be a matter for Broussais and those who followed his lead of identifying a point of convergent balance and calling that "health." A person in what they now called the "normal state" was located somewhere between the extremes, appropriately distant from both. The acme of perfect health was being replaced by a *range* of indications that could be considered normal. By definition, limited variety was now included within the normal.

In the middle of the twentieth century, Georges Canguilhem brought a quite specific philosophical perspective to the history of nineteenth-century medical thought. He argued in *The Normal and the Pathological* ([1966] 1991) that it had been a theoretical mistake to conceive of the normal in quantitative terms, as so many thinkers of that time had come to do and as people continued to do in the present. A true understanding of the concept, he said, needed to be properly grounded in biology. Most nineteenth-century medical thinkers had lost sight of the fact that any living organism was by definition in a dynamic relationship with its immediate environment. Living organisms tended by vital necessity to impose their norms on those around them, and that needed to be taken into account in theoretical writing. It was how life worked, and statistical approaches had failed to engage with this central fact. In Canguilhem's view, which owed some key elements to that of Jean-Baptiste Lamarck, life itself was normative. The normal was a literally vital topic.

There emerged in the nineteenth century two different ways of thinking about the normal that have never been effectively reconciled in medical thought. The first of them defined the normal in distributive terms, asking what was normal within a particular group. To take an example that continues to be influential today, the Belgian statistician Adolphe Quetelet calculated the relation of weight to height in people, naming that relation the body mass index (BMI). The point of his index was not to define some classical perfection of the human form: it served simply to identify the range of measures found across a population. A subsequent set of statistical moves developed a procedure for analyzing the range itself. Outliers could be defined as such—they were either so heavy or so light as to distort the average—and all those in between were distributed in such a way that mean and median values became evident. A middle group was thus defined by mathematical convention, and the members of that group declared all at once to be average, normal, and healthy—those terms now being mutually self-defining. But there was a second, quite different way of conceiving the normal. It was possible to understand normality in vitalist terms like those of Lamarck (and Canguilhem), as biologically normative for a given person. In clinical circumstances, the question became this: How might the individual's normal state, once characterized, be maintained or restored? Quetelet actually tried to imagine a personal application of the statistically normal. He suggested taking vital measurements from each patient in their "normal state" so that standards of good health could be established for that individual, thereby allowing any future pathological conditions to be identified by their distance from a calibrated personal average. That approach was not generally taken up in clinical practice. Even as population-based medical statistics received closer public attention in nineteenth-century Europe, especially during epidemics of cholera and typhoid fevers, many doctors eloquently resisted any application

of quantitative thinking in their own clinics, insisting that there were in fact no average patients and no utterly typical presentations of illness.

The tensions and slippages between these two understandings of the normal—as a distributed range that could be calculated in quantitative terms and as a dynamic or vital condition that must be assessed in qualitative terms—continue to inform the way the word is used in the present both in the context of the health humanities and within popular culture more broadly. It was only in the middle of twentieth century, however, that the word *normal* began to circulate in a significant way in popular discourse. Until then, the word largely remained what it had been in the historical narrative traced above: a specialist term used primarily in professional contexts, such as writing on medicine and statistics. It was a not a word heard often in everyday speech.

This began to change during the first half of the twentieth century. One of the key drivers behind this change was the increasing popularization of ideas and approaches first developed in the context of psychoanalysis and sexology. As these fields gave rise to new and popular markets in psychiatry, psychology, sexual science, and sexual advice literature, the word *normal* became ubiquitous. One reason for this was the new idea of the normal person and normal sexuality that emerged in the works of Krafft-Ebing, Freud, Hirschfeld, and others. Whereas the normal had previously referred to a particular state conceived as healthy, early psychoanalysis and sexology reconceptualized the normal as a general quality of the person and of their sexuality taken as a whole. In these terms, it could happen regularly—normally—that a person deviated from the normal understood as a kind of ideal condition: "In no normal person does the normal sexual aim lack some designable perverse element," Freud argued in *Three Contributions to the Sexual Theory* (1910, 571). No one was perfectly normal. Or rather, it was normal to be a least a little perverse. The normal and perverse were different in degree rather than kind.

This gave the idea of the normal a new purchase in the popular imaginary. Public figures such as Marie Stopes, author of the popular *Married Love* guide, found themselves inundated with letters from members of the general public, eager to know whether their sexual desires and practices were "normal." The normal, as it is used in medical, statistical, and popular contexts in the twentieth century, is a key example of what the cultural historian Ian Hacking (1995) has referred to as a "looping effect." A looping effect is one in which a particular diagnosis or medical classification has the effect of changing the identification or behavior of the person to whom it is applied. As the word normal moved out of the restricted spheres of medicine and statistics and entered everyday speech in the twentieth century, it exerted a powerful looping effect: eliciting in some a keen desire to identify or be identified as normal and in others an equally strong resistance to the term.

The semantic slipperiness of the normal, in which it names an average or healthy quality that is also an unachievable ideal, is evident in the public health research and education campaigns conducted in the middle of the twentieth century. It is primarily through the sphere of public health that the word normal came to enter popular discourse in a significant way. As the Second World War drew to a close in 1945, a wide range of public health initiatives focused specifically on the normal person and the need for normality. In 1944, the industrial engineer Lillian Gilbreth coauthored a practical guide with Edna Yost, titled *Normal Lives for the Disabled*, which encouraged persons with newly acquired disabilities to maintain a positive attitude in seeking employment and maintaining home independence. The following year, the physical anthropologist and eugenicist Earnest Hooton published a report on Harvard University's large multidisciplinary study of "normal young men," titled *Young Man, You Are Normal* (1945). In the same year, the public sexual health education campaigner Robert Dickinson exhibited two statues representing the average American male and female, which he called Normman and Norma. These were composite statues, modeled on the statistical averages of tens of thousands of young American men and women. To celebrate their display at the Cleveland Health Museum in September 1945, the museum held a nationwide search to find a living embodiment of Norma. Although a winner was eventually announced, it was noted that her bodily measurements were not a perfect match with the statue's and that "Norma remained a hypothetical individual" (quoted in Cryle and Stephens 2017, 323).

Here was a lasting discrepancy. The proportions of a statue representing young womanhood could only appear in idealized form precisely because they were strictly, formally average. No living woman actually had those exact dimensions. The distance between the strictly average and the routinely usual defines the space of normality as the word is used both in contemporary health discourses and in popular culture. Just as psychoanalysis and sexology argued that no one is perfectly normal, so that it is entirely normal to be at least slightly "perverse," normality names the distributed space or spectrum of possibilities between the average and ideal. The statues of Norma and Normman also make visible the extent to which the word *normal* was tied to a very particular set of characteristics that, as Julian Carter (2007) has argued, were often obscured by the apparently objective and neutral label of "normal": able-bodied, young, white, and heterosexual. The gap between an ideal normal and so-called average people allows the meaning of the

NORMAL PETER CRYLE AND ELIZABETH STEPHENS

word *normal* to slip from the descriptive to the prescriptive.

It is the prescriptive application of the normal that has made the word the subject of trenchant and sustained critique in recent scholarship in fields such as critical disability studies (Garland-Thomson 1996; L. Davis 1995), gender and sexuality studies (M. Warner 1999; Spade 2011), critical race studies (Carter 2007), and the medical and health humanities (Dreger 2004; E. Reiss 2009). In each of these contexts, the normal has been critiqued for the way it has primarily tended to function as a template or standard to which bodies should be made to conform. Rosemarie Garland-Thomson (1996) influentially referred to this, in a neologism designed to denaturalize its privilege, as the "normate" body. Such criticism has had a noticeable effect, most recognizably in recent efforts to destigmatize both bodily and behavioral diversity by drawing attention to the importance of the range within which bodies and their capacities are distributed: the development of new interpretative and diagnostic frameworks such as "neurodiversity" is exemplary of this. Such frameworks provide relief from the requirement to dwell within a very narrow range, even as they embed the idea of the normal as a distribution all the more securely within the contemporary health humanities.

44

Observation
Alexa R. Miller

Observation: from the Latin *observationem*, a watching over, "an action . . . performed with prescribed usage," as in the observation of a religious rite or a civic ritual expressing a patriotic ideal (*OED Online* 2021, "observation"). The ritualistic undertones point to the sacred nature of the everyday work of busy clinicians: seeing patients. Observation is crucial to diagnosis, to the creation of treatment plans, and to the promotion of healing. To do it accurately, unhinged from judgment, is an act of respect, healing, and mastery. For a patient to be accurately seen and heard is a major event in their journey—and too often a rare occurrence.

It is too simplistic to understand observation as the careful watching of a single phenomenon in isolation; rather, observation extends to its cause and effects as well as to its physiological, social, cultural, political, and linguistic context. It is not only the act of paying attention; observation is a fundamental means through which we know the world. It drives the interactive progression from novice to expert in the clinician.

Without observation, medical knowledge would not exist. The unique prowess of eastern medicine lies in its basis in three millennia of observing the human body. Western medicine, meanwhile, is storied to have begun with artists hungry to observe, so as to know, human form. Vesalius famously unearthed graves in secret so as to obtain prohibited access to bodies; his drawings released the study of human composition from religious confines, catalyzing the field of anatomy while triggering a renaissance of knowledge in science, art, and medicine.

Observation is not only the first step in the scientific process but also a continuous and basic aspect of the discipline of science, generating reliable knowledge in uncertain territory. The National Committee on Science Education Standards and Assessment (National Research Council 1996) describes "inquiry" as "a multifaceted activity that involves making observations; posing questions; examining books and other sources of information to see what is already known in light of experimental evidence; using tools to gather, analyze, and interpret data; proposing answers, explanations, and predictions; and communicating the results." This challenge is especially evident in diagnosis—a complex process of information-gathering and information-synthesis deriving from science principles and emergent by way of humanities wisdom.

A basis of both art and science, observation is where the scientific paradigm of medicine dovetails with the patient's distinct needs, goals, and lifeworld, tying scientific value to care and respect and forming the basis of a therapeutic alliance. With the humility required to see—really see—the clinician holds the stance not of the expert but of the expert learner, linking knowledge with compassion to enact a sacred respect for nature's complexity and for human life. As the poet Mary Oliver writes, "attention is the beginning of devotion" (Oliver 2019).

It sounds so simple—to observe—yet it is complex, situational, and adaptive. Just as dialogue can be defined as "listening deeply enough to be changed by what you learn" (H. Saunders 1999), observation is reciprocal, changing observers even as observers change what they observe. The combination of discovery and care that converge in the best practices of observation is the basis for expertise in health care. This connection to the world inheres in the etymology of the physician—*physica*, which means "relating to nature" (*OED Online* 2021, "physician"). Or, as William Osler declared, "the whole art of medicine is in observation" (Andrews 2002).

Careful observation is always a choice. Do we look up, again, or longer rather than default to what is already known—or to avoidance, apathy, hostility, or worse? Do we allow our engagement with the world to become automatic, or do we embrace the deliberate practice of clear-minded and empathic seeing? Do we see ourselves as human observers with cultural, social, and emotional dimensions, or are we best imagined as seeing machines? In medicine, this choice often represents the difference between poor care and medicine's best moments. It is the difference between the internist who orders ten tests and the internist who orders two after a careful exam, between the cardiologist who says, "I've never seen this before; I can't help," and the cardiologist who says, "I've never seen this before, perhaps because the specimens I learned upon were highly limited phenotypes; let's look and see." The conscious effort to see allows the emergency medicine team to avoid the pitfall of the most commonly missed fracture—the second one (Daniel et al. 2017). The treatment plan for a patient in pain may hinge on the humanity of an observer who attends to body language or facial expression. Rapid but careful observations determine the surgeon's ability to take in the entire situation of the room and make a decision quickly under pressure. In the same way handwashing takes a bit of time and radically reduces infection rates (Gawande 2004), astute observation is a conscious choice that can mark the difference between life and death.

We observe differently when we believe we already understand what we are seeing rather than commit to the perspective that there may always exist more to be seen. Visual arts can teach this lesson. As the work of art makes the familiar strange (Kumagai and Wear 2014), it teaches the receptive viewer to look with new eyes. It teaches attentiveness and liberates the viewers from stale perspectives. Such a humble and respectful approach to patients should be an aspiration (Blenkinsop 2005). Respectful observation is the first step in breaking from the insidious legacies of unequal treatment and harm in the US and abroad. Such respect, moreover, born in the context of human-human fellowship, or "affiliation" (Charon 2005), leads to greater accuracy. The meaning of accuracy is not, as we might think, a "correct" answer. Rather, accuracy is rooted etymologically in the idea of meeting or in "running together" (*OED Online* 2021, "accuracy"). As with diagnosis, the best care emphasizes the process that yields accuracy.

As observers, we cannot fully escape our biases, but we can become more aware of them; that awareness is crucial for the clinician. The structures, beliefs, experiences, technologies, and cultural codes of clinicians' upbringing and training—which, in the US, we can assume to be constructed of violent racist legacy—form a forceful undertow in swaying their choices: which observations seem "normal" or "weird" or "remarkable" or "wrong." Health humanities facilitates recognition of the biases, assumptions, and values that are endemic to social structures, such as those underpinning structural racism. In so doing, it contributes to the process bell hooks calls "deconstructing" racism through which, as she writes, "we both name racism's impact and help break its mold. We decolonize our minds and our imaginations" (hooks 1992). Such "critical consciousness" (Kumagai and Lypson 2009) starts with observing one's self, or introspection: what cognitive scientists and educators call "metacognition," Buddhists call "awareness" or "true perception" (Trungpa 2008), and high-performing athletes call "mental focus." It is what

artists know as the quiet place from where, for example, a painter paints. The state where her seeing becomes distinct from her judgment: a slowed-down place where well-held internal calm animates clarity and performance at its best.

Such self-observation can significantly improve the clinician's ability to observe the patient. It can help transform preconceived ideas that inflect an intuitive response, "fast thinking" or "System 1" (Kahneman 2011), into mindful cognition, "slow thinking" or "System 2" (Kahneman 2011). Mindful observation replaces *looking at* with *looking with*:

- Looking with high regard for the patient, believing they know their story best (D. Gilbert 2009), prepared to suspend belief (Scarry 1985).
- Looking with desire to develop self-awareness and pattern recognition by way of engagement and feedback.
- Looking with the perspectives of others, leveraging them as both a "forcing strategy" (Croskerry 2003) and a resource to discerning the best path forward.
- Looking with strategic pauses (Moulton et al. 2007).
- Looking with an unflinching gaze, just as "to be an artist means never to avert one's eyes" (J. Goodwin 2013).
- Looking with awareness of how fear, stress, and anxiety feel in her body—and how to progress with it.

Looking with is a posture—that of reliable clinical beholders—a stance from which they hold a space beyond transaction, a space that enables the cocreation of health.

Observation is at once medicine's core art and its central dilemma. Clinical observation requires time (Boudreau, Cassell, and Fuks 2008), while the increasingly fast pace of clinical medicine and increasing demands on the clinician—all part of "the business of medicine"—have turned time into the rarest of commodities. The lessons of health humanities make visible what masterful clinicians know and studies indicate: increasing demands on clinician attention prevent the best clinical practices (Simmons et al. 2006; Aiken et al. 2002; McDonald, Rodriguez, and Shortell 2018; ALQahtani et al. 2016). As medicine becomes more reliant on the ostensible empiricism of tests and procedures, health humanities offers a crucial reminder that the best medicine begins with the skilled and careful clinician's observational skills. We would do well to consider what health care today could look like if medical training included a consistent model for teaching and learning observation, rather than leaving it up to individuals and to chance. We would do well to imagine health care where the practices of close engagement with patients matched in value those of tests and procedures. We would do well—wellness to the point of a far more thriving society—to imagine what medicine could look like if the patient became the business of medicine and the business of medicine prioritized the clinic as a space of trained and careful looking at human life.

45

Pain

Catherine Belling

Indispensable and elusive, pain marks the limit of medicine's semiotic capacities. At this limit, where access to another's experience is most desirable and most difficult, the discursiveness of caring for suffering becomes inescapably manifest. Health care's struggle with the representation of pain emerges clearly in a recent definitional shift by the International Association for the Study of Pain (IASP; medical- and US-based) from "an unpleasant sensory and emotional experience associated with actual or potential tissue damage, or described in terms of such damage" to an "experience associated with, or resembling that associated with . . . tissue damage." This change eliminates the activity of description. The amendment is well intentioned, stemming from a fear that the original might be "interpreted as excluding infants, elderly people, and others—even animals—who could not verbally articulate their pain" (IASP 2017). But without representation, the definition is circular: we associate pain with tissue damage, and pain both is and resembles experience associated with tissue damage. The passive voice shuts down communicability further. (Who is "we"? Those in pain? Those who define, evaluate, or manage it?) In their concern about those whose pain may not find the right words (we might add those whose language the clinician doesn't understand or those who are ignored or demented or sedated), the IASP does away with communicability. For description is not necessarily verbal and articulate. Pain may be (descriptively) enacted without words; to reach beyond the self, we can describe our pain with screams, grimaces, curses, as well as precise histological metaphors.

The IASP's well-meant terminological contortion reveals pain to be an "epistemological nodal point," as Susannah Mintz puts it in her vivid and impeccably precise account of pain's literary descriptions—a work that belies claims, following Elaine Scarry in particular, that pain shuts down language (Mintz 2013; see also Jurecic 2012). Pain is the nodal point where subjective experience demands expression and description, both because its aversiveness sends the subject out beyond itself to seek help and because its corporeality forces the subject into a Cartesian-dualizing estrangement from the body felt both as a suffering site and as an object of (not necessarily medical) observation and description. If I cannot make of it a sign, pain takes root in my body, which is in turn reduced to a patho-anatomical object (of "association" and "resemblance"; of an abysmal metaphor where vehicle and tenor are identical).

Description is thus essential to defining the word *pain*, and description depends on what discourses (including nonverbal ones) are available. Introducing a pain-themed issue of the journal *Representations*, Rachel Ablow describes pain as "always already enmeshed in social life" and "representation [as] the means through which we can engage this imbrication" (Ablow 2019). Pain is an anthropological and ethical question of epistemology and discourse. Medicine's thwarted desire—encompassing patients as well as practitioners—is for it to be an unambiguously indexical sign. Pain is thus always a translational challenge.

In *The Culture of Pain*, David Morris calls for "a dialogue among disciplines" in response to medicine's tendency to "suppress or overpower . . . other voices that offer us a different understanding of pain" (1991, 2). While more of those voices are speaking and writing, nonbiomedical language still goes "unrecognized and unvalued in medical culture" (Jurecic 2012, 48). There is a danger: demedicalizing pain must not mean disembodying it. Reserve the word for what we think of as physical experience, by which I do not mean experience necessarily caused by or linked to observable physical injury but rather experience that, unlike other aversive feelings, is felt as if materially situated in one's body rather than in one's orientation out toward the world (despair, ennui) or back toward the past (grief, remorse) or forward to the future (anxiety, dread). Part of the translational challenge of pain may be that it is both spatially and temporally *present*. Pain is too physical for psychology and too subjective for somatic medicine. A valuable task for the health humanities is, then, to examine pain's role as a hinge between two experientially and disciplinarily dualized (yet interdependent) domains.

I'll risk a solipsistic effort to describe how, in pointing us toward our bodies, pain asserts an unsustainable distinction between self and body, a contact point where the word *pain* circulates as a signifier and where medicine sutures pain to lesions. As a small child, I had repeated bouts of appendicitis. What I can remember now is that my body was harming me. It took me and clenched me around my middle, knees to chin, then thrashed me about as if to shake the thing off, then curled me back in, and I could only say "it hurts" and "take it away." I did not know what "it" was. "Irritable appendix," the doctor said. I became afraid of my body. People didn't seem to know how much it hurt until one attack added a fever making me rattle the bed like the exorcist, and I was rushed to emergency surgery. Afterward, the surgeon gave me my appendix in a plastic bottle. That shaggy little thing was my pain, visible and harmless. I didn't feel pain like that again until years later, in labor, and then I knew what I was working with my body to expel, and that made a difference.

Later, during a root canal, I found pain's usual presentness temporarily brought into focus by the dissociation caused by nitrous oxide. I knew the drill was causing a sensation I could name only as pain—a sharp, clear-cut buzz in my jaw—and yet it was not hurting *me*. Because, drugged, *I* was not stuck in my sensitive body, the pain, now as objectified as my bottled appendix, had no emotional weight. My cognition artificially unhooked from sensation and affect, I was able to wonder at how hard it usually is to manage that subject-object relation to pain. Perhaps we need words to grasp our pain in the same way we need mirrors to see our faces.

Medicine wishes pain would stay attached by reference to a lesion (the burst appendix, the rotten tooth root) and be extracted with it. This means my acute experiences, the ones that make medicine happy, are terrible examples, because pain's referent is the phenomenological body rather than one medicine can anatomize. Sometimes the two coincide, often not. (Perhaps this is why an amputated limb can hurt and haunt despite having been literally disembodied.) Chronic pain, being nonindexical, undoes the language medicine relies on and demands a different language. To read pain as necessarily referential of, and proportional to, physical damage is to misrepresent both pain and bodies, a move egregiously exemplified in the legal definition requiring an act defined as torture to cause pain "equivalent in intensity to the pain accompanying serious physical injury, such as organ failure, impairment of bodily function, or even death" (Bybee 2002, 1).

Hence the trouble, too, with calling pain medicine's "fifth vital sign" after a campaign introduced in 1996 by the American Pain Society, validly reacting to undertreatment (N. Levy, Sturgess, and Mills 2018). Calling pain a "vital sign" made it an indication, not just in the grammatical sense (a verb's indicative mood claims objective fact), but in the clinical sense, where an indication is an imperative, not just to interpret but to act, with opioids or surgery, in response to reductive measurement scales. All despite the fact that in medicine's own language, pain—unlike temperature, heartbeats, and breaths—is not (despite those reassuring numbers from 1 to 10) an observable (or quantifiable) sign but a subjective symptom. Clinical access to symptoms is by definition dependent on the patient's representing what she feels. We cannot evade discourse.

Raymond Williams's keywords project emerged from the observation that "We"—speakers enmeshed in different contexts—"just don't speak the same language" (1976, 11). The *word* "pain," then, is an exemplary challenge to translation between medico-clinical and critical-colloquial dialects because, as felt phenomenon, as sign, and then as the name for a sign that can never be reduced to a single word, it demands specificity and interpretation rather than reductive positivism. Before it is a word, pain is already a sign pointing the self (and often the doctor) toward the body. Yet as the hinge where meaning and body meet, pain is also the extratextual and unspeakable Real that reminds us why we needed language to begin with: the discomfort that makes the infant cry and the mother respond and communication in every instance begin. Pain happens in the somapsychotic space where body and mind suffer together and, therefore, where language might have to do its hardest and best work.

This work has long been underway; as well as a growing list of monographs, several recent pain-themed collections of humanities research provide a map for this work (see, for example, Stoddard Holmes and Chambers 2005; Kall 2013; Goldberg 2018; Ablow 2019). Future work might expand our lexicon for pain, our languages for describing it, and the narratives with which we situate it. The health humanities' work may be to de-medicalize pain without foreclosing its diagnostic value and to open up the interpretive capacities of the health-care disciplines to the semiotic implications of pain, its descriptions, and the significance of what it indicates about the bodies we all have in our minds.

46

Pathological
Michael Blackie

In its search for the pathological in the human body, modern medicine found itself. The historical timeline of this discovery may be contested, but its reliance on "opening a few corpses" is certain (Foucault [1963] 1975, 124). To know the body, to diagnose and cure it, required evidence of deviance from the normal, which as a concept can only exist in constant proximity to shifting conceptions of the pathological (Canguilhem 1991; Foucault [1963] 1975; Foucault [1976] 1990; see "Normal"). For Foucault's mentor Canguilhem, whose work lays a foundation for future interrogations of the normal, to "discern what is normal or pathological for the body itself, one must look beyond the body" (Canguilhem 1991, 200–201). We cannot, then, know what is normal for the body (or the individual) before we establish what is pathological, and what is pathological depends largely on culture and context. Canguilhem, like Foucault, draws attention to the construction of normalizing institutions, like medicine, to highlight the tensions and oscillations between the pathological and the normal that reach beyond physiology into culture, from organic matter to social interactions. Notions of normalcy and pathology are, therefore, constructed and evolving. These insights expose the conceit that medicine is a science based solely on objectivity.

The relationship between the normal and the pathological has a history that is, like all histories, built upon subjective and contested foundations. The study of medicine and its cultural influence that is the subject of health humanities trace back to this line of questioning. Although approaching the body as an object of knowledge, intervention, and cure relies on a notion of normal that can only exist in pathology's shifting shadow, critiques of normalization do not discount the importance of a biopsy coming back negative, as in the case of cirrhosis of the liver. Cell deformation is real. Health humanities might nonetheless examine the material conditions that led to a particular outcome and the social structures influencing the afflicted individual's access to care. We can, then, question medicine's reliance on this ambiguous term and still look to it for useful disease categories and diagnoses. But even this caveat requires qualification. For whom is a diagnosis useful? For patients? Physicians? Pharmaceutical companies? The medical-industrial complex? These questions draw attention to the inability of the pathological to function as a stable term because of its vexed relationship with objectivity as recognizable to the dictates of the scientific model.

The wide circulation of *pathological* in medicine and culture relies on its different discursive meanings within different institutions (*OED Online* 2021, "pathological"). Historically, the use of *pathology* first appeared in the early 1600s to describe processes or disciplines that study disease. By the mid-1800s, *pathological* begins to function as a means of describing physical and mental disease states, such as "pathological depression." Even mathematics deploys the pathological to describe the "grossly abnormal in properties or behavior," a development that begins in the 1930s. Where we see the word becoming imbued with meaning beyond these specific deviations within norms of science and math is in colloquial speech, as in the use of pathological to refer to persons "exhibiting a quality or trait to a degree considered extreme or psychologically unhealthy," such as "he's a pathological liar." Although using pathological to characterize the feelings or emotions of individuals is now considered obsolete, at least by the OED's standards, it nonetheless continues to inform popular and medical perceptions of race, ability, and sexuality, among other categories of difference. In addition to *pathological*'s common use as an adjective, it can also be a noun. Certain individuals displaying particular behaviors become *pathologicals*, as in, "Plenty of pathologicals torment themselves . . . by worrying over imaginary sins" (*OED Online* 2021, "pathological"). This usage may be unique to the US, but the process of reducing someone to behaviors culturally marked as worrisome knows no borders.

Identifying worrisome behaviors relies on subjective and prejudicial definitions and diagnoses. Consider the emergence of shyness as a social anxiety disorder, treatable by psychotropic drugs (Lane 2008) or the pathologization of boisterousness as oppositional defiant disorder. In both cases, physical responses that once seemed unremarkable, like shyness, or behavior that seemed typical of childhood, like acting out in class, become pathologies. But these diagnoses are not equally distributed across populations. Black and Brown boys are far more likely to be diagnosed with oppositional defiant disorder even though their manifestation of boisterousness is no greater than that of white boys—the pathologizing of everyday behavior. Often identity categories, like race and class, are conflated within the health-care system, revealing the pervasiveness of bias. For example, doctors are more likely to prescribe antipsychotic drugs to children on Medicaid than children on private insurance, which speaks to the persistent assumption that impoverished children and children of color suffer from greater mental health problems and behavioral instability than their wealthier, often white, counterparts (Kafer 2013; Roberts 2012).

The history of schizophrenia, in particular, shows the influence of a prejudice, hence of culture, on the diagnostic process. Initially, schizophrenia was ostensibly a psychological malady primarily afflicting middle-class housewives who challenged the gendered expectations of that role (Roberts 2012), but during the Civil Rights Movement, it became a disease understood to disproportionately affect Black men (Metzl 2009). Through this diagnostic process, to protest racial inequality was to suffer from "delusional anti-whiteness" (Metzl 2009, xiv), which is a diseased state of mind best treated, the reasoning went, by incarcerating Black offenders in state facilities for the criminally insane (Roberts 2012). This biased and racist diagnostic process reaches back to the antebellum United States with *drapetomania*, a supposed mental disorder that described Black resistance to enslavement (Roberts 2012). Based on this diagnostic profile, to resist a cultural norm is to be deemed diseased, pathological.

Two fields of critical inquiry that have engaged longest and most productively with the relationship between the normal and the pathological are disability studies and queer theory. These fields have brought considerable attention to how individuals are reduced to behaviors and capacities by a dominant, able-bodied, heterosexist culture that relies on "embodied, visible, pathologized, and policed homosexualities and disabilities" to constitute itself as normative (McRuer 2006, 2). Efforts to combine disability studies with queer theory have had to contend with tensions riddling this shared past, between the lived experiences of individuals and communities that identify as either disabled or queer (with *queer* here designating a catchall for the LGBTQ spectrum) or both. Although "homosexuality and disability clearly share a pathological past" (McRuer 2006, 1), the sting of the pathologizing process matters for these groups differently. For so-called "sexual minorities . . . disability is all too often understood as something that queer sexuality has liberated itself from—the estranged sibling whose kinship threatens to reveal a shameful and pathologizing past" (Barounis 2019, 20).

Before the coining of *homosexuality* in the late 1890s, there were long-standing civil and canonical laws that forbade certain behaviors associated specifically with being gay, like anal intercourse, or sodomy (see "Sex"). But these strictures against such deportment only condemned individuals for behaviors—participating in these acts—and did not extend to the individual as an embodiment of that legal transgression. The invention of the term *homosexuality* was an act of pathologization. And what was once a "juridical subject" became "a personage, a past, a case history," "a species" (Foucault [1976] 1990, 43). To understand the homosexual in biological terms is to place a person squarely in pathology's shadow. In that shadow, movements, inclinations, and desires become signs of a pathological nature, which leads, in turn, to "an explosion of theories on the biological origins" of homosexuality (Eckhert 2016, 240).

It is tempting to see this development as potentially liberating, laying the foundation for contemporary claims of being "born this way," and in some ways it did, but not before medicine raised the possibility of curing homosexuals. One late-twentieth-century example is the reclassification of homosexuality from a mental disorder to a sexual orientation disturbance in the DSM-III in 1973, a renaming that resulted from "a compromise between the view that preferential homosexuality is invariably a mental disorder and the view that it is merely a normal sexual variant" (Spitzer 1981, 210). This diagnosis remained until 1987. But as Canguilhem makes clear, acts of identifying what is pathological are usually in the service of defining what is normal. *Heterosexuality* as an identity and category comes into existence only after the invention of *homosexuality*, which is not to say people did not engage in behaviors, sexual and otherwise, that we would attribute to being straight today; they certainly did. Rather, in the process of codifying homosexuality as a diagnostic entity, medicine and its adjacent institutions establish what it means to be a healthy heterosexual. Queer theory's challenge to the reliance of this nomenclature on a medical model of sexuality parallels the activist work of disability studies.

The medical model of disability that emerged in the nineteenth century continues to dominate cultural perceptions of disability as a corporeal state and to determine the quality of care people with disabilities receive (see "Disability"). This model sees "a dysfunction of a particular body" as something "to be prevented, cured, corrected, or rehabilitated" (Couser 2011, 22) and therefore "reduces disability to individual deficit" (Shakespeare, Lezzoni, and Groce 2009, 1815). Disability studies questions the narrow focus of this model on the individual by shifting attention to the social conditions that make a particular bodily impairment disabling—the absence of ramps into buildings and curb cuts for wheelchair users. Such a critique emphasizes how "culture (in all its dimensions, not just material) enables and empowers individuals with 'normal' bodies and dis-enables and disempowers those with 'deviant,' or 'abnormal,' bodies" (Couser 2011, 24). This binary does not hold up under scrutiny. As we have seen with other processes that pathologize specific behaviors and attributes, the definitions of abnormal—whether somatic, psychic, or both—in the medical model rely on subjective measures that reflect the biases of health-care providers. For example, people with disabilities often rate their own quality of life much higher than their doctors do (Shakespeare, Lezzoni, and Groce 2009). The gap between the life view of someone with a disability and the perception of health-care providers or other able-bodied persons undermines the claims to objectivity of the medical model.

Both disability studies and queer theory have begun to turn toward structural thinking. For disability studies, this has meant a shift toward understanding how class, race, politics, and geography determine whether a person can claim disability in the first place (Puar 2017). Theorists and activists likewise now recognize how the political gains of gay sex decriminalization and gay marriage legalization largely favor able-bodied white gay men and lesbians, leaving out intersectional communities for whom the sting of pathologization persists (Eng, Halberstam, and Muñoz 2005). In making this turn, both fields look beyond individual "constructs of normality and pathology" (Puar 2009, 165) to the larger structures that determine access to health care, housing, immigration status, and citizenship, to name a few. The health humanities began its own structural turn in distinguishing itself from the narrow focus of the medical humanities on the doctor/patient dyad. To riff on Canguilhem, future work for the field should move beyond definitions of what is normal and pathological to question the cultural and political institutions that benefit from maintaining those categories.

47

Patient

Nancy Tomes

The patient is the endpoint of medicine's core mission, which is to care for sick human beings. A sense that modern biomedicine has lost sight of that goal has inspired a quest for more "patient-centered" medicine over the past half century, which has contributed to the interdisciplinary field now known as the health humanities.

Derived from the same Latin origins as "patience," the word *patient* conveys the sense of a passive object of medical action (*OED Online* 2021, "patient"). Yet typically becoming a patient requires some degree of participation, first by feeling sick and then by seeking a healer. From ancient times onward, doctors recognized that some degree of patient cooperation was conducive to good medicine. Hippocrates' *Aphorisms*, a text widely used in medical training through the 1800s, had as its first principle, "It is not enough for the physician to do what is necessary, but the patient and the attendant must do their part as well and the circumstances must be favorable" (Chadwick, Mann, and Lloyd 1983, 206). But what it meant for patients to do their part remained a matter for debate and negotiation.

Starting in the late 1700s with the "birth of the clinic," a new kind of "clinical gaze" gradually transformed those debates in Europe and its colonies (Foucault [1963] 1975). Medicine became more scientific by literally and figuratively dissecting the human body into ever smaller parts. Gradually, physicians in these parts of the world listened less to patients' accounts of their illness and depended more on the results of physical exams and laboratory tests. Whereas once most doctors and patients shared a similar set of explanations for disease and its treatment, now they communicated across a steadily widening chasm of understanding (Charles Rosenberg 1979). In sum, scientific medicine's ethos required "eradicating the person of the patient from medical discourse" and making physicians achieve "a degree of detachment from the demands of the sick," in the words of sociologist Norman Jewson (Jewson 1976, 238, 240).

As medical specialization accelerated in the twentieth century, both physicians and patients expressed concerns about the loss of perspective on the "whole patient" (C. Lawrence and Weisz 1998). But those worries had comparatively little impact on the way physicians were educated or regulated until the 1950s. Wartime developments, including Nazi science's excesses and the atomic bomb's development, combined with a huge leap forward in medicine's technological capacities to deepen concerns about a growing "God complex" among both researchers and clinicians (D. Rothman 1991). Patients complained about the rising cost and uneven quality of medical care and the tendency to overtreat some (e.g., white, wealthy, often female patients) and neglect others (e.g., elderly, poor, and nonwhite; Tomes 2016). Criticisms of mainstream medicine's treatment of patients became even more radical in the late 1960s. Widely read public intellectuals suggested medicine had been captured by a "medical industrial complex" that put profits before patients. The sexist and racist foundations of the "white male doctor knows best" paternalism became a focal point of both the women's health and Black power movements (A. Nelson 2011; J. Nelson 2015). By the 1970s, the idea that medicine needed radically to revise its conception of the "patient" had become a commonplace of popular and policy discussion (Tomes 2016).

This upheaval led to calls to replace the term *patient* with a word less steeped in medical paternalism (Neuberger and Tallis 1999). Some advocated for the term *client* to convey a more person-centered approach to treatment, others for the term *survivor* to indicate both an overcoming of disease and the deficiencies of conventional medicine. What largely prevailed in the United States was referring to patients as "health care consumers," a shift that emphasized the economic terms of the medical encounter and the need for laypeople to become more active, informed participants in their care (Tomes 2016).

For help with their patient problems, elite medical leaders began to reach out to experts outside medicine. They did so for both moral and professional reasons, understanding that to retain its autonomy, medicine had to do a better job of regulating itself and communicating with patients. Thus, medical leaders consulted with scholars trained in religion, philosophy, and the law about issues such as informed consent, the right to refuse treatment, and the allocation of scarce medical resources (D. Rothman 1991). These discussions proved so useful that many medical schools began to include courses on what became known as "bioethics" (Martenson 2001). At the same time, bioethics took an individualistic, rational approach that did little to address the emotional and cultural distance between doctors and patients. To bridge those divides, medical educators turned to literary scholars to develop courses on medicine and literature using storytelling to cultivate medical students' empathy and cultural perspective (Charon 1986). This branch of what became known as the "medical humanities" emphasized the importance of listening carefully to patients: to "read them like a text" to advance both the science and art of medicine (A. Jones 1994).

Housed as they were in academic medical centers, the medical humanities tended to be doctor-centric in their concerns and restrained in their criticisms of biomedicine. But in the rest of academia, far more critical, patient-centered perspectives multiplied across both the humanities and the social sciences. From the 1960s onward, successive waves of scholarship problematized the nature of embodiment and the lived experience of illness as it varied by gender, sexual orientation, race, class, and illness. What began as an interrogation of Western medicine quickly widened to include the colonial and postcolonial reach of its influence (Adams 2010). This critical scholarship insisted that far from being value neutral, medical science was a cultural enterprise that reproduced the power and privilege of its time. In addition, it assumed patients were far from passive in this process, sometimes helping coproduce, sometimes resist this medical "imperialism."

In the late-twentieth century, disability and race emerged as particularly important categories for rethinking what it meant to be "the patient." Critical disability studies questioned overly simplistic oppositions between the abled and disabled and medical versus social models of "helping" the latter. As Lennard Wilson wrote, "the 'problem' is not the person with disabilities; the problem is the way that normalcy is constructed to create the 'problem' of the disabled person" (L. Davis 2016, 3). While raising questions about medicine's role in promoting reductionist notions of personhood, critical disability studies also emphasized the complicated relations that disabled people have with the concept of "cure" (Clare 2017).

Likewise, critical race studies challenged the health humanities to widen their attention to race. In the early 2000s, the Human Genome Project confirmed that at the genetic level, the categories of racial difference medicine had long promoted simply did not exist. The well-known racial disparities in health status and outcomes were the consequences, then, of race as a *social* construct. Critics suggested that since modern medicine and public health had played central roles in biologizing racial difference, they now needed to take a leading role in dismantling that difference, a task that required rethinking every aspect of health care (Roberts 2012). That included attending to the many ways patient "privilege" was denied to people of color. In the case of substance misuse, for example, white people ended up in private doctors' offices while Black people ended up in clinics and jails (Hansen and Roberts 2012; Herzberg 2020).

The health humanities provide an interdisciplinary space where such fundamental challenges to the concept of the "patient"—and patience—can be explored. But the "patient" is not an easy concept to define or survey. Just as biomedicine juggles competing perspectives from multiple sciences and specialties (genetics, biochemistry, oncology, psychiatry) and other health-care professions (nursing, physical therapy), so too the health humanities contend with the perspectives on human experience produced by many different humanities and social sciences. The health humanities wrestle with thorny questions as a result: What matters more, the individual experience or the social framing of that experience? How do we locate individual experience within the larger structural inequalities that pattern its expression? How do we track the many ways power and privilege work in the supposedly objective institutions of scientific medicine?

The ultimate challenge in this work is maintaining a *critical* perspective. Questioning biomedicine's relations with patients is complicated by the fact that many practitioners of the health humanities are embedded in the institutions they seek to explain. The health humanities have long faced questions of whether they function more as lapdogs than watchdogs when it comes

to promoting human values in biomedicine (Stevens 2000). Their commitment to critical inquiry is not necessarily welcomed by patients or health professionals. But the ways power and privilege shape the patient experience can and must remain at the heart of the health humanities.

48

Pollution

Sara Jensen Carr

The word *pollution* is derived from the Latin *pollutionem*, meaning "defilement." The *Oxford English Dictionary* also closely links the term to the tainting of spiritual purity as well, noting its Middle Ages use to refer to the "desecration of what is sacred" and later "spiritual or moral impurity or corruption" (*OED Online* 2021, "pollution") Today, the use of the word is primarily tied to the contamination of the physical environment, especially in relation to unchecked urbanization and its disruptions to the well-being of both humans and ecosystems. During the industrial revolution, the specter of pollution became associated with the contagious illnesses that also wracked early Western cities, cast as the generalized price paid for the sins of civilization, embodied in the diseases of its inhabitants. The idea of environmentally borne afflictions faded from public consciousness as their study and treatment turned to internal causes, but in the late-twentieth century, surges in chronic diseases such as cancer and asthma demanded a reexamination of the links between industry and illness.

Hippocrates' *On Airs, Waters, and Places* connected the health of the environment to the health of those who inhabit it. He described the difference between "wholesome" and "unwholesome" waters, the latter being "marshy, stagnant" and those who drank from them as having "large and obstructed spleens . . . bellies . . . hard, emaciated, and hot; and . . . shoulders, collarbones, and faces . . . emaciated." This connection had

wide acceptance well into the early twentieth century, most notably in the form of miasma theory. A landmark cartoon in *Punch* magazine showed Death, represented by a shrouded skeleton, rowing the polluted Thames River with the London skyline against a sky rendered in dark strokes, portending the grim inevitabilities of the polluted environment. Cities were transformed by waste infrastructure and zoning regulations, and the saying "the solution to pollution is dilution" guided planning development, with effluent dumped into the largest available water bodies and factories moved to the edges of cities. Although large swaths of the cities were improved, immigrants and communities of color, who also often lived at the margins and in the lowlands of urban environments, still bore the brunt of industry.

Metaphorical and direct thinking about pollution's effect on bodies guided the infrastructural design of many European and American cities, even as miasmic theories fell out of favor. Richard Sennett (1994) linked urban planning employed in 1700s and 1800s European cities such as Paris to William Harvey's seventeenth-century discovery of blood and oxygen circulation. Public sanitation in hand with the deployment of wide boulevards, public squares, and green spaces were meant to circulate healthy air through streets and rid them of dirt and grime. These strategies were in turn adopted in many Progressive-era American urban landscapes. Frederick Law Olmsted, the landscape architect of Central Park and Boston's Emerald Necklace, famously had a background in public health and used that expertise to evangelize the mechanical power of trees and green space to clean the air. Another driving force behind Olmsted's parks was to bring nature back into the city to rebalance health, especially to a working class that couldn't afford time or money to leave the city like the elites who were escaping to country homes and nature resorts to cure their respiratory and nervous afflictions.

The study of environmental health became increasingly supplanted in Western medicine in favor of germ theory and vaccines, although formative works like Jacques May's *The Ecology of Human Disease* (1958) continued to make a case for enumerating the medical geographies of illness and wellness. The connection between May's theories and contemporaneous environmental studies, such as Aldo Leopold's writings on "land health" and "land ethic," is the continued idealization of untouched nature and the human body as discrete but tethered self-regulating systems. Disease in both bodies and the land is a signal of disruption, most often in the form of urbanization and pollution. The work of Leopold and others underlaid the establishment of ecology as a scientific field in the 1960s. This paralleled the burgeoning environmental movement, boosted by books such as Rachel Carson's *Silent Spring* ([1962] 2002) and Murray Bookchin's *Our Synthetic Environment* (1962; written under the pseudonym Lewis Herber), written the same year. The reexamination of industry's harm on the environment also uncovered its connections to chronic diseases, particularly cancer, which at this time had become a leading cause of mortality in the developed world. Carson drew on scientific evidence and journalistic doggedness to show how sprayed pesticides, most notably Dichlorodiphenyltrichloroethane (DDT), posed harm far beyond the insects they were meant to control. Her descriptions of poisoned water, dead birds, and carcinogens circulating in bloodstreams and breast milk made the book a phenomenon. Bookchin's polemic similarly connected the rise of chronic diseases in the United States to the exploitation and contamination of the ecosystem. Both authors denounced the complicity of the American government in the production of toxic chemicals and the disregard for planetary as well as human health. "The needs of industrial plants are being placed before man's need for clean air," charged Bookchin. "The disposal of industrial wastes has gained priority over the community's need for clean water. The most pernicious laws of the marketplace are given precedence over the most compelling laws of biology" (1962, 26).

The charge has grown louder as the evidence has mounted and the threat to life has grown. It has become clear, moreover, that both the cause and risk of pollution-related illnesses are not equally distributed. Several decades after the publication of these works, it became increasingly clear that the concentration on the threat to elite white populations, or generalizing pollution's harm as hazardous to humanity as a whole, obscured its inequitable effects on migrant workers, the poor, and communities of color. Pollution has become the defining characteristic of places such as Louisiana's Cancer Alley, Flint, Michigan, or Richmond, California, as statistics make transparent the injustices wreaked on low-income, primarily Black or Latinx residents by industrial behemoths, often with government sanction. If in the early twentieth century municipal planners undertook massive efforts to green urban streets and spaces to breathe fresh air into neighborhoods, they also conscribed communities of color to landscapes of risk through covenants and discriminatory home lending, quarantining them downwind and downstream of industrial plants or cut off by freeways, leaving them to breathe the emissions of traffic overhead. These neighborhoods still bear the brunt of both pollution and our rapidly deteriorating environment; recent studies have shown that formerly redlined neighborhoods have higher rates of asthma, less green space and trees, and are becoming increasingly inhospitable urban heat islands. Julie Sze connects this slow choking of the environment to the physical brutality enacted on black and brown bodies, calling "the inability to breathe . . . a metaphor and material reality of political oppression, state violence, and ongoing legacies of racism" (2020, 17). The environmental injustices wrought by pollution also continue to mount; at the time of this writing, it is also becoming increasingly clear that the preexisting high rates of respiratory diseases in these neighborhoods also have a strong correlation with COVID-19 mortality.

A distinct subset of literature has narrated the dangers of environmental toxins through the desecration of women's bodies. Sandra Steingraber's *Living Downstream: An Ecologist's Personal Investigation of Cancer and the Environment*, for example, is an account of her own environmentally caused illness, and Richard Powers' novel *Gain* tells the parallel stories of an American soap company turned chemical conglomerate and a neighboring woman's ovarian cancer. Although *Silent Spring* omits autobiography, Carson's cancer diagnosis, received in the midst of her research and her death shortly after its publication, implicitly infuses her account.

Urban ecologist Kristina Hill (2005) posited the human body as permeable to physical flows of "energy, materials, and organisms" with both beneficial and detrimental effects on health. The same can be said of the social environments. In the twenty-first century, where pollution represents our most existential threats of climate change, racism, and late capitalism, these are inextricably linked. Pollution is the cause of the "unwholesome" airs and waters against which Hippocrates cautioned—but of society's own making. Rather than confronting systemic causes of pollution, instead it has historically been hidden at the edges of urbanization, where it thickens the atmosphere, taints the water, and lies buried in our soils until it becomes embedded in our most vulnerable and marginalized populations as well, prompting an urgent need to delineate and repair the complex web of connections between nature, cities, and bodies.

49

Poverty
Percy C. Hintzen

Poverty is popularly understood as a state or condition of material and financial "lack" or insufficiency that negatively affects the ability of a person or group (very broadly defined) to "satisfy their basic needs" consistent with a healthy existence such as food, shelter, clothing, and health (K. Thompson 2011) and/or an inability to meet "the minimum level of living standards expected for the place where one lives" (Crossman 2019). Poverty is often stigmatized, blamed on insufficiencies in the character of the impoverished, but it is in fact evidence of the failure of governance at all levels, and it is the cause of one-third of all human deaths.

In Medieval times, poverty might be a choice: a sign of Christian virtue, for example. Alternatively, it could be cast as evidence of unworthiness and justification for exploitation. Representations of poverty codified in early nineteenth century Britain viewed it as a "moral problem" resulting from the failure of the poor to exercise restraint—as in reduction of their fecundity or refusal to pursue initiative. Stigmatized for presumed irrational engagement in profligate consumption rather than adherence to an asceticism that supported investment for success, the impoverished were a "threat" to society. They were seen as the cause of generalized vice, misery, famine, starvation, disease, ill health, and even war (see Malthus [1798] 2015; MacRae 2019). Contrasted with the "moral restraint" exercised by the upper strata, their behavior justified the imposition of harsh penalties of sterilization, criminal punishment, forced emigration, and confinement in poor houses under conditions intended to induce "severe distress." As the benefits of industrialization began to support middle class lifestyles for the vast majority in the global north, these ostensible differences in morality came to characterize the divide between the rich developed and poor underdeveloped countries. The stigma of immorality continued to taint categories such as minorities, immigrants, the "working poor," and the "underclass."

Historically and globally, poverty has been the product of dislocation of rural populations from their means of sustenance, the denial of their rights, and dispossession from their material assets. It is integrally tied to political decisions accompanying a transformation to market capitalism, urban industrialization, and commercial agricultural production for profit, beginning with the industrial revolution in Europe and continuing in earnest with the geopolitics in the wake of World War II in which the inequities of colonialism were perpetuated with the construction of "the Global South."

Poverty is an issue of ethical concern pertaining to what Hannah Arendt ([1958] 1998) called the "human condition" that extends beyond the mere biological to conditions of production and consumption as activities and to rights pertaining to political collectivity. Surfacing at the conjunctions of production and consumption, basic needs, and rights, poverty is a "politically induced condition in which certain populations suffer from failing social and economic networks and disproportionate exposure to injury, violence, and death" (Butler 2009, 25). As a manifestation of precarity, "it induces an inability to adequately satisfy the material need for food, shelter, clothing, health care and other conditions of well-being" (Butler 2009, 25; Shaw and Byler 2016). The impoverished live on the very "borderlines" of the most minimal necessities for survival at

levels conventionally judged unacceptable by the standards of a community.

The precarious conditions of poverty include insufficiencies of food, shelter, personal security, access to health care, and other needs that impact health and well-being. The need to survive or provide for dependents leads to high-risk circumstances that affect health outcomes. The impoverished constitute a readily available pool of surplus labor that moves in and out of the formal economy. Many are seasonal or temporary workers or day laborers—such as sharecroppers or migrant farm workers in rural areas—or those living in urban environments, where working conditions are not well regulated or, in most cases, humane. Workers are likely to be exposed to anything from grueling hours to toxins as well as physical and emotional abuse and exploitation. They are often forced to endure dislocation from friends and family (for Africa, for example, see Olopade 2014). Frequently lacking access to education or forced to drop out to support families, they are often unskilled and functionally illiterate. Those who are not homeless may be forced to live in shanty towns or in the most impoverished sections of the inner cities. While some in the richer countries of the world can rely on public assistance for meagre income support, food assistance, medical care, and housing, these provisions are mostly absent in the poor countries of the Global South. As a result, many die prematurely from preventable diseases (Kendrick 2020).

Challenges to subsistence farming from a variety of factors, often produced or exacerbated by a changing climate, are a major cause of migration to urban areas, which in turn likely contributes to rather than mitigates the problem. Rapid increases in population densities that accompany urbanization and semiurbanization bring with them new challenges, including threats to public health. Displacement disturbs traditional practices of population control while increasing dependence on the income and labor of children for survival. The conversion of the rural peasantry into wage laborers and their rapid urbanization in search of jobs contribute significantly to the immiseration, destitution, and insecurity that are the hallmarks of poverty. Larger families universally constitute a "survival strategy" of the poor: while they provide an important labor force for rural families, in urban settings they are an effort to stave off many of the deleterious consequences of urbanization, including infant mortality and low rates of life expectancy. Paradoxically, however, those efforts produce dramatic increases in the population under conditions of food insecurity as they are displaced from their lives of rural subsistence production where their basic needs for sustenance are fully satisfied. The traditional use of barter for exchange in subsistence economies locates them outside of the monetized formal economy.

In urban settings, these factors catapult the impoverished into the crisis conditions of "bare life" that first appeared in Europe in the initial stages of industrial capitalism (Agamben 1998; see also Ong 2006, 21–25). As the crisis escalates, it places unsustainable burdens on governments, which typically respond by formulating and implementing policies and practices aimed at "punishing the poor" for what is seen as a product of their own irrationality (Wacquant 2009; Lees 1998; Quigley 1996). A "politics" of poverty emerges as a consequence of exclusion from the ostensible "rights" of citizens. The impoverished suffer from forms of "graduated citizenship" where their rights are subjected to different degrees of compromise depending on how useable they are to a formal economy that privileges "growth and productivity" (Ong 2006, 78–84; Ferguson 2006, 38–42).

While poverty is a universal phenomenon, differences in the concentration of resources between the industrialized "developed" countries of Europe and North America and the countries in the formerly colonized nations of the Global South have significant effects on their respective rates of poverty. The latter have significantly reduced opportunities for betterment, in both qualitative and quantitative terms, available to the majority of the population. In 2014, the richest eighty-five people in the world living in the Global North were worth more than the poorest 3.5 billion living primarily in the latter countries (Sutherby 2014). These differences determine the way economies across this global divide function. Economies of the former colonies compel dependence on export production based on cheap labor. Such a dependence has created a global system of "unequal exchange" by forcing a reliance on the availability of a large reserve pool of cheap labor constituted by the poor (Amin 1976; Amin 1980).

Powerful companies headquartered in the Global North are drawn to the "superprofits" resulting from this cheap labor. Conditions of poverty are exacerbated by their consequent domination of the economy and exercise of undue power as well as extraction of the profits (Amin 1982). This phenomenon severely limits the home countries to provide for the health, education, welfare, and well-being of their exploited populations, which augments their vulnerability to disease, chronic debilitation, and death.

The promise of a middle- and upper-class lifestyle was the justifying trope that catapulted the decolonizing nations into adoption of modern forms of industrial capitalism with its consequences of immiseration after the end of World War II. The peasantry of these countries, comprising two-thirds of the world's population, were deemed, by this standard, to live "in poverty, squalor, and misery" (H. Wilson 1953, 11; see also Escobar 2012, 21). This "discovery of mass poverty" in Asia, Africa, and Latin America provided the rationale, under a global project of "national development," for the transformation of the population ideally into an industrial labor force as "modern" producers and consumers (Escobar 2012, 21; see also A. W. Lewis 1950; and A. W. Lewis 1979). But the resulting conditions have not delivered on the promises, instead forcing the impoverished—in both the Global North and the Global South—into behaviors that pose risk to their health and well-being, including forced migration; unhealthy and crowded living and working environments; inadequate sanitation, nutrition, shelter, and access to health care; and compromised immune systems. Blamed for what are actually failures of governance, the impoverished are stigmatized collectively and individually through practices that become structural as they are transformed into legalized restrictions affecting their rights and opportunities (James Livingston 2013, 9; see also Corrigan et al. 2005; and McCrudden 1982).

Of the top forty-five countries with the highest HIV/AIDS rates, all but eight are located in Africa (the remaining eight are in the Caribbean). While "African AIDS" gets worldwide attention, people in Africa die mostly from preventable diseases. Such discrepancies among geopolitical regions attest to conditions of extreme health inequities resulting from the inadequacies associated with poverty and to a clear relationship among poverty, precarity, inequity, and stigma. The relationship extends to every aspect of the human condition. It emerges at the intersection of precarity and poverty. What is most extraordinary and disturbing is that this relationship is the ineluctable condition of capitalist modernity out of and for which it was produced.

50

Precision
Kathryn Tabb

Precision medicine, personalized medicine, P4 medicine, individualized medicine, stratified medicine—broadly speaking, these terms refer to an aspirational set of transformations in biomedical knowledge (see Tutton 2014, 4–6; and Hedgecoe 2004, 16–20). After these transformations, it is imagined, clinicians will use biomarkers (such as genetic signatures, blood products, or neural maps) to categorize patients instead of their superficial features—their signs and symptoms. Therapies will no longer be applied helter-skelter through a process of trial and error but on the basis of causal understanding and predictive power. While in much of the English-speaking world the term *personalized medicine* has dominated, in the United States, the label "precision" has become increasingly popular. Following the 1990s vogue for precision warfare after the Gulf War, since the early 2000s there has been an enthusiasm for medical interventions that minimize collateral damage, and make efficient and effective use of costly, innovative technologies. Compared to "one-size-fits-all medicine," its apologist Francis Collins once claimed of precision, "it's a smart bomb" (Juengst et al. 2016, 24; for more on this metaphor, see Kenney and Mamo 2020).

The uneasy jostling of these various terms reflects some conceptual confusion about the new paradigm. As De Grandis and Halgunset note, future-oriented concepts like these, "aimed at mobilizing initiatives and building networks, are bound to be fluid and contested" (2016, 8). Taking the terms together, questions arise: is the vision one in which each patient has truly personalized care, prescribed on the basis of, for example, the unique features of their genomic profile? Or is the paradigm one in which revised strata of patients are demarcated by newly discovered biomarkers or drug responses—an era of "mass customization" (Tutton 2014, 162)? Or is the point not about the patient experience—individualized, personalized, or stratified—but rather about disease entities themselves? Is it *they* that are to be made precise? These questions do not have established answers; but as Kenney and Mamo argue, "although precision medicine has not been fully realized, the *promise* of precision medicine shapes biomedical research in ways that often go unnoticed" (2020, 194).

While the precision paradigm has been applied to medicine writ large, its signature successes have been within a few specific clinical areas—most of all, within oncology. Here the extraordinary results of monoclonal antibody treatments have allowed for the sort of transformations in biomedical understanding and patient outcomes associated with the precision revolution. A common poster child is trastuzumab (brand name Herceptin), an anticancer drug that is significantly more effective than traditional chemotherapies in treating tumors that overexpress the HER2/neu receptor (for detailed discussion, see Hedgecoe 2004, chaps. 6–8). Such tumors may be located in the breast, the stomach, or the esophagus—the new stratum crosscuts traditional classifications based on anatomy. Once the genetic signature of a tumor is known, advocates claim, it is immediately clear to the clinician if trastuzumab will be an effective therapy.

Maël Lemoine (2017) has argued that the development of monoclonal antibodies is unusually able to bring about the changes in medical research and therapies to which the new paradigm aspires. Indeed, this technology—focused on the genetic profile of the tumor—differs from the original promise of pharmacogenetics, which was envisioned as personalizing medicine on the basis of the inherited genotype (Tutton 2014, 155; Hedgecoe 2004, 24). Together Lemoine and I have compared oncology to psychiatry and shown how differences between the two disciplines mean that precision medicine's successes in oncology are only faintly reflected in psychiatry as ideals (Tabb and Lemoine 2021). Psychiatry currently lacks the basic biological foundations, and theoretical consensuses, to enable the discovery of precision treatments based on biomarkers. Psychopharmacology thus remains an exercise in "drug cartography," the drawing of disease categories on the grounds of therapeutic responses discovered through trial and error, as opposed to the rational drug design that has led to the development of precise chemotherapies (Radden 2003). The case of psychiatry should remind us that for most areas of medicine, precision remains an ambitious dream, a narrative written in the optative mood.

Insofar as the analysis of dreams and of narratives is the domain of the humanist, it is appropriate here to consider some conceptual questions about precision that are tethered to central concerns in the ethics, politics, and hermeneutics of medicine. To the extent that participants increasingly walk away from medical encounters with new personal bioinformation—or, as direct-to-consumer genetic testing takes off, acquire it for themselves—a different medical imaginary will take shape (Levina 2010). People may participate in precision initiatives because they think getting their genetic information will increase their capacity to make informed health-care choices. But given the complexity of predicting future outcomes on the basis of genetic profiling, personalized medicine is not something most of us can do for ourselves. The suggestion otherwise becomes nefarious when, far from providing a benefit, the giving over of health information ends up recapitulating biomedicine's historical exploitation and abuses of minority populations (S. Lee 2011; Matthew 2019). Another worry stems from the fact that precision medicine often stratifies patients not into disease categories, but risk categories. As Nikolas Rose has noted, "the very act of designating an individual 'at risk' changes not only their own self-perception, but also that of others . . . such designation, even if false, may lead to stigma or to an individual regarding every small event as indicative of impending doom" (2013a, 347). The massive effect diagnoses have on self-narratives has long been a site of attention from the health humanities. Precision medicine requires reconsidering these effects in light of the particular psychological challenge posed by information about the self that is dilatory, uncertain, or contingent.

Why does it matter if the language of personalization is indeed hyperbolic (Doz, Marvanne, and Fagot-Largeault 2013)? First, there are repercussions of this rhetoric for the ethics of consent. For precision medicine to work, millions of people are required to give up their health information to massive data recruitment efforts. In the United States, the government's "All of Us" initiative uses a rhetoric that appeals not only to people's general sense of civic duty but also to their more specific desires to help their own communities (Neuhaus 2020). However, the assumption that precision medicine's new strata will reflect meaningful social categories is likely faulty, despite its usefulness for the commercialization of precision findings (S. Lee 2011; Tutton 2014). Indeed, it has been argued that the explicit attention paid to racial categories by initiatives like All of Us has resulted in the reification of races as biological entities, while they are better seen as constructed proxies for the complex social and economic inequities driving health disparities (S. Lee 2011; Callier 2019). As Matthew has argued, "precision medicine's basis in genome science may be misused to resurrect the backwards and hateful assertions of racialized science" (2019, 630).

Returning to the semantic question of whether "precision" and "personalized" amount to the same thing, it is worth observing that there is strong sentiment among certain clinical constituencies that they do not (Tutton 2014, 157). Some practitioners resent what they see as the appropriation of person-centered language; they see advocates for precision as "exploiting its rhetorical force and emptying it of its critical potential to oppose narrow and reductionist approaches to medicine" (De Grandis and Halgunset 2016, 7). Personalized care, person-centered medicine, patient-centered medicine, and other such terms have traditionally captured medical ideals that seem diametrically opposed to those of the new paradigm. They have referred to practices that treat patients holistically, rather than reducing them to their dysfunctional systems or parts (Doz et al. 2013), and that foreground the clinician-patient relationship by emphasizing the importance of interpersonal skills and joint decision-making (D. Rosen and Hoang 2017). Precision medicine, on the other hand, can be seen as attenuating patient choice by relying on decision-making algorithms based on big data (Juengst et al. 2016, 25; N. Rose 2013a, 344).

I will conclude by noting that the second half of the term, seldom considered by critics—*medicine*—is also a possible site for critical attention. It may well be the case that what is revolutionary for our scientific understanding of disease is not particularly impactful in the clinic (Hedgecoe 2004). Returning to the case study of psychiatry, as enthusiasm for precision medicine has grown within the US's National Institute of Mental Health, resources have flowed away from clinical research, including epidemiology and psychopharmacology, and toward the basic sciences like genetics, biochemistry, and especially neuroscience (Tabb 2020). Nonetheless, precision psychiatry's findings have not translated into significant clinical advances. As Teachman et al. have written, it has rather "prioritized potential long-term gains at the expense of more immediate gains, and hampered our ability to link biological processes to the human environments, social factors, and behaviors that shape and define mental illnesses" (2018, 12). The new paradigm is a boon for translational researchers working at the frontiers of biomedicine, but can feel inhospitable to clinical researchers, epidemiologists, and those working in global and public health (Chowkwanyun, Bayer, and Galea 2018). As Kenney and Mamo put it, in medicine as in warfare, precision "is a sociotechnical fiction that conceals what falls outside of its official targets" (2020, 195).

Advocates of precision medicine may frame their preferred paradigm against clinical approaches they see as *im*precise or *im*personal. But imprecision and impersonalization have their defenders. With *individualized*, we might contrast the solidarity at the heart of health ethics, which generally considers medical care as a collective right rather than a private resource (Neuhaus 2020). Against the reductive division of clinical populations into parts, we can counter public health's traditional emphasis on the whole, with its recognition that only at the level of emergent structural factors such as entrenched poverty, systemic racism, and inequitable environments do the causes of morbidity and mortality become visible (Chowkwanyun, Bayer, and Galea 2018; Matthew 2019). Advocates of anonymization believe it requisite for the just distribution of health-care resources, regardless of one's utility to the market, or one's purchasing power (N. Rose 2013a). The stratification of populations can often mean more efficient health-care spending rather than more effective care (Kenney and Mamo 2020, 196); in this sense, the best antonym for precision medicine may well be "general" medicine or "public" health care. In other words, the rise of precision as a virtue for state-sponsored medical research may indicate that medicine's goals are being reimagined as individualistic rather than universal (see Tutton 2014, especially chaps. 1–2). Critical attention to "precision," "personalized," "P4," and the like should not distract us from this fundamental and provocative semantic shift.

51

Psychosis

Angela Woods

Psychosis names states in which so-called normal or neurotypical modes of thinking, feeling, perceiving, communicating, and being a self "at home in the world" become disrupted in ways that might be experienced as frightening, painful, destabilizing, and isolating. Psychosis is sometimes, but not always, synonymous with what in nonclinical contexts would be called "madness" and sometimes, but not always, used in place of the arguably more fraught and certainly more contested "schizophrenia." Clinically, psychosis can be acute or chronic; episodic or enduring; attributed to specific proximal stressors, injuries, or intoxicants; or regarded as arising from the complex interplay of traumatic and adverse life events, structural inequalities, underlying vulnerabilities, and biopsychosocial factors. Experientially, psychosis can be profoundly difficult to articulate and to make sense of, as Henry Gale explores in his 2013 animation "Psychosis Is Nothing like a Badger." Within an academic context, Magi, Jones, and Kelly drily observe of psychosis that "certain modalities, experiences, versions or variants of 'symptoms' are regularly privileged or fetishized—and those who control these terms and constructs and their academic lives, are rarely if ever themselves mad" (2016, 148).

Psychosis is important to the health humanities because the suffering it names arises from and impacts on every level of our existence—from the folds of the paracingulate sulcus to our divergent views on what constitutes a self—and because, despite one hundred and seventy years of scientific inquiry, its definition, meaning, and treatment remain deeply contested.

First used in medicine and psychology in the late 1840s to refer to "any kind of disordered mental state or mental illness," psychosis came over the latter half of the nineteenth century to refer more specifically to "severe mental illness, characterized by loss of contact with reality (in the form of delusions and hallucinations) and deterioration of intellectual and social functioning" (*OED Online* 2021, "psychosis"). Today, the term remains stubbornly imprecise and conflicted in its operation. The American Psychiatric Association DSM-5 Task Force (2013) and World Health Organization (1992) define psychosis narrowly through the presence of hallucinations and delusions, symptoms that can occur across a large number of psychiatric and neurological conditions. By contrast, the UK's National Institute for Health and Care Excellence guidelines use the term to refer to a "group of psychotic disorders that includes schizophrenia, schizoaffective disorder, schizophreniform disorder and delusional disorder" (2014). The British Psychological Society, in its landmark report *Understanding Psychosis: Why People Sometimes Hear Voices, Believe Things That Others Find Strange, or Appear Out of Touch with Reality, and What Can Help,* is more expansive still in looking beyond diagnoses or disorders toward the particular experiences "that are usually thought of as 'psychosis', 'schizophrenia', 'mental illness', 'nervous breakdown' or sometimes 'madness'" (Cooke 2017, 10).

Psychosis is not frequently considered a keyword in health humanities contexts. But the set of experiences it names and the relationship of those experiences to the societies in which we live; the organisms and entities we understand ourselves to be; and the regulatory, therapeutic, and hermeneutic systems in which we place our faith *are* central concerns of the field. In order to see psychosis in operation in the health humanities, we need first to look sideways and back, at "madness," "schizophrenia," "hearing voices," and "unusual beliefs."

The work of French philosopher Michel Foucault has been extremely influential in the way madness has been conceptualized, investigated, and valued by scholars across the humanities and social sciences for over half a century. Charting major shifts in the way that madness was understood and managed across Europe from the medieval period to the birth of the asylum in the nineteenth century, *Madness and Civilization* challenged the scientific and moral authority of psychiatry, its taxonomies, and its practices:

> As for a common language [between the "mad" and the "sane"], there is no such thing; or rather, there is no such thing any longer; the constitution of madness as a mental illness, at the end of the eighteenth century, affords the evidence of a broken dialogue, posits the separation as already effected, and thrusts into oblivion all those stammered, imperfect words without fixed syntax in which the exchange between madness and reason was made. The language of psychiatry, which is a monologue of reason about madness, has been established only on the basis of such a silence.
>
> I have not tried to write the history of that language, but rather the archaeology of that silence. (Foucault [1961] 2001, xii)

In an analysis that resonated powerfully with the antipsychiatry movements of the 1960s and 70s, Foucault offers a vision—and valorization—of madness as something fundamentally distorted by and inaccessible to medical and scientific understanding.

Reclaiming madness from psychiatry and finding ways to attend to its truth became urgent undertakings for scholars working in the disciplines we would now recognize as contributing to the health humanities. Research inspired by Foucault has demonstrated the inadequacies, inconsistencies, and ideological underpinnings of psychiatric classification; traced the differential effects of psychiatric power on bodies and communities; and proposed new ways of attending to the articulations of madness including what they reveal about trauma, oppression, suffering, and the structure of subjectivity. Following Sandra Gilbert and Susan Gubar's *The Madwoman in the Attic* (1979) and Elaine Showalter's *The Female Malady: Women, Madness, and English Culture, 1830–1980* (1985), madness became a focal point of Anglo-American feminist literary criticism. The UK-based Madness and Literature Network went on to play an important role in making literary and cultural representations of madness, and their analysis, central concerns of the newly defined health humanities, with Showalter a keynote speaker at "Madness and Literature: The First International Health Humanities Conference" in 2010 (Madness and Literature Network 2021). Addressing madness—as distinct from mental illness or a particular clinical disorder—explicitly signals a scholarly starting point outside psychiatry, frequently one that entails a greater attentiveness to individual experience. In this, many literary, cultural, and historical analyses of madness paralleled and in the same contexts drew inspiration from disability and mad studies, even if they did not advance the same political claims as scholar-activists in these fields.

A very different scholarly trajectory is opened up by the term *schizophrenia*. Engaging primarily with psychoanalytic accounts of psychosis, Gilles Deleuze and Felix Guattari's *Anti-Oedipus Capitalism and Schizophrenia* (1977), Fredric Jameson's *Postmodernism or the Cultural Logic of Late Capitalism* (1991), Avital Ronell's *The Telephone Book: Technology, Schizophrenia, Electric Speech* (1989), and Louis Sass's *Madness and Modernism: Insanity in the Light of Modern Art, Literature and Thought* (1992) all explicitly link aspects of what is distinctive in the structure of "schizophrenic" experience to the social and material conditions of modernity and postmodernity. As philosophers, psychologists, phenomenologists, and critical theorists, it is doubtful that these authors would recognize themselves as working within the health humanities; however, critics who analyze how, why, and with what effect clinical terms such as schizophrenia come to be deployed within cultural theory most certainly do situate themselves within this field (see Woods 2011). Schizophrenia is also located at a fraught intersection of clinical and cultural spheres by Jonathan M. Metzl. Metzl in his 2009 book *The Protest Psychosis: How Schizophrenia Became a Black Disease* analyzes multiple clinical, institutional, pharmaceutical, and historical sources to reveal how diagnostic racism and corporate and medical interests transformed the way schizophrenia was defined, diagnosed, and treated in the USA. Psychosis becomes a prism through which to interrogate and challenge structural racism and the role of psychiatry in perpetuating inequalities.

A third vein of scholarship in the health humanities focuses not on the global changes to self and world that are implied by the terms *psychosis*, *madness*, and *schizophrenia* but rather on specific aspects of experience understood as existing on a continuum stretching from "normal" to "pathological." Health humanities scholars have embraced work by cultural theorists Grace Cho (2008) and Lisa Blackman (2001) and anthropologist Tanya Luhrmann (2012), which understands the experience of hearing voices within specific cultural and religious contexts, and the decade-long research project Hearing the Voice is a strong example of how scholars from across the humanities and social sciences collaborate with psychologists, clinicians and experts by experience to enrich our knowledge about voice-hearing, its

origins, meanings and effects (Woods, Alderson-Day, and Fernyhough 2022). Research published under the banner "imperfect cognitions" has similarly used insights from philosophy and the social sciences to shift our collective understanding of what distinguishes "unusual" beliefs in a clinical context (Imperfect Cognitions Network 2021). Research of this kind also contributes to the broader political project of denaturalizing psychiatric taxonomies, questioning their definition and highlighting their differential operation in the lives of individuals and communities around the world.

If we can only fully see psychosis at operation in the health humanities by looking first at the terms *madness*, *schizophrenia*, *hearing voices*, and *unusual beliefs*, we must also recognize that this scholarship variously encompasses, reframes, or sits alongside research primarily identified in other fields and subdisciplines. Medical and health humanities perspectives on psychosis draw on insights from the history and philosophy of psychiatry, mad studies, disability studies, cultural and critical theory, gender studies, queer theory, trauma and memory studies, phenomenological psychopathology, psychologically oriented research in anthropology, geography and sociology, and the psy sciences.

So what, if anything, is distinctive about the way that psychosis is approached within the health humanities? What does the health humanities contribute to the study of psychosis, and what does psychosis, in turn, do within and for the field?

"I get a sense of vertigo when talking about psychosis," writes one pseudonymous blogger of her efforts to "explain the inexplicable" (zedkat 2021). Addressing the communicative challenges posed by experiences of illness is a cornerstone of health humanities scholarship and a key area in which the field seeks to demonstrate its utility, especially within clinical settings (here, the celebrated autobiographies by Saks [2007] and Jamison

[1996] have been a focal point). Like pain (Scarry 1985) and trauma (Caruth 1996), psychosis is often experienced, by individual and interlocutor alike, as severely disrupting the cognitive, linguistic, and narrative capacities on which communication typically is thought to depend (Roe and Davidson 2005). So if the health humanities is to heed Foucault's warning not to perpetuate a "monologue of reason about madness," then greater attention will need to be paid to the multiple, messy, embodied, and discursive renderings of psychosis (Woods 2013); to its lived reality within specific sociopolitical as well as clinical contexts; and to experiences of marginalization, stigmatization, discrimination, coercion, and trauma within and outside of mental health services. Learning from the pioneering work of survivor researchers and mad studies scholars and activists, the health humanities is increasingly centering the research and wider contributions of people with lived experience of psychosis (Magi, Jones, and Kelly 2016; Kalathil and Jones 2016; Faulkner 2017). This is not simply a question of proliferating analysis but of engaging with fundamental questions about the politics and ethics of how knowledge about psychosis is produced. The consequences of doing so are far-reaching—epistemically, ethically, practically, and institutionally—and I hope it is a challenge to which the field can rise.

52

Race
Rana Hogarth

Race is a fluid term lacking a single agreed upon definition. It boasts a long history, inextricably linked to health, medicine, and the body. As it refers to the parsing of people into groups, tribes, or clans, race has origins rooted in medical antiquity. In his well-known treatise *Airs, Waters, and Places*, Hippocrates of Kos, the so-called Father of Medicine, apprehended distinct races of people and posited their differences in physical appearance as a product of their customs and the geography and climate of the places they inhabited (Hippocrates 1849, 213, 218; Painter 2010, 9). While the Hippocratic notion of race is very different from our modern version of the term, both versions of the word group people based on their physical features (though we no longer attribute physical features to climates or habits). Today, consciously or unconsciously, we rely on assumptions that certain races of people have shared characteristic skin color, hair texture, eye color, eye and nose shape, and other phenotypical features. This mapping of race onto a person's body by virtue of their physical features can be a matter of simple observation, but it paves the way for oversimplifications about entire groups of people. More to the point, it can harm, for it facilitates racial profiling and stereotyping. For example, criminality and athleticism—traits that have been "associated with Black American men" are more strongly associated with people who have so-called Afrocentric features—dark skin, a wide nose, wide lips, and coarse hair (Kleider-Offutt, Bond, and Hegerty 2017, 28).

Rather than trying to locate or create an ideal definition of race, this essay instead explores how race came to be mapped onto the body and why that approach for parsing race endures. It also interrogates how we arrived at the taken-for-granted associations between race and health that circulate in medical and scientific discourse and national discussions. Looking at race in this way is instructive for revealing the subtle and explicit ways we still think and talk about it with vocabularies rooted in biology, hence assumptions that race is tangible—a biological fact—rather than a social construction. It is important to recognize the pull of history—the difficulty of accepting new insights, even when they are supported by science—in order to understand why physicians, scientists, and those in allied health fields (groups ostensibly trying to improve health outcomes) still talk about race as biology in ways that can be harmful or in the very least to sanction the dangerous idea that there are innate biological differences between the races. Indeed, that history—and the urgency in challenging it—explains the centrality of race as a keyword for health humanities.

When François Bernier, a French physician and traveler, published *New Division of the Earth* in 1684, he elevated the role of the body in determining race. Indeed, Bernier pointed to corporeal features like skin color, lip shape, and hair texture as useful for classifying different types of humans into groups. This practice of explaining race via the human body was a departure from the conventional reliance on Biblical interpretation and conjecture, which was common in western Europe (Koslofsky 2014, 796). Some scholars have credited him with sketching out a hazy notion of the modern concept of race (Stuurman 2000, 2, 4, 5). Bernier's influence, however, was but one of the many factors in the process of making and defining race; the concept Western medicine has inherited was (and is) a multisited, subjective, and collective process.

From the seventeenth century onward, European naturalists, physicians, and those in allied fields compared nose and skull shapes of one group against another, dissected layers of African skin, and displayed nonwhite peoples in European courts (Schiebinger 2013, 370; Koslofsky 2014, 799). This ability to see and parse race through the body was not only the purview of European thinkers on the continent. Joyce Chaplin compellingly demonstrates that while English settlers to mainland North America may not have invoked the modern concept of race, they relied on "bodily differentiation" among themselves, Native Americans, and the sub-Saharan Africans they encountered. There was already a practical way of seeing racial difference through comparison well before any kind of formalized corporeal definition of race emerged (Chaplin 2003, 193). The settler colonialists of the New World saw their bodies as situated between the weakness of Native bodies and the supposed hardiness of African bodies at a time when they were gaining control over North America and relying on slavery to do so. Racism may well, paradoxically, have preceded race as the justification for treating a needed labor force as less than human. Seeing and sensing race was tied up with conquest and commerce. Both brought different groups of people together in unprecedented ways that put the examination and comparison of bodies in the service of perceived social and economic exigencies.

With more access to different bodies came more strident claims that race (and by extension differences between races) was observable. Resulting in part from the work of physicians and anatomists, assumptions that race was an element of the human body became remarkably durable. Proslavery English commentator and one time resident of Jamaica, Edward Long encapsulated this sentiment in his 1774 *History of Jamaica*: "It seems now to be the established opinion, founded upon anatomical observations, that the black complexion of Negroes proceeds entirely from a reticulum mucosum, or dark colored network spread immediately beneath the cuticle of their bodies" (Long 1774, 49). Here was proof that Black racial traits existed and could be easily detected. As he detailed the features of an albino child, born to two Black parents, Long noted the complexion was of a "dead dull white," but the "features" were "truly of the negro cast," "the nostrils wide and lips thick and prominent" (Long 1774, 49). On the view that racial differences existed, Long quoted an ableist turn of phrase penned by the antislavery French philosophe Voltaire: "None but the blind can doubt it" (Long 1774, 335–36). For Long, and others (regardless of their stance on slavery), to say that race was discernable on the body was to state the obvious.

Much has changed over the course of three hundred or so years. Race is an arbitrary way of grouping people; many scholars across the humanities and sciences have repeatedly demonstrated that there is no biological basis for it. That said, how we understand what race is, how we account for the very real ways people perceive race and feel raced in their interactions with others, still carries strong associations with biology and the body. And the durability of these associations between race and biology is still too often sanctioned by modern biomedicine. Published scientific and medical research not only bears out this persistence but also reveals how race has become a precision term used to offer predictive insight into one's health as well.

Its precision is implied in its use for the collection of important health data and vital statistics (Braun et al. 2007). Drug trials, medical research, mortality and morbidity, and disparities in health outcomes rely on race to bring clarity to trends found in data. In these contexts, it should be noted, capturing race does more to capture racism's insidious influence on one's health than

illuminate any meaningful links between one's race and their biology. Medical decision-making has also validated the notion of a biological basis for race. This is most evident in race correction algorithms in medical practice. The *estimated glomerular filtration rate*, or eGFR, which measures kidney function, has race correction built into it. Black patients have their results "corrected" due to data from 1999 that suggested that self-identified Black people had higher levels of creatinine. Measuring serum creatinine levels is an accessible way to estimate kidney function; higher detected creatinine typically signals a low eGFR. Low eGFR suggests deficiency in kidney function. For Black people, a multiplier is added, boosting the eGFR value. The result of this race correction is "higher reported eGFR values (which suggest better kidney function) for anyone identified as black" (Vyas, Eisenstein, and Jones 2020, 875). A growing number of scholars, across disciplines, have seized upon the very problematic nature of this assessment. "A patient with one Black parent and one White parent" would have different eGFR readings depending on whether or not they identified as White or Black; if they identified as both, the clinician would make the call (Amutah et al. 2021, 4). Not only does this example underscore what little precision race offers, but it also reveals how race harms rather than helps. In this case, a higher eGFR might suggest higher kidney function in a Black patient, potentially obscuring their illness—a concern that has been noted by practitioners in the medical profession, and other allied health fields (Vyas, Eisenstein, and Jones 2020, 875; Roberts 2021, 18). The attempts to replace eGFR and the larger questions about assessing what race an individual is bode well for sundering these associations between race and biology.

Confronting the historical associations drawn between race and the body helps to reveal the process of race's social construction in a way that recognizes the less abstract ways the term came about. It is a way of acknowledging that race is not an element of biology, despite people mapping it onto the human body in the past and present (i.e., identifying someone as a "person of color" or POC to describe them). It is a way of showing its paradoxical existence as something geneticists and scientists will say has no biological basis and a thing that clinicians still use to make medical diagnoses and decisions. Reorienting our way of perceiving race is necessary, as many have argued, but it will be no small feat (Wald 2006). In the meantime, however, we can try to perceive race less as a real part of our biology and more as a proxy for illuminating the real effects of racism in our society.

53

Reproduction
Aziza Ahmed

The word *reproduction* has always exceeded the biological. Its meanings range from the act of bringing into existence again, the formation of new tissue, the act of being productive in the economy, and the action of recreating a memory (*OED Online* 2021, "reproduction"). *Reproduction* is particularly useful for scholars in the health humanities because even its biological meanings are always inextricably bound up with the term's social, cultural, political, religious, and economic dimensions.

As Michel Foucault ([1976] 1990) revealed most famously, reproduction is not simply an act. Rather, since at least the sixteenth century, reproduction has been a locus of state power. It was at that time, Foucault teaches us, that at least in France, government shifted from wielding power over death alone to controlling life. He called this *biopolitics*, a term that describes the state's turn toward managing the life and reproduction of populations, especially through demographic tools like birth rate and mortality. Many scholars have followed, conceiving of reproduction as a site for thinking about the relationship between population, governance, and political economy as well as the representational tools, rhetorics, sociocultural dynamics, religious ideologies, and structures of power shape how reproduction is understood and managed in given times and places, shaping the future of population health (Hartmann 2016; Kline 2010; Roberts 1999; Bridges 2011).

Biological reproduction has been a site of intense focus because many societies invest in the idea that future generations carry with them another form of reproduction: the process by which values, tradition, culture, and religion are carried forward. The figure of child, then, distills and carries with it the social, cultural, religious, and political elements that will be reproduced, if with alterations, for future generations. In this sense, the health humanities have a key role to play in uncovering the sociopolitical role that medicine, medical practice, and innovation in medicine play not only in determining the biological characteristics of future generations but in reflecting and promoting values and ideologies that shape the very processes of biological and social reproduction. For example, who has access to an abortion or to fertility treatments are not simply biological questions but at once reflect and, in turn, promote political, social, and religious values. Health humanities work is crucial, then, because it challenges medical framings of reproduction that would render the term largely a natural process, if not, according to some proponents, *the most natural* biological process. The danger of investing in rhetoric that reduces reproduction to a natural biological process (itself an ideological position) is that it hands control of reproduction over to scientific experts in arenas like the law rather than considering and foregrounding reproduction's significant and knotty sociocultural complexities.

A health humanities perspective on reproduction can help counteract the failure of the current health-care regulation to address issues of health inequality where the current legal regime favors some people over others under the guise of objective, scientific consideration. In assisted reproduction, for example, most states in the United States do not mandate that insurance cover new technologies. This means that people who cannot afford assisted reproduction are unable to access it even if they need access to these medical procedures to have children. In that sense, reproduction is not simply biological but contingent on class. LGBTQ people may also face challenges to access because of contemporary definitions of infertility, which require those seeking care to prove they have attempted to reproduce on their own repeatedly for a set period of time. Understanding how definitions of reproduction influence medical knowledge, practice, and regulation allows us to see these limitations as discriminatory, which is the first step in addressing inequality.

Health humanities can thereby help make visible the sociopolitical biases hidden in the regulation and implementation of new technologies. A focus on the sociocultural dimensions of reproduction as well as the kinds of narrative, rhetorical, historical, and ethical understanding the health humanities brings to bear on the term is necessary as we seek more just outcomes for our reproductive futures. Feminist and critical race theorists working in health humanities have been vigilant in uncovering medical science's biased centering of the white man's body as the anchor for research. The "gods eye view" of the world—that there can be an objective way to "know" the world—offers a limited perspective (Haraway 1988). As Sandra Harding argues, knowledge derived from marginalized people produces a more nuanced—hence, more accurate—view than that produced by those who wield most power, especially for "explaining the limitations of standard accounts of nature and social relations" (1998, 163).

Despite the popularity of this viewpoint since the 1980s, courts in the United States have continued to use a positivistic understanding of science and expertise in the domain of reproduction. Even as the court began to liberalize abortion laws, they reified the idea that science and medicine should lead the way and that the law should follow (Ahmed 2015). In *Roe v. Wade*, the 1973 decision that decriminalized abortion in the United States, Justice Blackmun famously turned to medical science as a way to avoid the controversies surrounding abortion including population control and environmental issues. By starting down the path of the right to abortion as rationalized by scientific truth and progress as the Supreme Court did in *Roe*, the Court shut down the possibility that science itself might be politically constructed, hence reflect the sociopolitical environment. It enabled the rise of a conservative "science" that aimed to depict abortion as harmful to women and painful for the fetus. By treating this evidence as on par with other claims made by abortion and antiabortion advocates the Court gave these claims legitimacy. As disturbing challenges to *Roe* have mounted in the courts, leading to the recent *Dobbs v. Jackson* ruling that overturned *Roe*, it has become more important than ever to challenge the sociopolitical dynamics that legitimate the potential to outlaw abortion. Rather than viewing the court as a mere recipient and neutral adjudicator of legal, moral, and scientific assertions, humanities-oriented scholars demonstrate law plays a role in legitimating some claims over others (Ahmed 2015; Jasanoff 2015).

An uncritical reliance on medical facts concerning reproduction independent of context and other factors extends beyond the period between conception and birth, where childhood and parenthood are likewise used to sociopolitical ends. For example, the claim that "crack" use was producing "crack" babies in the 1980s resulted in the incarceration of Black women and the separation of families. The crack-baby narrative also enabled an ongoing vilification of Black women and the poor as irresponsible and undeserving of welfare. For these Black women, reproduction was framed as a liability to the state, producing more individuals as dependents. The Reagan administration narrated the problem as a story about Black women—framed as "welfare queens"—exploiting a system for economic gain

(Roberts 1999; M. Goodwin 2020). The narrative turned the public's attention away from the conditions that produced widespread drug use (not limited to any race or gender) and its ramifications and toward an excuse for the dismantling of the welfare state. This strategy is on display in the 1980 case *Harris v. McRae*, for example, in which plaintiffs seeking to challenge the application of the Hyde Amendment—the ban on federal funds to reimburse the cost of abortions under Medicaid—for medically necessary abortions for the indigent. The Court upheld the amendment with the explanation that "although government may not place obstacles in the path of a woman's exercise of her freedom of choice, it need not remove those not of its own creation. Indigency falls in the latter category" (Harris v. McRae, 448 US 297 [1980]). In other words, the government does not cause poverty; women are poor of their own making. When a woman is poor of her own making, the government has no obligation to pay for her abortion. Health humanities scholars have had and continue to have an important role to play in placing these decisions in context and dislodging them from a formalist understanding of lawmaking, shedding light on the relationship between law, reproduction, and the state.

Humanities perspectives on reproduction in its various meanings, uses, and entanglements not only offer opportunities to explore how society understands health in a variety of contexts—individual, social, economic, political, cultural, and religious—but also suggest ways to intervene in the political uses of the natural and the scientific that claim to be outside of or above politics or ideology. By asking questions about the history, rhetoric, narrative, and ethics of reproduction, scholars in the health humanities can play an important role in recontextualizing assumptions about the nature of reproduction and, in so doing, helping reveal the complexity of the politics surrounding it.

54

Risk

Amy Boesky

The word *risk* came into English in the late medieval period from the Italian (*riscio*, "danger") and the French (*risqué*). Its initial sphere was economic, used "as a description of uncertain commercial transactions" (Itzen and Muller 2016, 9). The new term was linked to new aversions: Niklas Luhmann suggests it was associated with apprehension, as older ideas of Fortune (allegorical and religious) gave way to a newly monetized idea of risk emphasizing human agency (Itzen and Muller 2016, 10). Whereas earlier ideas of danger had belonged to the realm of the divine, modern "risk" fell in the human domain. One aspect of this shift was the sense *risk* was something that could be hedged against or avoided. Maritime ventures changed both the vocabulary and the practice for assessing gains and losses, helping to create a new (and antithetical) social value of "prudence" (Itzen and Muller 2016, 9–10). Emphasis on being careful emerged as modern ideas of risk were taking shape. Both ideas eventually found themselves projected onto other fields, including medicine and, in the twentieth century, the emerging field of public health. Connections between risk and personal responsibility may pose challenges for health and health care, but they also offer opportunities, particularly in charting transdisciplinary ventures.

Risk is often represented in quantitative terms. We measure risk: someone has, say, a 30 percent chance of contracting a certain disease; heart attack risk increases based on a lipid profile. While risk pertains to the individual, its measurement is comparative, depending on a statistical norm based on population.

The connection between health and statistics has a long history. The eighteenth century made advances in mathematical modeling (Laplace, Bernoulli, Graunt, Quetelet, Ferr, Condorcet) including censuses, probability studies, and medical topographies. From 1830 to 1870, a "flood tide" of such studies appeared (G. Rosen 1958, 147). In the mid-1800s, Adolphe Quetelet developed the concept of *l'homme moyen* (the average man), produced by a systematic study of statistical tendencies (G. Rosen 1958, 149). This "average" could distinguish those without known health risks from those with vulnerabilities.

Quetelet's "average man" demonstrates that assessing risk is never simple. Which population is studied? Who is omitted? How are disparities weighted? Moreover, quantitative representations occlude the subjective experience of risk. Why do some people experience a statistical propensity for disease differently than others? What does risk feel like? To answer these questions, we must include qualitative as well as quantitative materials. If, for instance, you are a woman in the United States, your (statistical) odds of developing breast cancer may be as high as 1 in 8, increasing as you age, and those chances may increase based on family history, environmental exposures, race, or ethnicity. But how you experience risk will be shaped by individual experiences: what is "high risk" to one person may be imperceptible to someone else. Risk has a subjective as well as a statistical value. As I write, in the "messy middle" of the global pandemic, responses to spikes in COVID-19 across the world have ranged from nonchalance to terror. The subjective sense of risk posed by the virus is as varied as its symptoms and outcomes.

From the qualitative perspective, risk involves agency and control. Risk, after all, is not the same as danger.

Risk is more abstract; it is future-oriented, an adversity or hardship feared to come later rather than a challenge faced in the here and now. You can, and often should, do something about a known risk. Still, associations between risk and control, especially in medicine and public health, can be problematic. People believed to be at high risk for poor health often experience discrimination: eating a high-fat diet, using drugs, or having unprotected sex are all seen as risky choices, and individuals are often judged as deserving the negative consequences of such behaviors. Health vulnerabilities, however, rarely track to a single cause. Individuals may inherit health risks or may be more susceptible to disease by virtue of both biological heredity and inherited social conditions. Health risks are often socially constructed and too frequently misunderstood or overlooked.

The desire to quantify risk is often part of a larger desire to control it. Yet our criteria for measuring risk remain crude. In my study of genetic subjectivities, for instance, I found people describe heritable risks for conditions such as deafness, early-onset Alzheimer's, breast cancer, or Huntington's Disease in strikingly different ways (Boesky 2013). Statistics are experienced across a spectrum. Is 1/100 big or small? A heritable risk for a potentially fatal condition may feel insurmountable to one person, leading to avoiding marriage or having children, yet is perceived as manageable for someone else. Cultural narratives also shape risk and its perception. Medical professionals often describe having a baby with Down's syndrome as a "risk" to parents when weighing genetic testing. Yet the discourse of risk presumes a host of nested ideas about norms and disabilities. Health policies rely on representations of risk that presume shared underlying assumptions about what constitutes "health."

Ideas of risk are also historically inflected. Sociologists Ulrich Beck, Anthony Giddens, and Niklas Luhmann argue risk is tied to industrial modernization. Beck writes that a "risk society" emerged in late-twentieth-century culture, shaped by the threat of unpreventable large-scale disaster (nuclear accidents, pollution; Beck [1986] 1992, 21). Giddens emphasizes the temporality of risk: its most important characteristic is projecting danger into the future. And Luhmann highlights the distinction between risk (connected to human behavior and choice) and danger (which implies an external threat).

Contemporary ideas of health risk have been strongly influenced by the rise of insurance companies working to understand relationships between health hazards and cost of treatment early in the twentieth century. The compound word *risk group* dates from 1912, around the emergence of "the first extensive movement for a comprehensive system of compulsory sickness insurance" (G. Rosen 1958, 265). *Risk group* shifts the sense of hazard from individuals to populations believed to share vulnerabilities based on age, race, ethnicity, or "unhealthy" behaviors. Early epidemiology relied on classifying and studying such "risk groups" to better understand determinants of disease. Classifying "risk groups" can usefully inform public policy and health reforms, but such groupings often stigmatize or delegitimize minorities, the elderly, people living in financial precarity, or people with physical or cognitive disabilities. Stigma is compounded when health insurance companies monetize risk, using actuarial charts to determine how life expectancy might increase or decrease based on the risks carried by an individual. Health risks in these terms are costly—the larger group "carries" those who are vulnerable. (Though "sickness coverage" dates from the late-nineteenth century in the United States, modern health insurance really began to emerge in the 1920s and '30s.) While identifying individuals at elevated risk is fundamental to public health, these groupings can shore up ableist constructions of "health" and stigmatize groups deemed most vulnerable. As risk groups are formed, differences get reified, and while "risk groups" may benefit from public money, programs, or outreach, they may also become targets of stigma, penalized for risk factors in the workplace, education, and wider aspects of social and cultural life, a problem created by an overreliance on quantitative representations of risk.

We can counter this tendency by thinking about health vulnerabilities qualitatively as well as quantitatively. Conceptions of risk challenge us to think about individuals and groups simultaneously. Thinking carefully about risk beyond our own individual experiences may open new opportunities for research and clinical care: recognizing that transgender youth may be at increased risk of depression, for instance, or studying risk factors for breast cancer in regions associated with high toxicities from pollution can improve care. Considering who is at risk and what risks have not yet been explored may engender more compassionate models for future care work.

We might also fruitfully reevaluate risks experienced by health-care workers, whose sacrifices are often deemed "heroic" by cultural narratives that appear to privilege providers while instead erasing their needs (and their humanity). Providers' legitimate risks of burnout, compassion exhaustion, and chronic fatigue could more usefully be addressed through reconsiderations of clinical education, while protective workplace measures could mitigate unnecessary risks that, however "heroic" they may be, are not consistent with best practices. We cannot and should not try to live entirely without risk, for that would rule out development, growth, adventure, creativity, and connection. In the health humanities, however, we do well to expand our understanding of risk, even as we remember its histories.

Not only should we be attuned to subjective and qualitative experiences in addition to relying on data, but we would also be well served in remembering that notions of carefulness emerged in response to the opportunities (and hazards) risk engenders.

55

Sense

Erica Fretwell

Crosscutting the cultural, political, and epistemological coordinates of health, sense has been hiding in plain sight: elemental to organic life yet an elusive object of humanistic study. For much of the twentieth century, neuroscience dominated the study of sense. At the turn of the twenty-first century, the formation of the interdisciplinary field of sensory studies served to push back against dominant scientific accounts of sense as a universal phenomenon reducible to the brain and to instead demonstrate that sense is a lived experience—and therefore historically conditioned, culturally variable, and socially constructed. The value-laden contexts of *how* and *why* we perceive shape *what* we perceive (Howes 2003). This critical reconfiguration of sense furnishes key insights into how the intricacies of bodily life, living, and livelihood are managed and imagined at the microlevel of perception and feeling. Following the Western philosophical and scientific genealogy of sense can illuminate the colonial logics that historically and continuously govern the uneven distribution of humanity and health. Only by decolonizing sense might we forge a new "sense" of health organized around the in*ter*dependence, rather than independence, of all bodies and things.

Sense encompasses body and mind, yet Western philosophy has framed the component parts of sense as mutually exclusive. *Oxford English Dictionary* presents sense as relating to "meaning, intelligibility, [and] coherence" and to "any of the faculties of sight, hearing, smell, taste, and touch . . . as opposed to the intellect, spirit, etc." (*OED Online* 2021, "sense"). Sense is either ideal *or* material, spiritual *or* corporeal, rational *or* emotional. Lexical bifurcation divides bodily experience into two parts—mind and matter—and then pits them against each other.

This opposition dates back to classical antiquity. Aristotle famously likened sense to pressing a gold signet ring into a block of sealing wax, which transfers the ring's design (form) but not its gold (matter); sense is the form or "impress" the object world leaves on the mind. But not all sense impressions are born equal. Aristotle split the perceptual faculty into five senses, then hierarchized them based on their proximity to reason: sight, hearing, smell, taste, and touch, respectively. Sight, hearing, and smell were "rational" senses because they place distance—requisite for reflection, the basis of ethics—between body and world, and taste and touch were "emotional" senses because they put the body and world in contact. This mind/matter distinction further differentiated humans from animals: human consciousness favors rational senses that subordinate the body to ethical values, whereas animal consciousness relies on emotional senses that activate the unruly urges and primal pleasures of the flesh. The classical sense hierarchy doubled as a hierarchy of organic development.

Aristotelean psychology influenced Western liberal philosophy's conception of Man as a rational subject—a notion that, since the seventeenth century, helped fuel racial capitalism (born of settler colonialism, the Atlantic slave trade, and imperialism) and justify the genocide and oppression of "primitive" people. Indeed, the cornerstone of John Locke's empiricism (all knowledge comes from the senses) and Adam Smith's theory of moral sentiment (directing our perceptions toward feeling for others) was a newly materialist model of sense; scientists revealed that the nerves mediate consciousness by transmitting sensations to the mind, which then direct the body. Imagined as a "body politic" whose health depends on "fellow feeling" among citizens, the liberal state required *sensibility*, the neurophysiological capacity to cultivate raw sensations and transform them into refined feelings like sympathy. The civic ideal was a "sensible self": a porous body that absorbs sensations but that is tempered by a mind agential enough to turn those sensations into sentiments that guide autonomous action (Knott 2009). At the nexus of physiology and philosophy, sensibility biologized social life by delimiting civic membership along the bounds of mental acuity and bodily vitality.

In the teeth of liberalism and empiricism, sense became a concept of universal reason that secured colonial hierarchies of humanity. "Having" sense meant having the ability to regulate the bodily senses, "to perceive and observe in normal ways," which made one a sympathetic and rational subject—and made it possible to "[be] considered human" (Ogden 2013, 425). And as the science of sensation came into contact with emergent theories of heredity in the nineteenth century, the anatomopolitics of sensibility (targeting the body of the self) gave way to a sentimental biopolitics (targeting the body of the species). This biopolitics turned on the neo-Lamarckian theory of impressibility: the survival of a species depends on its ability to acquire sensations and transmit sentiments over generations.

Sensibility and impressibility were vectors of racialization, shaping how the health of peoples and populations was managed. Race scientists and social reformers held that impressibility was unevenly distributed among human beings—civilized races more impressible than primitive races—and hence key to determining which populations were biologically "fit" enough to make live and those the state ought to let die (Schuller 2018a). Groups allegedly unable to feel

pain were treated as objects of research for improving white people's health, such as the gynecological experiments that J. Marion Sims performed on enslaved Black women without consent and without anesthesia (Cooper Owens 2017). Eugenics policies—from antimiscegenation laws to the forced sterilization of "feebleminded" white and nonwhite people—were a response to fears that white people's decreasing reproduction rate would cause "race suicide." And the US government "revitalized" indigenous tribes by kidnapping and "rehoming" indigenous children to teach them the cultivation of sentiment (Wexler 2000). Liberal conceptions of sense thus underpinned the disposability of "insensible" peoples, which ensured the protection and preservation of the civilized white body.

While the dominant liberal philosophy held that "the newly defined 'other' did not perceive, experience, or sense the world as it was," racialized peoples have long been theorizing and practicing alternate kinds of *sense*—with decidedly anticolonial effects (Gómez 2017, 116). The Afro-Caribbean belief system Obeah, for instance, comprises a "set of bodily responses to the world" directly opposed to the "objective forms of sense perception that were gaining traction in the Enlightenment" (Jaudon 2012, 716). The Obeah worldview sees humankind as situated within a web of agential objects; sense is not "internal" to any one body but is *distributive*, a perceptual experience that takes shape among bodies and things. Obeah deregulates the senses, insisting that the sensory body's attachments to (rather than its dominion over) the natural world is the basis of individual health and collective survival. For enslaved Black people, this entanglement of spiritual and physical worlds upended Lockean sense, the epistemological perch upon which "the political order of colonial things" rested (Stoler 2009, 9). As such, Obeah was an "essential form of slave resistance" that deployed a desecularized, "fugitive" empiricism to estrange enslavers from the common sense they wielded against their subjects (Hogarth 2017, 84).

Obeah highlights the limitations of Western medicine, organized around liberal conceptions of the self-enclosed body. When sense is something one does or does not have—not what draws human and nonhuman bodies into relation—all that is external to the self becomes a threat. In the nineteenth century, for example, scientists developed the medical notion of nervous sensitivity. Because of its elastic nerves, the civilized white body was an "open body," receptive to external stimuli (Murison 2011, 3). Yet this receptivity might make the white body *too* open to the world. Susceptibility to modern civilization's panoply of stimuli expressed "physiological refinement, development of the nerves, and consequently evolution in terms of civilization as 'sensitivity'" (Strick 2014, 72). But it also could mark the devolution of the sensible self into a nervous self. US physician George Beard claimed that sensitivity caused "neurasthenia," a debilitating nervous disorder involving fatigue, insomnia, and irritability that plagued bourgeois white women. Neurasthenia was a mark of racial and class distinction—up until, Charlotte Perkins Gilman's story "The Yellow Wallpaper" (1891) shows, it tips over into the pathologically female mental illness called hysteria. The white woman's body required medical intervention to ensure that sensibility did not become sensitivity, a raw state of feeling that leads away from, rather than toward, rational sense.

While environmental stimuli had the power to sicken the civilized body, the senses were also diagnostic tools for distinguishing health and disease. Prior to the turn-of-the-twentieth-century bacteriological revolution, the miasma theory of disease ("bad air" from decomposing matter spreads disease) dominated medical science. As a result, smell was thought to indicate the spread of contagion—and a person's social class. Given the importance of circulating clean air, the systematic control of odors (e.g., hygiene codes) became central to public health policy. With the consequent conflation of poverty and disease, the "bourgeois emphasis on the stench of the poor and the bourgeois desire for deodorization were inseparable" (Corbin 1986, 144). But even as the epistemic value of smell waned with the ascendance of the germ theory of disease (the theory that pathogens spread illness), the olfactory sense mapped onto the uneven geographical conditions that determine health. The link between air quality and health that smell registered once was material, but today this link is structural. From urbanization to postindustrialization, air is "an uneven medium of physical and mental health" that has enabled "sociability in some places, while inducing asthma and exhaustion in others" (H. Hsu 2016, 794, 789). Although in the case of odorless toxins smell does not always index pollution, it nonetheless points to the structural inequities—for example, the housing crisis that forces a family to live in an asbestos-laden apartment—that produce racialized health disparities. In contrast to the Victorian women whose nervous sensitivity made them "naturally" vulnerable to their environment, specific senses like smell materialize the slow violence visited upon those who *are made vulnerable* to their environment.

These genealogies help us recognize that *sense* names the conceptual and material problem of the body's physical and emotional vulnerability, its entanglement with a world it cannot control. Disability studies scholarship helps us imagine new possibilities for health humanities because it approaches complex embodiment and neurodiversity as a phenomenological orientation and a world-making capacity. Autistic consciousness, for instance, is marked by a "susceptibility to overstimulating situations" that powers "ways to imagine alternative disability universes," ultimately re-making sense itself (D. Mitchell and Snyder 2015, 201). Addressing issues of caregiving, Janet Price and Margrit Shildrick consider touch its own kind of medical ethics, for it is a sense that "demands recognition that our sense of self, and how we orientate ourselves to the world, is irrevocably tied up with the bodies of those around us" (2002, 63). Today, against the backdrop of medical and carceral institutions that involuntarily or coercively ad-minister psychotropic drugs to deaden people's senses, the call for more touching and feeling, for a decolonial and nonableist configuration of sense—a robust, em-bodied sense—is a matter of shared survival. How might human and nonhuman health be reimagined when we regard sense as a zone of contact rather than an indi-vidual capacity?

56
Sex
René Esparza

The English word *sex* has multiple origins, from Old French *sex* and Latin *sexus* (possibly from *secāre*, "to cut"), and locates the first English usage in the fourteenth century, referring to the divisions of humans and many other living organisms between male and female on the basis of genitalia and other physical organs involved in reproductive functions.

The term evolved, in the commonsense Western us-age, to index an identity and a practice. One has a sex (a specific set of genetic, chemical, and anatomical charac-teristics that mark one as "male" or "female"), and one has sex (based off the heterosexual or homosexual at-traction one has to others). Beginning in the late 1800s, Western science and medicine proliferated a series of narratives in which sex was vested with "truth" about human bodies. These narratives imposed upon sex an intensified system of classification, observation, and intervention.

The poststructuralist turn in the humanities and social sciences in the 1970s and 1980s introduced new ways of thinking about sex and its engagement with power and modes of governance. Experts in the hu-manities and social sciences refuted the dogma that outwardly observable behavioral attributes (gender) corresponded with biological or anatomical features (sex; Karkazis et al. 2012). Queer theory and disability studies have since interrogated the role of biomedical knowledge in the discursive production of sex, show-ing how medicine, far from scientifically objective, has authored the criteria through which bodies are (and continue to be) classified as "normal" and rewarded as such—or diagnosed as "abnormal" and punished accordingly.

The two-sex system of categorization, although institutionalized as universal, cannot capture the full spectrum of human sexuality (Fausto-Sterling 2000). Intersex people, for instance, are born with sex characteristics that do not correspond to dominant notions of biological maleness and femaleness. Estimated to occur roughly once per two thousand births, intersex births attest to the breadth of human physical variance (E. Reiss and McCarthy 2016). No single physiological or biological feature enables simple demarcation of people into male or female (Jordan-Young 2011; Karkazis 2008); indeed, none of the markers of sex—chromosomes, gonads, hormones, secondary sex characteristics, external and internal genitalia—are present in all people labeled male or female. Nonetheless, by the 1950s, experts in medicine and psychology prioritized external genital morphology as the determining factor in how to treat people with intersex traits (E. Reiss 2009). Psychologist John Money and his colleagues at Johns Hopkins University standardized gender "corrective" surgery after reasoning that matching the genitals of the child with the gender chosen by doctors would ensure parental and child psychological well-being (Meyerowitz 2002). But as intersex activists have countered, many of these infants have since grown into adults who reject their surgical gender assignment (Carpenter 2016). As a result, pediatric endocrinologists, urologists, and psychologists have reexamined the practice of early genital surgery, with some countries now banning the practice and health advocates deeming it a human rights violation (Human Rights Watch and InterACT Advocates for Intersex Youth 2017).

By ensuring that genitalia were deemed appropriate for adult heterosexual performance, doctors' medical decision-making was shaped by "compulsory heterosexuality," the assumption that men and women are innately attracted to one another emotionally and sexually (Rich 1980). The belief that heterosexuality is the universal norm underscores the prominence of the seemingly stable relations between the concepts of biological sex, gender, and erotic desire that Judith Butler (1990) calls the "heterosexual matrix." Yet the very concepts of "heterosexuality" and its corollary, "homosexuality," are recent (Katz 1995; Rubin 1984). Although men and women have been having sex, marrying, and establishing families for millennia, there was no special name for their acts or desires. That changed on May 6, 1888, when Austro-Hungarian journalist Karl-Maria Kertbeney used the words *heterosexual* and *homosexual* in a letter to German sexologist Karl Ulrichs (Blank 2012). Within a few short decades, those words would be etched into the collective psyche by medicine and psychiatry as the bywords for "normal" and "abnormal" sexual acts and desires.

In *The History of Sexuality*, Michel Foucault ([1976] 1990, 34) traces how sexuality, beginning in the eighteenth century, underwent an "incitement to discourse." Far from being repressed, sexuality was endlessly discussed for the purpose of identifying, managing, and/or correcting "abnormal" sexual expressions. Foucault shows how industrialization prompted a shift from the sovereign power of preindustrial societies—where rulers had the power of life or death over their subjects—to a more diffuse form of power spread out through society like a network and in which the goal is to optimize *certain* forms of life, which he calls "biopower." This new form of power brought individuals under surveillance from multiple directions at once: law, science, and medicine. And, argues Foucault, it accounts for the emphasis on bodily discipline and normativity in modern capitalist societies, which led to the emergence of sexuality as an identity category. Although prior to the 1860s homosexual acts were treated as criminal or sinful, they did not indicate a person's innate proclivities. With the institutional rise of medical discourse and the emergence of new fields of study, including psychiatry, homosexual acts became aligned with a type of person: the homosexual. Under this modern regime of sexuality, homosexual people would be subjected to medical treatment for the purpose of "curing" them of their "perverse" desires.

This biomedicalization of sex in the late 1800s coincided with the rise of eugenics as a philosophy and social movement that advocated the selective reproduction of "desirable" populations. As Siobhan Sommerville (2000) shows, methods popular in the medical and scientific literature of eugenics, such as anthropometry—the measurement of the human body—proved instructive for early sexologists. A pioneer of sexology, the scientific study of human sexual behavior, Havelock Ellis assumed that the sexual "invert" was distinguishable from the "normal" body through anatomical markings like physical differences mapped onto race. Focusing on the reproductive anatomy of female sexual inverts, Ellis insisted that enlarged clitorises were somehow a mark of sexual excess, hence degeneracy. Given the imprimatur of science, eugenics ascended as one of the main instigators behind practices that sanctioned the abuse, discrimination, and at times death of "biologically inferior" populations: people of color, queer people, and people with disabilities (McRuer 2006).

Medico-scientific rationales likewise certified the expansive regulatory powers of public health in the late 1800s and early 1900s. With the license to survey and monitor cities and their inhabitants, public health authorities instituted protocols of personal hygiene and public sanitation. In their mandate to remove any medical menace, however, public health authorities harnessed the medicalized language of racialized sexual deviance to name and contain threats. Sex became a means of regenerating race and an instrument of white supremacy. In the late-1800s San Francisco, for example, as Nayan Shah (2001) illustrates, health officials characterized Chinese female sex workers as vectors of disease who endangered white families through the transmission of syphilis. This medicalized construction of Chinese people as disease-ridden amplified a fervent anti-Chinese animus that resulted in exclusionary immigration laws, including the Page Law of 1875, which banned the immigration of "prostitutes" from China, Japan, and "any Oriental country," essentially shutting down the immigration of unaccompanied Asian women.

The perceived sexual excess of women of color also facilitated rampant sterilization abuse. In the 1927 case *Buck v. Bell*, the US Supreme Court upheld the state of Virginia's right to forcibly sterilize anyone labeled "unfit," providing legal precedent for other states to enact compulsory sterilization laws (Lombardo 2002). As many as seventy thousand Americans were involuntarily sterilized throughout the twentieth century. People who were labeled "mentally deficient" as well as those who were deaf, blind, mute, epileptic, and even alcoholic were sterilized, usually without their consent and often without their knowledge. The state of California alone sterilized approximately twenty thousand people (Lira and Stern 2014). At Pacific Colony in Pomona, California, Mexican-origin women were sterilized at rates out of proportion to their population, often for violating white middle-class norms of respectability, such as "promiscuously" having children out of wedlock. The biomedicalization of racialized sexuality likewise sanctioned and naturalized colonial power. Under the Indian Health Service, as many as 25 percent of Indigenous women between the ages of fifteen and forty-four were sterilized by the 1970s (J. Lawrence 2000).

Medicalized discourses that frame racialized sexuality as deviant have similarly legitimated medical experimentation on bodies of color. The Tuskegee Syphilis Experiment, for instance, was based on a belief that Black people were far more lascivious than white people. Yet 61 percent of syphilis cases in Macon County, Alabama—where participating Black male sharecroppers lived—were congenital, nonvenereal syphilis (Washington 2006). In Puerto Rico, where a third of all Puerto Rican mothers ages twenty to forty-nine had been sterilized by 1965, doctors conducted clinical trials for Enovid, the first oral contraceptive, on Puerto Rican women at a public housing development (L. Briggs 2002). The women were administered a hormone dosage ten times what is administered today, resulting in dire side effects, including three deaths (Cacchioni 2015).

Queer and feminist health activists of the 1960s and 1970s challenged the use of biomedical knowledge to "correct" so-called sexual abnormalities. Aided by Alfred Kinsey's midcentury surveys of sexual behavior in the United States, LGBTQ activists under the banner of the Gay Liberation Front (GLF) challenged the dominant belief that homosexuality was an illness when, in 1970, members of the Chicago chapter of the GLF distributed "A Leaflet for the American Medical Association" to doctors present at the convention of the American Medical Association (A. J. Lewis 2016). The activists argued that LGBTQ people experienced mental distress not because they were sick but because they were subject to pervasive homophobia, legitimated by the scientific authority of the medical establishment. In 1973, the American Psychiatric Association removed homosexuality from the *Diagnostic and Statistical Manual of Mental Disorders*, replacing it, in 1980, with the new diagnostic category "gender identity disorder in childhood" (GIDC).

Queer and feminist health activism remains more pertinent than ever as racist and able-bodied discourses around normative sex continue to shape public health and welfare reform policies. As Dorothy Roberts (1999) shows, because politicians regard the so-called hyperfertility of women of color as the culprit behind poverty—not state racism or neoliberal capitalism—policy responses focus on reforming the sexual practices of women of color. In 2020, reports about the unwanted hysterectomies performed on immigrant women detained by Immigration and Customs Enforcement (ICE) reminded the public about the continued devaluation of reproduction among certain populations.

Because medical science has historically treated nonwhite, queer, and disabled populations as diseased or deviant, medical humanities would benefit from deeper engagement with queer theory and disability studies. Queer theory deconstructs traditional notions about gender and sexuality, questioning the embrace of heterosexuality as the universal norm and the insistence of rigid binaries. Disability studies, meanwhile, identifies the deleterious effects of normalization on people's experience of their bodies and desires. Critical medical humanities would, in turn, challenge what is prescribed as "normative" and instead recognize human variety in corporeal embodiment and erotic desire—disentangling the biopolitical linkage between "normal" sex and health.

57

Sleep

Benjamin Reiss

For much of its run through history, sleep was understood as a state that temporarily released the soul from the body. Virtually all religious traditions view dreams as a vehicle for accessing spiritual visions (Bulkeley 2008). In ancient Greece, dreams could yield either a magical inward sight or a message from the gods (Hacking 2002); reports of Hopi and Ojibwa dreams also reveal high spiritual content (P. Burke 1997). In early modern England and France, the sleeping body was popularly viewed as a battleground in which divine or demonic forces could seize the soul, prefiguring its ultimate destiny after death (Handley 2016, 77). But little medical attention was paid to the lumpish, nondreaming aspects of sleep other than how to manipulate it through hygiene, diet, or potions (Kroker 2007, 25–29, 60–64). According to the Aristotelian tradition, which persisted through much of early modern thought, while dreams could carry dreamers into the empyrean, sleep itself put human flesh on a par with plants and animals (Sullivan 2012). Recently, this leveling has extended to computers and other machinery that are said to be in "sleep mode."

In the age of sleep science and sleep industry, slumber has lost most of its spiritual associations and has been conjoined to a dizzying array of biomedical concepts, practices, technologies, and institutions. Since the second half of the twentieth century, *sleep* has become the first term in a proliferating set of compounds: sleep disorders, sleep centers, sleep clinics, sleep research, sleep

science, sleep aids, sleep hygiene, sleep trainers, sleep trackers. The content of dreams has been of relatively little interest during this period—a blip in the long history of sleep. Denuded of spiritual or metaphysical content, sleep is valued as a marker of health, efficiency, and productivity: both as fuel for economic activity and as a magnet for entrepreneurs, researchers, and hucksters who claim to hold the keys to its kingdom.

"Sleep science" had its legendary start in the 1930s with the research of Nathaniel Kleitman: famed as a codiscoverer of REM state, he also authored important studies on fatigue and wakefulness. William Dement later established the first sleep clinic and taught the first course on sleep in a medical school in 1972 (Kroker 2007, 222–36). The field, now often referred to as "sleep and circadian science," has hit boom times. The Emory University Libraries list twenty journals with *sleep* in the title; over 2,500 sleep clinics are in operation in the US alone; over five thousand researchers and clinicians attend the annual meeting of the Associated Professional Sleep Societies; and sleep research flourishes in neurology, psychiatry, dentistry, epidemiology, pulmonology, endocrinology, sports medicine, and pharmacology. The *International Classification of Sleep Disorders* (the first edition of which was published in 1990) describes over seventy disorders from insomnia to exploding head syndrome. Notwithstanding this proliferation, sleep researchers often complain about the lack of public awareness about—and relative lack of funding for—sleep research as opposed to research on addiction, nutrition, or pain management.

Connections between sleep and "health" go well beyond medicalization. "Healthy sleep" is understood to promote resistance to disease and efficient recovery or recuperation, but it is also linked to wakeful efficiency, peak levels of concentration, reduced stress and anxiety, and avoidance of the risks associated with fatigue.

Healthy sleep may be abetted by medical means—pills and respirators, for example—but also by advice books, training systems, online chat forums, and a dizzying array of commercial products.

The economization and commodification of sleep works in several directions: products are designed to produce, maintain, or customize it; other products, like cell phones and video games, are said to block or warp it. It is treated as fuel for optimal performance in school, work, sport, and the military, and sleep deprivation is often measured in economic terms of lost productivity. The economic impact of sleep loss is a matter of concern not just for individuals but for corporations and even nations (Hafner et al. 2016). Yet sleep is also one of the last great freely available, if unequally distributed, resources (Crary 2013).

The term *sleep health* can apply both to individuals and to whole populations that experience sleep disruptions or disturbances as a result of social inequities, rough living conditions, traumas, or discrimination. This parallels recent use of *debility* to refer to impairments or disabilities that are experienced broadly within populations exposed to environmental hazards, labor risks, or traumas of war or punishment (Puar 2017). The journal *Sleep Health* features research devoted to sleep and population health, including articles on sleep issues facing refugees, veterans, minoritized populations, teens, disabled people, bus drivers, and caregivers, among others.

As medical and scientific attention to sleep has risen, sleep talk is also saturating culture. The ProQuest newspaper database shows close to two million articles with sleep in the title over the past ten years. Memoirs, novels, and films have been a little slower to catch on, in part because sleep—other than the dreaming part—is seemingly antithetical to narrative. Nonetheless, films like *Inception* (2010) and *The Science of Sleep* (2006)

lavishly picture the world of dreams, and novels like Karin Thompson Walker's *The Age of Miracles* (2012) and *The Dreamers* (2019) and Karen Russell's *Sleep Donation* (2014) tell dramatic stories about sleep's ruination in an off-kilter world. Ottessa Moshfegh's unsettling *My Year of Rest and Relaxation* (2018) is an allegory of post-9/11 history viewed through the barely open eyes of a woman trying to drug herself into virtual hibernation. Despite making these inroads into fiction for adults, sleep's most successful attempt to colonize literature has been in the genre of children's bedtime books. Their pages—or boards—are inherently tied to rituals of bourgeois sleep: they frequently conclude with scenes of children, or barnyard animals, overcoming fears agreeing to go off to bed, alone in their own rooms (Wolf-Meyer 2012, 129–44)—a plot device akin to the weddings that resolve the plots of nineteenth-century novels. The lullaby is the musical genre associated most clearly with sleep, but recent high-concept instrumental and electronic works such as Max Richter's eight-and-a-half-hour-long *Sleep* (2015), Moby's *Long Ambients 1: Calm. Sleep* (2016), and new-agey playlists like "Healing Piano" and "Sleep Waves" intentionally induce slumber wordlessly, with sonic competition coming from the producers of hundreds of white-noise apps. Mumbling, whispering, and cooing, rather than singing or chanting, seem to be the preferred vocal soporific modes for adults: podcasts, in particular, are rich in blurry sleep talk, including the deliberately boring shaggy dogistry broadcast by Drew Ackerman in *Sleep with Me* (2013–) and the ASMR-influenced "whispered readings and ramblings" of *Sleep Whispers* (2020–). One of the few artworks to critically explore sleep and population health is the Indian documentary *Cities of Sleep* (2015), chronicling the black market in improvised sleeping accommodations for homeless residents of Delhi. Another is an exhibition/performance piece by

Navild Acosta and Fanny Sosa called "Black Power Naps" (2019), an installation of moodily lit resting stations designed for Black, indigenous, and migrant people to rest, sleep, or play. Acosta and Sosa see their installation as a response to the "sleep gap" experienced by people of color since the harsh sleeping conditions of transatlantic slavery and the traumas of colonialism (S. Burke 2019; B. Reiss 2017a, 2017b).

For all this cultural, scientific, and commercial fuss about sleep, it has gotten surprisingly short shrift in the humanities. There are no regular conferences or journals devoted to the cultural, social, and historical meanings of sleep. Yet excellent sleep-related research in the humanities exists, albeit in scattered or isolated form. The concept that history is not solely populated by people who are awake prompted both Kenton Kroker's sweeping history of sleep research, from antiquities to the turn of the twenty-first century (Kroker 2007), and A. Roger Ekirch's famous article "Sleep We Have Lost" (later incorporated into his book *At Day's Close*), which made the case that sleep patterns are subject to dramatic change over time (2001). Disrupted sleep can prompt both social conflict and economic exploitation. The historical significance of this phenomenon drives both historian Alan Derickson's exploration of sleep deprivation in relation to changes in labor formations in the twentieth century (2014b) and art historian Jonathan Crary's (2013) investigation of how globalization and neoliberalism are commodifying the final frontier of the sleeping body and blunting the social imagination. Sleep always happens *somewhere*, and a trio of recent books detail the history of the surprisingly recent invention of the bedroom, which helped establish modern notions of domesticity and privacy (Handley 2016; Perrot 2018; Fagan and Durrani 2019). Sleeplessness on the battlefield, and the broken sleep of veterans, prompted Franny Nudelman's powerful account of Vietnam-era

"sleep-ins" as a protest against military experiments in mind control (Nudelman 2019). And while sleep always happens to some*one*, its apparent unraveling of human identity has inspired philosophers and writers from early modern Europe to postmodernity (Sullivan 2012; Nancy 2009). Questions of how, when, where, and with whom we sleep—depending on who the "we" might be—propel anthropologist Matthew Wolf-Meyer's book (2012) on the social meanings of sleep's medicalization and regimentation as well as my own book on the development of Western sleeping norms and the anxieties, conflicts, and disparities they produce (Wolf-Meyer 2012; B. Reiss 2017b).

Of this work, Ekirch's finding about the prevalence of biphasic sleeping in early modern Europe has had the greatest impact on medical approaches to sleep difficulties, resulting in some changed clinical recommendations about what constitutes "insomnia" and what might be a "normal" sleeping pattern. Some historians and anthropologists, however, have questioned whether the segmented model is actually the default for *homo sapiens* (Handley 2016, 9; Yetish et al. 2015). Ekirch (2015) himself has revisited and qualified his earlier thesis.

Some of the most important concerns of humanities research today might naturally attach themselves to sleep: a biopolitical approach can explore how sleep is regulated and commodified; studies in gender, sexuality, and race can detail shifting cultural expectations, power dynamics, and inequities associated with managing the sleep/wake cycle and arranging marginalized and socially privileged sleeping bodies in space; scholars in science and technology studies have a vast array of cyborgian apparatuses to ponder. Postcolonialists can examine the implications of European regimes of efficient and private sleeping among the populations they ruled and the ways global capitalism deranges sleep schedules in the decolonizing world, while ecocritics can study how sleep configurations and technologies depend on and exploit natural resources. Histories and theories of time, architecture, sound, labor, childhood, war, capitalism, religion, disability, transportation, and urban planning all can benefit from studying the sleeping body's role in these systems as well as the waking one.

Health humanities can put this work in conversation with research in the health sciences. Exciting new scientific findings—such as the detection of the glymphatic system, which washes the brain clean of toxic proteins that build up during waking hours—are opening up new frontiers in the biomedical understanding of sleep. Humanists can interrogate the social meanings of those findings and the new technologies and treatments they will inevitably lead to as well as the cultural transmission of emerging scientific knowledge. More broadly, a humanist sense of contingency and variability concerning expectations and rules around sleep can help scientists understand the situatedness of their own investigations. Yet the relation need not be oppositional: humanistic cultural relativism versus scientific search for species-wide norms and mechanisms. Evolutionary anthropologists, for instance, point to the flexibility and variability of human sleeping arrangements and timing mechanisms as one factor that allowed human societies to flourish in so many different environments (Samson and Nunn 2015). The practice of sleep may be changing as dramatically as the science. In our productivity-fixated world, sleep tends to get wrapped around waking activities such as work, school, travel, and commerce. And when these activities are disrupted, as in a pandemic or widespread emergency, it is always fascinating to watch—often with the blurred vision of sleepless eyes—how sleep itself responds.

58

Stigma
Allan M. Brandt

Stigma has attracted attention within the health humanities in large measure because it relates to core human emotions and behaviors about disease, disability, and the body in historically and culturally specific ways. Exploring stigmas associated with various conditions and their effects on individuals and groups—through humanistic and other qualitative approaches—offers insight into fundamental questions of suffering, caregiving, social relations, health disparities, ethics and values, as well as health-care outcomes. The health humanities, broadly construed, offer important approaches and methods for understanding how stigma is generated and functions, the harms it produces, as well as strategies to mitigate its impact.

Although the word *stigma* has deep historical and theological lineage from ancient Greece to early Christianity, the modern centrality of the study of stigma as a critical concept and problem is rooted in the period from the mid-twentieth century to the present, a time of examination of universal human rights and civil rights around the globe (Hunt 2007; Donnelly 2013; Allport 1958). As a result of disease-related stigmas, people and populations have found themselves subject to prejudice and demoralization, abuse and discrimination, isolation and segregation, as well as harassment and violence. The powerful moral and pejorative judgments about those who have stigmatized conditions generate additional suffering and poor health for individuals and populations.

Diseases that are highly stigmatized—leprosy, epilepsy, HIV, mental illness, obesity, addiction, among many others—inflict multiple harms on those who find they suffer from these ailments (Schneider and Conrad 1992; Hinshaw 2007; Corrigan 2019; Farrell 2011; Herek 2007). It also has profound effects on access to services, the quality of health care, as well as health systems and economies in the United States and around the globe. Despite concerted efforts by patients, professionals, and the public to reduce disease stigmas over the last century—and especially in recent decades—they continue to impact patients and remain a major obstacle to medical and public-health efforts to improve health. Fundamental inequities that center on class, ethnicity, race, gender, and sexuality are often augmented by stigmatized diseases. Those affected by stigma suffer a double jeopardy of bodily pathology and social judgment. In this respect, the phenomenon of stigmatization is *biosocial*; the biological experience of illness cannot be fully addressed without attending to important social constituents of diseases and their moral meanings. As a result, stigma is an *embodied* harm.

Stigma materializes the impact of biases, which often ascribe disease to personal responsibility, the result of an essential moral failing. The health humanities have investigated the problem of disease stigmas to demonstrate the social and cultural processes by which individuals and groups are held accountable and blameworthy from the perspective of disease, the body, and social identities. There can be no stigma without two parties, the stigmatized and the stigmatizer. Stigma is often associated in the health humanities with the term *othering*. To "other" constitutes a process in which a person or group actively "others" another person or a group with a particular disease, condition, or identity. "Othering" is the process of creating the division of "them versus us." Stigma is therefore "produced" in particular historical and social contexts, the result of both ideas and feelings about those who are ill or suffering, those who are fundamentally excluded and devalued, and the causes of their plight. Those who actively stigmatize often express a range of affects that include fear, anger, rage, and hate. The expression of these emotions may be implicit or explicit, silent or vigorously voiced, hidden or purposeful. Those who are stigmatized often experience shame, guilt, and humiliation as well as resentment and anger. Through the examination of literature and drama, historical texts, and the arts, among other approaches, the health humanities have contributed to the identification of stigma and its implications, especially for those who experience its toxic consequences (Thornber 2020).

Although the problem of stigma has been recognized across time and cultures, its modern-day investigation is often marked by the publication of two highly influential books. Sociologist Erving Goffman, in his pathbreaking book *Stigma: Notes on the Management of Spoiled Identity*, published more than a half century ago (1963), used ethnographic methods and formal interviews to explore the experience of those who endured the indignity, isolation, and reproach of stigma. Goffman centered his assessment of stigma on "tribal" practices, the character of perceived differences, and the everyday experience of what he labeled the "spoiled identity" of those who are subject to stigma. He viewed stigma as a largely fixed, chronic social status; his essays centered on how affected individuals "managed" the shame and humiliation associated with their conditions, often through strategies of concealment and isolation (Yoshino 2006). As Goffman explained, "By definition . . . we believe the person with a stigma is not quite human." As a result, "we normals" knowingly or unknowingly reduce the life chances of those who are stigmatized (Goffman 1963,

5). Goffman defined stigma by this process of discreditation and dehumanization.

Literary critic Susan Sontag began where Goffman left off. In a series of essays central to the evolution of the health humanities, *Illness as Metaphor* (1978), she directed her attention—and antagonism—to the use of disease as a literary metaphor (Sontag 1978, 1989). She centered attention not on strategies for avoiding the impact of stigma and derision but on the experience of being stigmatized and the character of the suffering it produces for patients. She contended that the widespread use of disease metaphors caused material harm to patients with stigmatized diseases. Sontag centered attention on the meanings of tuberculosis and cancer, principally drawing on drama and fiction to explore the shifting meaning of these two prominent, life-threatening ailments. Although unacknowledged in these essays, at the time of writing, Sontag was being treated for breast cancer and had received a poor prognosis (Moser 2019). The book registered her anger at being stigmatized by the metaphors and meanings associated with cancer, especially by the perception that cancers originated as an aspect of repressed emotion.

To explain some of the profound differences in the stigmatized identities of tuberculosis and cancer patients, Sontag turned to the rise of scientific medicine. She argued that the emergence of successful biomedical understandings of TB and the development of effective antibiotic treatments at midcentury purged the disease of specious cultural beliefs, irrational fears, and victim-blaming. In short, stigmas expressed in works of drama and fiction could only be reduced through scientific and medical *progress*. According to Sontag, only the rational instrumentalities of biomedicine and the development of effective therapeutics could herald the end of persistent stigmas. This line of reasoning—centered on what is widely referred to as *medicalization*—drew considerable criticism, since it presented a positivistic view of science while ignoring the considerable evidence that medical authority and power have often been the source of formidable stigmas (take, for example, obesity). Further, Sontag did not address the question of why many diseases with effective—if not curative—treatments remained so persistently the object of stigma. As a number of studies of stigma would make evident, medical authority and cultural assumptions could also give rise to stigmatization.

In recent years, the health humanities have elaborated how stigma operates at several specific but related levels. In addition to the well-recognized harms of stigma for individuals and its characteristic *interpersonal* effects, it has also become clear that stigma has deep *sociostructural* characteristics (Pescosolido and Martin 2015). Structural stigmas have often been difficult to make visible, since they are embedded in cultural assumptions and practices, sometimes hidden or unconscious (Link and Phelan 2001; Link and Phelan 2014; Major, Dovidio, and Link 2018). Often those who stigmatize are not aware of these processes, but they account for aspects of separation, isolation, and segregation. Finally, stigma also serves powerful political and economic interests. In the process of *politicostigma*, othering is intentionally used as an explicit tool for the assertion of particular political identities, authority, and power. In this context, fear and anxiety are manipulated to enhance ideas of difference. Xenophobia is utilized to emphasize "us vs. them," a central aspect of the "tribal" stigmas that Goffman pointed to in his early treatise. In this modality, stigma serves the prevailing interests of the status quo through the subordination of the "other" (T. Morrison 2017; Tyler 2020).

Within the health humanities, the study of stigma offers important opportunities for comparative analysis across nations and cultures. While stigma may be a universal and transhistorical process, it nonetheless is expressed and produced in historically and culturally specific ways that the health humanities may potentially illuminate. A number of stigmatized diseases, conditions, and identities have become the focus of evolving fields within the humanities over recent decades. These fields constitute important approaches to understanding a range of marginalized and oppressed communities. For example, gay studies and queer theory, disability studies, crip theory, and fat studies, among others, reflect humanistic and interdisciplinary investigation into fundamental aspects of identity, prejudice, cultural identity and practice in the face of ostracism, segregation, and forms of oppression linked to stigma.

Finally, it has become clear that stigmas may change as a result of a number of cultural, social, and political forces; new stigmas may be attributed to diseases, or in some instances, stigmas may be moderated or reduced. Understanding these shifts in meaning are central to current studies in the health humanities. The term *destigmatization* is widely used to describe this process and the instrumental efforts deployed to mitigate persistent stigmas. Over recent decades, the historical stigmas associated with most cancers have been significantly reduced. Similarly, scholars have documented important shifts in stigma and social tolerance of people with AIDS and the wider gay community. Few would have predicted the evolution and protection of marriage equality in the US from the perspective of the early years of the AIDS epidemic. These changes are the result of diverse actions and activism, political and social change, as well as the enhancement of medical treatments and effective therapeutics. Understanding these processes offers the potential to reduce persistent stigmas associated with many other diseases, where irrational moral judgment has been so difficult to resist.

59

Stress
David Cantor

There are three accounts of the origins of contemporary ideas, practices, and experiences related to stress. The first focuses on the etymology of the word. According to the *Oxford English Dictionary*, the term *stress* comes from *strictus*, past participle of *stringere* (tighten, draw tight) and also the source of the Old French *estrece/estrecier* (narrowness, compression, oppression) and the Old English words *distress* and *strict*. In the fourteenth century, the words *estrece/estrecier* and *distress* mutated into *stress*: the noun *stress* meant a form of hardship, adversity, force, or pressure and, from the sixteenth century, physical injury; the verb *stress* meant to subject (someone or -thing) to force or compulsion. The noun and verb *stress* thus both referred to a quality of the environment, something external that affected a person or thing. An exception was the adjective *stressed*, which also in the sixteenth century opened the possibility of an internal condition, referring to something or someone as afflicted or distressed. Then in the seventeenth century, the noun *stress* also came to refer to an internal quality, and in the nineteenth century, to a mix of outside pressure and inner reactions. From thereon, all three meanings—external, internal, or a mix—were used, setting the stage for modern ideas of stress as they emerged in the nineteenth and twentieth centuries.

The second account focuses on the consequences of industrial-urban modernity (M. Jackson 2013, 21–55). In this story, experiences of stress in Western societies since the eighteenth century were shaped by new routines of industrial work and leisure, new technologies, and the pace of life in the rapidly growing cities. Scientists and physicians sought to explain such experiences in laboratory studies of physiological and emotional balance. And industries and governments sought ways to counter the threat that stress posed to industrial productivity and military efficiency. In such narratives, neurasthenia, fatigue, anxiety, diabetes, and insanity, among other ills, came to be seen as penalties of progress, and the concept of stress was deployed to describe the environmental circumstances responsible for triggering them. For example, during and after the First World War, commentators used the idea of the "the stress of battle" to discuss the fear, fatigue, sleeplessness, and sense of responsibility that the pressures of trench warfare fashioned. It followed that the entry of stress into the lexicon of discourses of about modernity, and the multiple meanings and uses of the term, reflected the complexities of modern urban-industrial society; the variety of different scientific approaches to the condition; and the varied experiences of those subject to the demands of new occupational routines, military operations, technologies, cities, and the bureaucracies and structures characteristic of emergent nation states.

The third account of stress focuses on the Second World War as the major transition point (Cantor and Ramsden 2014, 121–85). In this story, stress—as experience or object of knowledge or practice—was the product not so much of the long-term development of urban-industrial modernity but of the war and subsequent social, economic, and cultural developments. In this narrative, the flood of servicemen experiencing neurotic symptoms during the war started a trend to psychologize stress. Military psychological researchers described a general susceptibility to develop neurotic symptoms under the strain of combat—everyone had

a point at which they would break—and their research helped to popularize *stress* as applied to the general population, which was later also adapted to physiological models of the condition. Whereas *stress* had been deployed periodically before then, its use really took off after the war in the medical and popular literature (M. Jackson 2013, 141–80; Cantor and Ramsden 2014, 49–70): the *Index Medicus* first included the term as a subject heading in 1950, and the *Reader's Guide to Periodical Literature* listed it in 1951. Indeed, the term was mobilized to explain a host of issues: rising levels of sickness absence, executive burnout, suicide among university students, a reluctance among women to bear children, and a multitude of stress-related illnesses such as depression, heart disease, gastroenteritis, hypertension, diabetes, and rheumatoid arthritis among others, generally chronic ills then gaining growing attention. Stress thus attracted interest as a way of talking about the challenges to human health in the military, the factory, the city, and in everyday life, linking such challenges to a wide variety of bodily and of the mental ills. By the 1980s, scientists and journalists argued that people were overwhelmed by an epidemic of stress caused by the constant effort of adapting to the insecurity, unpredictability, changeability, and pace of the postwar world (M. Jackson 2013, 2–11). The postwar self was a stressed self.

These seemingly contrasting accounts of the history of stress—one focusing on long-term etymological changes, another on the social and cultural developments associated with urbanization and industrialization, and another pointing to a key moment of change during and after and the Second World War—raise a variety of issues for the health humanities. (For an introduction to some of the health humanities literature on stress, see Crawford, Brown, and Charise 2020.) In the first place, the last two especially highlight a long-term interest in the relationship between stress and the social, cultural, economic, and physical environments in which people live. In some of these accounts, stress is seen as a positive force, a stimulus to improvement, evidence of people's ability to work productively, and a measure of technological and social progress (M. Jackson 2013, 266–67). Others see it as a negative force, reflecting limitations in people's capacity to cope with modernity or postmodernity. Yet others see it as somewhere in the middle, a cause of both illness and resilience. This last model came to the fore after the Second World War, supplanting earlier models that saw stress as primarily depleting the body's limited amount of inherited nerve force with physiological models that saw stress as both depleting the body and (paradoxically) enhancing it. Too much stress at once or over a long period could damage health, while a small amount over a short period could improve the body's resilience (M. Jackson 2013, 75–88, 99–140).

Studies in the health humanities have tended to focus on the negative consequences of stress: the stress faced by patients undergoing medical intervention, the poor or dispossessed confronted by intransigent bureaucracies, women and minorities subject to the thousand small aggressions of the day among other groups. There has, however, been a division between those who focus narrowly on the therapeutic encounter and those who focus on broader structural causes of stress. Much research on the therapeutic encounter, for example, has examined the role of the humanities and arts—gardening, music, storytelling, poetry, literature, art—in helping combat stress and increase resilience within a clinical setting. Cultural critics, however, argue that attention should look beyond the clinical encounter to the broader social, economic, and cultural causes of stress: how they lead to illness and social disadvantage, how structural reforms might combat stress and improve resilience, and how we need a better engagement with critical theory; queer, feminist, and disability studies; activist politics; and other related fields. Stress in this formulation is a product of contemporary society, economy and culture, much as earlier scholars saw it and its forebears as a consequence of urban-industrial modernity or modern warfare.

In the second place, accounts of stress also highlight how it has come to be a way of discussing a host of issues associated with modernity and postmodernity by reference to their effects on the peoples subject to them. From this perspective, stress provides a means of talking about an almost countless range of topics: the quality of the built environment; the problems of the city; and the experiences of poverty, social disruption, war, work, unemployment, migration, housing, race/ethnicity, gender, sexual orientation, and social class among many other topics. Indeed, sometimes social concerns have been embedded in models of stress themselves and their forebears, such as in the work of the physiologist and sociologist Lawrence J. Henderson on adaptive stability, inspired in part by his conservative belief in the importance of scientific management in times of economic crisis in the 1920s and 1930s, or the work of the physiologist Walter Cannon on physiological stability—homeostasis—inspired by his belief in the liberal values of freedom and democracy (M. Jackson 2013, 65–75). For the health humanities, stress thus offers an opportunity to understand (e.g., through narrative analysis) how different people and groups use it to talk about other issues. The discourses of stress, from this perspective, are much more than discourses about health narrowly conceived as the absence of illness. They are also political, economic, social, or cultural commentary or critique.

Finally, for an interdisciplinary field such as the health humanities with different approaches to health and healing, such histories highlight the need for engagement with the many different meanings of this chameleon term (Cantor and Ramsden 2014, 4–9). At times, such diversity has undermined interdisciplinary conversations, prompting disagreements over what constitutes stress and how it affects those subject to it. Yet this diversity also ensured that concepts of stress thrived since World War II, in part because they provided opportunities to create conversations between different specialist fields. Clinical medicine, biology, physiology, endocrinology, neurology, biochemistry, psychiatry, the behavioral sciences, ethics, and more recently, health humanities have all engaged with one another through the medium of stress. They often mean different things by stress, but given its place at the intersection of all these fields, the term has also offered occasions to exchange ideas and practices, to create new professional networks, and to engage in public and disciplinary discussion. Indeed, stress is on the boundary not only between the health humanities and other fields but also among the different disciplines that make up the health humanities itself. The challenge for the health humanities is how to reconcile this diversity of approaches to and meanings of stress, to engage with the ways in which stress is used to talk about other issues, and to decide whether to focus narrowly on the clinical encounter or on the structural causes of stress and by extension the social, economic, and cultural transformations needed to ameliorate its negative consequences.

60

Technology

John Basl and Ronald Sandler

Technology combines the Greek roots *tekhnē*, which entails making—as in art, skill, and craft—and *logia*, the speaking or telling. Historically, technology has had a range of meanings, referring variously, according to the OED, to "a discourse on an art or arts," "the scientific study of the industrial or practical arts," "a branch of knowledge dealing with the mechanical arts and applied sciences," "the application of such knowledge for practical purposes," and "the product of such application." While contemporary usage often orients us toward thinking about specific objects, the roots of the term highlight the ways in which technology not only is an object for use but also partly defines and constitutes the practices that rely on the objects we typically identify as pieces of technology.

Medical practice is permeated by technology, from training and research to diagnostics and therapeutics. Medical experiences of patients involve serial engagement with technologies (both bureaucratic and clinical), and medical systems are built upon them (e.g., electronic records, telemedicine, billing systems). Individual, particularly novel, medical technologies are frequently subject to critical evaluation and robust debate—for example, gene therapy, machine learning-based diagnostics, IVF, algorithmic triage, electroconvulsive therapy. So, too, are particular technologies in particular contexts—for example, the use of psychopharmaceuticals in children, genetic diagnosis in embryos, and large doses of pain management medicine at end of life. Less discussed, but no less important, is critical evaluation of the role technology as such plays in medicine.

Instrumentalist View of Technology

Medicine is a value-oriented field. Medical practice aims at health and quality of life. There is considerable discussion about how to conceptualize and operationalize these—that is, what exactly constitutes health or quality of life, and how those metrics can be effectively measured. However, the aims are not in themselves in question. Medicine has a goal, an end, toward which both the field and the activities of individual practitioners—researchers, technicians, clinicians—are oriented. Furthermore, the norms and values that govern the appropriate attainment of the ends of medicine are entrenched. Foundational values of respect for autonomy, doing good while avoiding harm, and justice are operationalized as specific norms, policies, or requirements—such as requirements of informed consent or patient privacy policies—that govern both medical practice and research (Beauchamp and Childress 1979).

Because the ends and guiding values of medicine are so strongly and deeply established, medicine lends itself to an *instrumentalist conception of technology*—that technologies are essentially means to accomplishing sought-after ends. This is sometimes referred to as the *technology-as-tool view*. The technologies do not themselves have agency, aims, or ends; they are implements or means that agents use to achieve their goals.

The instrumentalist conception of technology has an allied evaluative perspective, which holds that technologies are neither good nor bad but ethically neutral. Medical technologies are evaluated against the backdrop of foundational values and norms.

Opioid pain medications and psychopharmaceuticals, for example, are good when they are prescribed for the right reasons to the right patients under the right circumstances—when they are used properly. The same is true of laser eye surgery, neuroimaging, machine learning algorithms, genetic diagnostics, and so on. On an instrumentalist conception of medical technologies, critical evaluation focuses on considerations related to safety, effectiveness, justice, equity, and autonomy: Is the technology effective in promoting health outcomes in comparison to the alternatives (if any)? Is there equity in access to the technology among patients and populations? Are the appropriate standards of informed consent by patients met when the technology is used? What are the risks and potential detrimental side effects for patients from using the technology?

One concern related to evaluating emerging medical technologies, especially those deploying recent advances in big data and artificial intelligence, such as in smart health devices and medical diagnostics, is that the long-established norms in medical practice and research are unresponsive to the particular ways these technologies relate to key values. For example, no established norms for protecting patient privacy accompany the power to reliably track and make predictions about individuals without the use of typically protected identifiers (Barocas and Nissenbaum 2014) or the ability of some algorithmic systems to essentially de-anonymize data (Rocher, Hendrickx, and Montjoye 2019). Appropriate evaluation of technology in an instrumentalist conception of technology requires attending closely to the relationships among the technologies, foundational values, and the ways in which those foundational values are operationalized into the concrete norms that govern medical practice and research. Such evaluation may require the development of new conceptions of consent and privacy, among other concerns (Dwork et al. 2006; Barocas and Nissenbaum 2009; Nissenbaum 2011).

Technology as a Form of Life

Philosophers, sociologists, and others who study the role of technology in human life and in social systems typically regard the instrumentalist view of technology as inadequate. Technologies are not merely means but partly constitute the form of human life. On the form-of-life perspective of technology, technologies are sociocultural phenomena that structure the material and social conditions of human experience. They expand agency, enabling new visions for how the world can be. They offer new approaches to resolving problems while raising novel ones. In so doing, they alter relationships—including power dynamics—between people. They change what people care about, who people interact with, and how those interactions occur. They modify our physical spaces and change our physical experiences and movements. They influence our expectations, values, and behaviors. Technologies often reshape us, even as we use them, and this metamorphosis often occurs in ways that make the influence of technologies invisible to us.

The standard illustration of how technologies can restructure human experience is the automobile. If one considers cars and trucks only as more effective ways than horses and wagons to move people and goods around, it obscures all the ways in which they are socially, culturally, personally, economically, and environmentally transformative (Leopold 1949; Winner 1983). Similarly, home appliances helped transform family dynamics and the workforce. Social media platforms have altered social experiences, relationships, and skills, as well as how people receive, access, and share information about the world, from current events to product availability. Synthetic fertilizer changed food systems, agriculture, and diets. Personal computing and the internet revolutionized educational systems, practices, and models. In each of these cases, technologies shape our expectations, aims, motivations, desires, and the ways in which we apply social concepts.

Technology in medicine has also been transformative. Consider, for example, the introduction of genetic research, diagnostics, and therapeutics. It has contributed to a reconceptualization of health, disease, and illness. It has led to new ways of conceiving of health challenges and problems. It has created new possibilities—such as through preimplantation genetic diagnosis or BRCA screening—that raise novel questions, choices, powers, and possibilities. Genetic medical technologies are means, but they also reconstitute aspects of medical practice, medical experience, and medical systems. Similarly, microscopes, antibiotics, medical imaging, anesthesia, vaccines, robotic and remote surgery, machine learning, and numerous other technological advances have not only promoted good health outcomes but also transformed medical practice, expectations, experiences, the knowledge and skills that are required, the social structures that support it, who is empowered in it, and what is involved in delivering it. Medical technologies and technological systems are *forms of life* in the sense that as they "are being built and put to use, significant alterations in patterns of human activity and human institutions are already taking place" (Winner 1983).

The evaluative concepts associated with considering technology as a form of life are different from those associated with considering technology as a means. The form-of-life perspective brings into focus issues such as power, meaning, relationships, perspectives, and values (Leopold 1949; Winner 1983; Borgman 1984; Sandler 2014). To see the difference, consider the concerns that have been raised about genetic selection and modification in human reproduction. Instrumentalist concerns include such things as the health and well-being of the child, informed consent by the parents, access and potential implications for inequalities and injustice, and sufficient oversight mechanisms. However, these do not exhaust the evaluative issues. Other concerns are connected to how these technologies might transform reproductive practices with implications for how parents approach childbearing and child-rearing, their expectations and attitudes about parenting, the child-parent relationship, and even social attitudes about ability and disability (President's Council on Bioethics 2003; Sandel 2009; Savulescu and Kahane 2009; De Melo-Martin 2014; Nuffield Council on Bioethics 2016).

A sufficiently robust and comprehensive evaluation of medical technologies—which is crucial to responsible development and deployment of them—requires considering them from both of the above perspectives, both as tools for accomplishing our ends and as things that shape and transform our worldviews in myriad ways. If we restrict our attention to only one perspective, we close ourselves off to critical questions about technologies essential to realizing their promise while avoiding their pitfalls.

61

Toxic
Heather Houser

Pervasive yet differential. These descriptors fit numerous twenty-first-century phenomena affecting human and more-than-human vitality, from the COVID-19 pandemic to climate crisis and toxic exposure. While individual immunity varies, no population is fully immune to COVID-19. No one is fully protected from impacts accompanying global warming. No one is untouched by the countless vectors for toxicity, even beings in Earth's remotest regions. Yet experiences of toxic threats, like experiences of the COVID-19 and climate crises, are not uniform across individuals, communities, and ecosystems. For this reason, the framework of the toxic offers the health humanities a crucial intervention into social injustices correlated to gender, wealth, geography, race, and ethnicity. We cannot sufficiently understand and redress health disparities keyed to these identity positions without accounting for industrial and petrochemical toxins. The toxic is at the nexus of identity, health, and environment and also rests at the nexus of varied epistemologies, from positivist science to environmental justice and queer and feminist materialisms. It demonstrates the value of entangling epistemologies that might otherwise conflict with one another.

The English word *toxic*, denoting the poisonous, has Latin roots and appears in the seventeenth century, but its usage takes off in the mid- to late-nineteenth century, neatly aligning with growing industrialized mining and manufacturing that corresponded to increased affluence and convenience in Western Europe and the United States (*OED Online* 2021, "toxic"). Today, however, the term's connotations have expanded such that *toxic* has become an all-purpose description of the present. Toxic securities brought down the financial system in 2008; toxic masculinity signifies gender norms underpinning rampant misogyny, homophobia, transphobia, and violence; a toxic relationship denotes any "bad" personal relationship that damages one or both of the parties. These twenty-first-century terms of art spanning finance, psychology, sociology, feminism, and queer studies retain the sense of *toxic*'s Latinate origins but also signify contamination, proximity, and pervasiveness. The sphere of influence for the toxic—whether an asset or a person—lacks fixed boundaries. It contaminates whatever it approaches or, as with polychlorinated biphenyl (PCBs) and financial securities, what is less physically near than enmeshed in the systems of which it is a part.

Notions of pervasiveness and contamination are cornerstones of twenty-first-century creative and humanistic scholarship on toxicity, especially from within feminist, queer, and critical race studies. The environmentalist bromide that "when we try to pick out anything by itself, we find it hitched to everything else in the universe" (Muir 1911, 211) becomes at once situated, raced, and gendered through these intellectual approaches. Ideas of interconnectivity gain a politics that refutes the masculine and white-supremacist positionality John Muir and many of his conservationist descendants have held (Finney 2014; Guha 1989; Guha 2005; S. Ray 2013; D. Taylor 2005).

Reimagining this idea of "hitching," a figure that differentiates the two objects that link up, materialist scholars have offered figures of permeability and vulnerability. Stacy Alaimo's approach to embodiment and toxicity highlights the "trans-corporeality" of bodies and other matter: "the material interconnections of human corporeality with the more-than-human world" that "often revea[l] global networks of social injustice . . . and environmental degradation" (Alaimo 2010, 2, 15). Literature and films by Susanne Antonetta, Todd Haynes, Meridel LeSueur, Audre Lorde, Sandra Steingraber, and others elucidate the gendered trajectories of toxins through incidence of cancers, reproductive ailments, birth abnormalities, and chemical sensitivities that biologically female women experience at high rates. Mel Chen expands on the transcorporeal through their theorization of "animacies," the pathways of "interabsorption of animate and inanimate bodies" (Chen 2012, 11). Their study details how race, sexuality, and ability shape who and what counts as animate and the valuative coding attached to this designation. For Alaimo and Chen, as for their fellow travelers (Alaimo and Hekman 2008; Barad 2007; Bennett 2010; Braidotti 2002; Houser 2014; Langston 2010; Nash 2006), toxicity indicates bodily "nonintegrity" and the inexorable intimacy between animate and inanimate, human and more-than-human agents (Chen 2012, 11).

These materialist arguments show the extensiveness yet unevenness of vulnerabilities to materials like lead, silica dust, airborne pollutants, and the slurry of synthetic chemicals appearing in consumer goods. Yet they also celebrate bodies' imbrication in the environments they coconstitute. Both aspects of Alaimo's and Chen's toxic consciousness—as a source of injury and as evidence of imbrication—dismantle Enlightenment conceptions of human exceptionalism and bust the false binaries of nature-human, human-animal, death-life, and nature-culture. In an era of pervasive toxicity and risk (Beck [1986] 1992; Buell 1998; Heise 2002), this consciousness also dismantles the idea of "safe" spaces (Haynes 1995; Langston 2010; Puar 2017). Though demonstrating pervasive bodily vulnerability and boundarylessness, materialist takes on toxicity also amplify positions within environmental justice and disability studies on differential risk and immiseration. As Chen writes, "we can . . . claim toxicity as already . . . a truth of nearly every body, and also as a biopolitically interested distribution . . . to deprivileged or already 'toxic subjects'" (Chen 2012, 218).

Indra Sinha's novel *Animal's People* (2007) vividly narrates the transcorporealities and animacies of toxins and positions toxic "distribution" in transnational capitalism and its damage to poor people of color in the Global South. Sinha fictionalizes the aftermath of the 1984 explosion and gas leak at a Union Carbide factory in Bhopal, India. The ecological and medical disaster killed thousands of residents, and hundreds of thousands more people live with injuries ranging from blindness to birth abnormalities as fights for compensation, health care, and other reparations wend through courts. Animal, the novel's ribald, clever narrator, embodies the poisons that seeped out "that night" of catastrophe when he was an infant: his spine is torqued such that he cannot walk upright, and he travels on hands and feet through the streets (Sinha 2007, 5). He epitomizes the nonintegrity and porosity of the body as he absorbs not only the poisons but also the languages, idioms, and narrative perspectives of his neighbors. Animal also engenders the "interested distribution" of toxicity resulting from imperialist capitalism. The factory produces chemicals for pesticides that bring great profits to Union Carbide (now, Dow) executives and shareholders and staggering risks to low-wage workers and residents living in the slums adjacent to the plant. Corporations externalize toxicity onto destitute parts of formerly colonized nations where labor costs are lower and accountability for industry's deleterious effects is reduced through distance, time, lax regulation, and lack of mechanisms for redress (R. Nixon 2011, chap. 1).

Animal's People embodies these conditions while dramatizing how grassroots activists work against "toxic postcoloniality" through environmental justice struggles (Mukherjee 2011). Environmental justice (EJ) scholar-activists fight against the outsized exposure to environmental pollutants in postcolonial locales and Black, Indigenous, and people of color (BIPOC) communities in the US (Allen 2003; Bullard 2000; Bullard et al. 2008; S. Lerner 2010). Julie Sze elaborates on EJ as a response to environmental racism: "environmental racism can be defined as the unequal distribution of environmental benefits and pollution burdens based on race," while EJ refers to resistance to this form of racial oppression through activism, creative interventions, and scholarly analysis (Sze 2007, 13). While there are undoubtedly class and gender dimensions to toxic burdens, race and ethnicity are leading predictors of environmental health in the US and determine the imperialist offloading of poisonous industry and waste onto formerly colonized nations. A few disgraceful statistics will stand in for many that substantiate this point for the US: African American households with annual incomes of $50,000 to $60,000 live in more polluted neighborhoods than poor whites making $10,000 (Washington 2019, 70). The life expectancy in Houston's 77026 zip code, which is over 84 percent Black and Hispanic or Latinx, is 69.8 years; in the predominately white 77007 zip code only eight miles away, the figure rises to 89.1 years (Watkins 2019). Drinking water in Navajo Nation contains uranium concentrations at least five times higher than the allowed level (Morales 2016).

Although snapshots of a moment in time, these statistics reflect entrenched racist practices affecting where certain people live, what infrastructural supports communities receive, and whether polluting extraction, manufacturing, and waste are proximate to their homes. For this reason, apprehending and eradicating racialized toxic risks exceeds the bounds of traditional scientific disciplines such as hydrology. It requires the intelligence of historians, anthropologists, urban planners, and cultural studies scholars. Understanding and mitigating the toxic requires entangled epistemologies (Houser 2020). We cannot rely solely on empiricist and quantitative analyses of toxic pathways but must integrate positivist epistemologies with ways of knowing rooted in embodied experiences that often occupy states of ambiguity, speculation, and unknowing. Sicknesses associated with toxicity typically involve "contested medicine" that pits Eurowestern scientific authority against lived knowledge of body and place (Di Chiro 1997; Houser 2014; Kroll-Smith, Brown, and Gunter 2000; Kroll-Smith and Floyd 1997; Sze 2007). Even when a source of toxicity is identifiable, tight causal connections between a poison—whether a carcinogenic chemical in water or an endocrine disruptor in plastics—and its effects are notoriously elusive. When the holders of this embodied knowledge are women, the impoverished, and/or BIPOC, those in power discredit it more readily. Disbelief from medical, government, and business authorities is often interested. Acknowledging that effluents from a mining operation or emissions from a coal-fired power plant harm neighbors, ecosystems, and in some cases, the Earth writ large can harm balance sheets and fuel legal and public relations attacks on polluting industries.

As I argue elsewhere (Houser 2020), literature, film, performance, and visual culture record the environmental racism engendered by toxic harms but also envision responses to them through entangled epistemologies. Percival Everett's *Watershed* (1996), like *Animal's People*, exemplifies cultural intervention into toxicity. The novel muddies distinctions between fact and fiction and features a protagonist drawn into an EJ battle against the poisoning of a Native group. Everett envisions a fictional tribe, the Plata, inhabiting an eponymous mountain range in Colorado. Robert Hawk, a Black hydrologist who escapes to the region for solitude and fishing, becomes embroiled in a detective plot: determining why two white FBI agents were murdered and why Plata Creek has been diverted into the tribe's reservation. The answer to both puzzles originates in an illegal military depot of biological weapons north of the reservation. As in Sinha's novel, powerful groups discredit toxic experience and its sources in environmental racism. Both texts braid scientific ways of knowing with contested histories and local knowledge through their formal choices. *Animal's People* is polyglot, seamlessly sliding between English, Urdu, Farsi, French, and various argots, while *Watershed* incorporates hydrological data, medical discourse, fishing manuals, geological documents, and tribal treaties with the US government.

Whether originating in materialist thought or EJ art, scholarship, and activism—or at their fertile intersections—twenty-first-century approaches to toxicity illustrate the interdependence of race, gender, health, and environment. Apprehending and redressing toxicity, while remarkably complex, offers ways to remediate damages that cross the social and ecological. Moreover, it offers ways to coordinate the intelligence of diverse peoples, disciplines, and ecoregions; the arts and humanities are especially well equipped for this task of coordination.

62

Trauma

Deborah F. Weinstein

What does it mean to be traumatized? Like other contested medical keywords with which it is intimately intertwined, such as *pain*, the concept of *trauma* has raised, and continues to raise, complicated debates over relationships between medical diagnoses and broader cultural categories, between events and memories, and between individuals and collectives. Within the health humanities, questions of trauma have tended to concentrate on studies of formal diagnostic criteria—that is, what defines real trauma and who gets to count as authentically traumatized. And as is more broadly the case with medical categories, definitions and diagnoses of trauma are specific to time and place. Indeed, contrary to some clinicians' depictions of "trauma" as a universal and transhistorical phenomenon, scholars in the health humanities generally seek to locate trauma, its meanings, and its treatment within particular historical and cultural contexts. Ongoing debate over those meanings highlights the continuing power of medical authority.

According to the OED, the word *trauma* entered the English language in 1684 as a way to describe physical injury, specifically "a Wound from an external Cause." The shift to apprehending trauma not only as a readily perceptible physical wound but as psychological harm came later, in the closing years of the nineteenth century. The OED credits William James with the first such use of the concept, characterizing psychic *traumata* as "thorns in the spirit, so to speak" (*OED Online* 2021, "trauma"). It also gave rise to what Ruth Leys has

characterized as controversy and confusion over the concept of trauma, whose unstable meanings have oscillated ever since (Leys 2000, 6).

As indicated in the movement from acute injury to "thorns in the spirit," the concept of trauma intersects with larger, intractable questions in Western biomedicine concerning the relations between mind and body—including epistemological questions about biomedical evidence (Harrington 2009). From nineteenth-century railway spine to contemporary traffic accident injuries, modern technology has contributed to the interface of psychological and somatic experiences of trauma (Micale and Lerner 2001; Solomon 2022). Like many other categories of suffering, certain kinds of trauma cannot be readily assessed by a blood assay or X-ray. As a result, even observable physiological effects that might be attributed to trauma, such as facial tics or mutism, have at times been minimized and devalued: as *just* hysteria, *mere* nervousness.

Just as diagnoses and associated criteria of trauma have been contested, so too is the matter of to whom diagnoses of "trauma" should, or should not, be applied. Crucially, early approaches to the topic of psychological trauma in medicine, and in the medical humanities, focused on the experience of trauma in war and specifically on the experience of male European and British soldiers during the Great War. An extensive literature on shell shock in the First World War explores the links among trauma, male hysteria, and war neuroses, such as those expressed in the wartime poetry of British writers Siegfried Sasson and Wilfred Owen. Humanities scholars often place gender at the center of these analyses, examining the psychological breakdown caused by war as a challenge to modern white masculinity that found parallels in female hysteria of the nineteenth century (Barker 1991; P. Lerner 2009; Reid 2014; Showalter 1985).

Disputes over the meanings and parameters of trauma only intensified with the advent of the diagnostic category of post-traumatic stress disorder (PTSD). First entering the third edition of the Diagnostic and Statistical Manual (DSM) in 1980, the disorder's connections to older categories of mental illness, such as shell shock or combat fatigue, have been alternatingly asserted and challenged. With the advent of the clinical—and cultural—category of PTSD, historians, literary scholars, novelists, and other humanists began wrestling with whether shell shock and combat fatigue might be considered the precursors of the new, post-Vietnam syndrome (e.g., Micale and Lerner 2001; Shephard 2001; A. Young 1995). Debates about the diagnosis of PTSD also reflect the broader contentiousness of the DSM itself, including the authority of professional psychiatric diagnosis to limit or curtail designations of "real" mental illness or psychic suffering (Horwitz 2002; Charles Rosenberg 2015; W. Scott 1990). Even as the DSM and related diagnostic criteria narrowed and specified the characteristics of PTSD, uses of the word *trauma* increased markedly after 1980, often used to evoke lasting psychic wounds in a more general, figurative sense.

If trauma came to be defined within the humanities, in part, through the shell shock associated with male military veterans, a counterpoint appeared in literatures focused on sexual trauma. Influenced by the women's and feminist movements of the 1970s and in line with the diagnostic category of PTSD, sexual violence and assault increasingly became framed as traumatizing and linked to the societal harm of gender inequity (Herman 1992). Many feminist advocates, wary of adopting the language of "victimhood," advocated use of the word "survivor" to describe individuals who had endured sexual trauma and its aftermath (Dunn 2004). Historians have further contextualized understandings and experiences of sexual and gender violence, including

their racialized stratifications and their lasting political aftereffects (Block 2006; McGuire 2011; H. Rosen 2009).

Central to trauma's movement out of the clinic and into wider political use is the concept's evocation of temporality. Trauma implies longevity: while a wound suggests an event, a discrete form of violence and harm to the body, trauma tends to imply a longer-term, perhaps even ceaseless experience. As such, the concept invokes the looping causality of memory, forgetting, and embodied pain (A. Young 1995). Accordingly, memory has been central to the literature on trauma—both the trauma of certain memories and the failures of memory itself, since amnesia and flashbacks are key symptoms of PTSD.

Equally central to trauma's wide cultural purchase is the concept of collective trauma. Clinicians and social scientists use collective trauma to describe the impact of adverse events that happen to a group of people, who then maintain intergenerational collective memory of the traumatic event (Hirschberger 2018). Sociologist Kai Erikson's analysis of a 1972 catastrophic flood in a mining town in West Virginia defined the disaster's impact in terms of the community's collective trauma that outlasted individual experiences of the flood (Erikson 1976). In their analysis of social suffering, Arthur Kleinman, Veena Das, and Margaret Lock note that responses to political violence or other atrocities that focus only on psychological or medical trauma can mistakenly cleave individual from social levels of analysis, or as they write, "The standard dichotomies are in fact barriers to understanding how the forms of human suffering can be at the same time collective and individual, how the modes of experiencing pain and trauma can be both local and global" (Kleinman, Das, and Lock 1997, x). Subsequent scholars have reflected on events like Hurricane Katrina, the terrorist attacks on 9/11, and myriad other calamities through investigations of communities and groups, not just individual sufferers. As Didier Fassin and Richard Rechtman note, the traumatic victim has become a viable political category—one applicable to domestic violence as well as state violence (Fassin and Rechtman 2009).

To these conversations about collective, shared trauma, humanities scholars have encouraged critical reflection on the nature of collective memory—including whether such a thing exists, and if so, how it may differ from written history. Questions about the limits of representing or understanding trauma have been particularly foregrounded in historiographical debates about the Holocaust as well as in psychoanalytic studies of the complex relationship between trauma and memory (Caruth 1995). Some scholars consider the implications of such profound trauma for writing history itself (LaCapra 2001). For them, trauma appears less as a medical or clinical category than as a historical category of analysis. Others have examined how trauma became a relevant clinical category for understanding the continuing effects of the experience on the suffering of Holocaust survivors (Herzog 2017). More recently, scholars across a range of disciplines including history, literary criticism, and anthropology have underscored the importance of moving beyond the Eurocentrism of early trauma studies in order to foster global, postcolonial analyses of trauma (Bond and Craps 2020; Buelens, Durrant, and Eaglestone 2014; Hinton and Good 2015; Micale and Pols 2021).

Such debates focus on collective trauma and question whether the historian *can* adequately represent violence of such an incomprehensibly vast scale, whether the historian *should* attempt to represent such violence, and whether "trauma" is a suitable register to account either for its immediate or intergenerational effects. Does "collective trauma" instead pathologize what might better be understood as structural violence? Particularly in debates concerning the historical representation of US racial slavery, scholarship has increasingly emphasized its intergenerational effects. The pushback on treating intergenerational harms as a matter of collective trauma has been that it risks psychologizing the effects of ongoing structural violence, thereby reinforcing a pathology of deficits and damage (Kendi 2016; Daryl Scott 1997). Recent literature on the afterlife of slavery attends to the structural lineage of contemporary racial violence and to the potential retraumatizing effects of witnessing photos and reenactments of graphic violence proffered on therapeutic or educational grounds (S. Hartman 2008; C. Sharpe 2016).

The keyword *trauma* speaks to the aftermath of violence and other kinds of harm as well as to the events themselves. Over the past century and a half, medicine, psychology, and psychoanalysis have been central to defining what counts as traumatic and who suffers from trauma, including who is endowed with (or saddled with) an official diagnosis. Humanities scholars have highlighted the importance of narrative and memory in their analyses of trauma, recognizing that the collective dimension of trauma raises thorny questions about memory, narrative, and healing, and about the limits of clinical approaches to recovery (e.g., Cvetkovich 2003). At stake, then, is not whether certain events or circumstances pertain strictly to individual psychology or broader structural forces but how those scales—the psychic and the structural—are mutually activated or imbricated. The concept of trauma therefore resonates with wider debates about medicine's role in pathologizing or legitimizing particular human experiences and suffering (Metzl and Herzig 2007).

63

Treatment

Keir Waddington and Martin Willis

Although standard dictionary definitions of *treatment* emphasize the medical or surgical remedies given to a patient for an illness or an injury, what is meant by treatment is historically, socially, and culturally contingent. This not only is true now within health humanities scholarship but is also the critical consensus within contemporary histories of medicine. In a medical sense, the term *treatment* was first recorded in 1744, rooted in the Latin *tractare*, meaning "to deal with." Until then, *cure* or *remedy* were used (Berkeley 1744). *Treatment* came into common usage in the nineteenth century—a shift in language that paralleled a new categorization of knowledge and medical practitioners' claims to possessing the primary expertise in the management of illness. At the same time, *treatment* as understood within medical spheres contains the traces of earlier definitions that identified the word with negotiation and the striking of bargains. There remains considerable evidence that medical treatments are dialectical: constructed by arriving at agreed settlements between active participants. Nevertheless, what is signified by treatment varies temporally and also between medical cultures in the Global North and Global South.

Over the past five-hundred years, what constitutes treatment in Western societies has come to mean many different things: it has encompassed everything from bloodletting and running repairs on the body undertaken by barber surgeons in early modern surgery to the patent medicines sold via quacks and newspapers in the eighteenth and nineteenth centuries. In the twentieth century, the range and efficacy of treatments expanded to cover everything from over-the-counter medicines, talking cures, psychopharmacology, and chemotherapy to key-hole surgery and acupuncture, while in the twenty-first century, experimental gene therapy offered new forms of treatment. Just as the nature of treatment has expanded, ethical questions about the nature, efficacy, and use of a range of different treatments (and when to give, suspend, or even withdraw, treatment) have attracted increasing attention from practitioners, policymakers, and patient advocacy groups. Treatments are often regarded as progressive forms of medical intervention that improve over time. Yet such narratives of modernity conceal continuities that lead to treatments working as a palimpsest of overlapping procedures and practices as well as how treatments in the Global South blended different approaches from different medical traditions. Equally, while treatment is often framed in scholarship as an active response to an illness or injury, the boundaries between cure and prevention have been blurred as suggested by the use of warfarin to treat and prevent blood clots. What is meant by treatment has hence often been highly malleable and always caught up in wider narratives of biomedicine, professionalization, and patient-led perspectives.

In a range of humanities disciplines, the approach to treatment has moved from hagiographic representation to rigorous critical examination, with scholarship increasingly exploring treatment from sociocultural and political-economic perspectives or through patient narratives. Older studies tend to highlight innovation, the experimental, or the dramatic. Treatments, those discovering and administering them, and those receiving them, could all be cast as heroic. Surgery acts as an exemplar here. Surgery is often framed in these terms whether it is the mastectomy Frances Burney underwent in Paris in 1811 or in modern accounts of cancer surgery and personal struggle as seen in the pink-ribbon culture that dominates presentations of breast cancer in Western societies (Gibson, Lee, and Crabb 2014). This framing supported surgeons' claims to professional power and partly accounts for the self- and popular image of the surgeon, which has been reinforced in a range of cultural representations from the paintings of Georges Chicotot or Thomas Eakins in the nineteenth century to Ian McEwan's *Saturday* and the Mills & Boon novels. Unsurprisingly, connections have been made between treatment and the professionalization of health-care workers and with the concept of medicalization, often through a Foucauldian framing of knowledge and power. Yet ideas of the medical marketplace embedded in scholarship on early modern health and medicine serve to remind us that treatment has always had a commercial side (Jenner and Wallis 2007). Such scholarship also highlights the importance of thinking about the plurality of actors who sought a foothold in treatment practices. For instance, the heroic treatment Frances Burney received for breast cancer between 1810 and 1812 saw negotiations between Burney, her husband, and a range of medical practitioners, including the four doctors present for her mastectomy. A very different form of surgery as treatment—plastic surgery—illuminates the more critical-evaluative approaches that are emerging in recent medical humanities research. Examinations of contemporary plastic surgeries undertaken as forms of performance art, for example by the French artist ORLAN, draw attention to medical treatments that ask ethical questions of normalcy, of bodily (self-)control, and of the complex web of relations between the economic infrastructures of treatment and their biopolitical formations (K. Davis 2003).

Scholarship has equally drawn attention to those treatments that have been framed as bizarre or brutal to modern eyes. For instance, Isaac Baker-Brown's advocacy of certain surgical procedures, including clitoridectomies as purported cures for epilepsy and hysteria in his female patients, feature prominently as an example of the brutal regulation of female sexuality, while Silas Weir Mitchell's "rest cure" has been similarly framed as deeply damaging to women. What is often at the center of this interest in the brutal or seemingly bizarre is how treatment reveals the interconnections among gender, class, and medicalization. Nor is a focus on such treatment limited to the treatments given to women. In the history of psychiatry, the interwar period is associated, in Andrew Scull's words, with a 'Gothic tale' of madness and medicine (Scull 1987). Here accounts emphasize the introduction of various shock therapies, such as ECT, and invasive life-altering treatments such as lobotomies. When shorn of their historical or social context, these treatments are easy to misread as examples of medical barbarism, but they raise important questions about agency, power and authority, and adoption. For example, shock therapies were rapidly introduced during a period of desire for new somatic treatments as a radical counterpoint to the therapeutic nihilism that had characterized psychiatry since the 1890s. Likewise, these treatments reveal how therapeutic innovation and practitioner zeal could become problematic, destabilizing narratives of progress. For instance, morphine moved from a miracle cure popularized by medical practitioners in the 1860s to a source of alarm around morphinomania in the 1880s and 1890s. Similarly, in under five years in the 1950s, thalidomide went from being widely prescribed to being considered a treatment nadir.

A concentration on the experimental, the dramatic, the pioneering or bizarre, even on the dangerous, provides only part of the picture and obscures other forms of treatment, even if such a focus does important psychological work about the value of contemporary medicine. For instance, a focus on innovation over-looks how many surgical treatments remained linked to preexisting practices into the twentieth century. Frequently, the ordinary has been overlooked. One strand of cultural studies asserts that the "power of the ordinary" not only brings to the foreground experiences marginalized by dominant groups but also draws to our attention ways of "making visible the question of power" (McCarthy 2006; Osborne 1999, 59). Historians have equally drawn on Michel de Certeau and Henri Lefebvre to explore how the everyday sheds light on lived experiences (Highmore 2002; Joe Moran 2005). The everyday can be seen in L. T. Meade's *Stories from the Diary of a Doctor*, serialized in *The Strand Magazine* from July 1893 to December 1895. Although the stories focus on the heroism and medical-detective work of Clifford Halifax, MD, and explore topical socio-medico concerns of the period, they also reveal the everyday nature of medical encounters from the role of pharmacists to the prescription of medical compounds for commonplace complaints. If drama is central to these stories, they also tell us much about quotidian forms of treatment: of the role of practitioners in providing reassurance and restoratives in the sick room (K. Waddington and Willis 2021). Neither heroic nor at the center of bioethical debates, such mundane treatments reveal yet another discourse that contributes to the complex cacophony of competing treatment narratives.

Notwithstanding interest in patient advocacy groups, in writing about treatment there is often a tendency to assume that interventions are practitioner-led. While scholarship on patient narratives helps reveal the agency of the patient in medical settings and the subjectivities that surround treatment, scholarship on the early modern period draws attention to the importance of being more attuned to examples of self-medication and self-treatment. If sensitivity to self-medication can tell us much about the everyday, as seen in the estimated 6,300 tons of paracetamol being sold each year in the UK, it can also reveal resistance to practitioner- or state-led treatments (Moore 2016). There is a long history of patients resisting advice from their practitioners. Vaccination offers one of many examples. For instance, in the eighteenth and nineteenth centuries, some saw the introduction of smallpox via vaccination into another body as impious, a view that was the subject of a thunderous sermon in 1722 by the London clergyman Edmund Massey, which was widely reprinted. Nearly three centuries later, the evidence that 60 percent of the French population are likely to reject the vaccine for COVID-19 not only highlights the endurance and extent of opposition to some treatments—exacerbated by a series of medical scandals since thalidomide in the 1950s—but also illustrates how resistance speaks directly to a wide range of socioeconomic and cultural concerns that medical treatments engender (Willsher 2021).

Definitions of treatment can hence conceal as much as they reveal. In thinking about treatment, scholars need to be aware of the sociocultural and political-economic contexts just as they need to be sensitive to alternative narratives beyond biomedical accounts. Scholars need also to consider treatment's pluralities, its performativity, its elements of sensation and of the everyday, its sources of conflict and tension. To say this is to admit that treatment as a category has an evolving biopolitics that requires ongoing attention to both its histories and present practices.

64

Virus

John Lwanda

The polysemous *virus* carries a number of in-built contradictions for such a critical keyword. Yet it seems "intuitive" in all its senses, from malign to benign. Although *virus* is a keyword in diverse fields, from science and medicine to popular culture and technology, despite different meanings, the underlying concepts are similar: viruses suggest uncontrolled proliferation, as in the "viral" spread of disease and the "viral" contamination of computers.

Even as the science of virology has progressed from earlier filtration studies in the 1890s, through the 1920s complement fixation, the 1940s tissue culture, the 1970s monoclonal antibodies, 1980s polymerase chain reaction (PCR), and the current high throughput sequencing that can more accurately identify and isolate viruses, the meaning of the word has become diffuse. Etymologically, according to the *Oxford English Dictionary* (OED), beginning with its Middle English roots in snake venom (from the Latin "slimy liquid poison"), it has mutated to suggest anything from "a living thing, too small to be seen without a microscope, that causes disease in people, animals and plants" or "an infection or disease caused by a virus" as in "He has a virus . . ." to "a harmful or corrupting influence" or a piece of corrupting code (*OED Online* 2022, "virus").

Viral illnesses can be mild and self-limiting, like the common cold, or lethal, like smallpox, rabies, and Ebola. The human immunodeficiency virus (HIV) in the twentieth century and the two coronavirus pandemics in the twenty-first century have caused personal, communal, national, and international changes in human behavior and economy in more recent times, as did measles and influenza in earlier times. Some viruses such as herpes, rubella, hepatitis C and B, and HIV can lie dormant or cause chronic infections. Viruses like hepatitis C and B and the human immunodeficiency virus can also cause cancers. Some viral illnesses can be easily clinically recognized, for example chickenpox or measles, by their effects on the skin. Others, like hepatitis C, may reveal themselves more gradually. Medical technology may be required to diagnose some viral infections. The spread of viruses is usually a social affair, via respiratory, enteric, and sexual secretions. It is here that virus takes on its adjectival form: viral.

The History

Although our current scientific understanding of these entities emerged more sharply beginning with the work enabled by the invention of the electron microscope in 1931, the idea of a malign substance or force—a slimy liquid or poison that caused illnesses like smallpox (recorded in Egyptian mummies from 3000 years ago and Chinese literature from the tenth century BC), yellow fever (recognized in Africa for centuries), and plant diseases—was suspected for centuries (Fenner et al. 1988). Viruses proliferated with human settlement and agriculture, manifesting the intimate relationships among animals, plants, and humans. Early medical knowledge imagined the body as the site of this "poison production," and that idea remains strong in many cultures.

The Dutch microbiologist and botanist Martinus Willem Beijerinck, one of the founders of virology, first used the term to name an agent that could not be removed by the finest filters of the time. Since that time, the word has crossed cultural and linguistic boundaries, not always following Beijerinck's particulate concept; some cultures translate *virus* as "a little beast," manifesting a reluctance to relinquish the tendency to animate a viral enemy (Lwanda 2003). Other cultures have regarded what would now be viewed as "viral causes" of disease as "spiritual causes" (cf. B. Brock et al. 2019).

The struggle between medical science and the virus is a tale of how "folk and foreign" remedies can translate to the "orthodox" medical arena, often by trial and error. Campaigns by the farmer Benjamin Jesty and better-known doctor Edward Jenner to use cowpox serum as a vaccination against smallpox have become medical legends (Gross and Sepkowitz 1998). The idea of vaccination traveled most likely from Asia and Africa to Turkey, from whence Lady Mary Montagu carried it to Europe (Behbehani 1983). During the Boston smallpox outbreak of 1721, an enslaved African, Onesimus, told his enslaver, Cotton Mather, about his own and his culture's experiences of variolation, which was commonly practiced then, and still is in some forms, in Africa (Imperato and Imperato 2014; Hurford 2010). This early attempt at vaccination is also described in an early Indian Sanskrit text (Behbehani 1983).

The small size of viruses imparted the sense of a more "occult" or "secretive contamination" than the more easily identified bacteria. This motif of a secretive agent has infused not only medicine but the viruses of computers and social science. Since viruses are packets of information, it is not surprising that the term would travel to computer and social sciences. The body politic is evidently as susceptible to viruses as individuals, an idea that circulates widely and rapidly has "gone viral." The idea of "computer viruses" dates back to the 1940s, when scientists postulated that "computer programmes could reproduce" (Rosenberger 1997). The term illustrates what the field of artificial intelligence

has reinforced: the tendency to use the human body as a reference point for our machines. Computer scientists use words like "inoculation, disinfection, quarantine and sanitation" and tally "disinfection and antivirus" programs (Motola 1997). While the potency of the viruses that infect living organisms are measured by their virulence (noun), however, computer viruses are measured by a newer noun: their virality (Hemsley 2011).

Culture and Imperialism

Viruses have been "witting" or "unwitting" tools of conquest and imperialism as well as resistant to both. Smallpox entered Europe with the eighth-century Moor invasions, having been endemic in Egypt and China long before that (Behbehani 1983). Viral plagues that came with invaders and traders alike, such as the bubonic plague (Black Death of 1348–50), reversed urbanization as it ravaged Europe (Whittaker 2017).

Viral illnesses were effective colonizing and genocidal agents, accompanying armies and slavers to the Americas, Australia, and Oceania and seeding epidemics among the Indigenous People who lacked immunity to these illnesses (Whittaker 2017, 458). Measles wiped out roughly a quarter of Fiji's population in 1875, including the majority of the chiefs. Christopher Columbus decimated the Taino people by bringing measles, smallpox, and influenza to Hispaniola. The effects of these diseases led colonizers to harness them as bioweapons (Fenner et al. 1988); millions of indigenous Mexicans and Aztec Indians succumbed, accidentally or otherwise, to viral diseases brought by Europeans (Fenner et al. 1988). The devastation of societies and economies by the human immunodeficiency virus in the late twentieth century and by the current COVID-19 virus, SARS-CoV-2, have shown just how significant viruses are in human evolution and survival.

The Past and the Future

Because of these dramatic effects, the destructive potential of viruses has received the bulk of medical and popular attention. Especially during a pandemic, the media treats the public to graphic depictions of how viruses enter cells and assume control of nuclei to spread their "information" throughout the body. While human dependence on "good" viruses such as bacteriophages, which destroy harmful bacteria, may not get the same attention, they are well known to scientists and those involved in the agriculture and food industries, among others. Some scientists, such as the Dutch virologist Jaap Goudsmit, have even speculated that humans could have evolved from viruses (2004, 156). Human bodies are designed to offer entry, denial, and destruction to viruses, and the idea that viruses are symbiotic agents that are more often benign than malignant has gained increasing traction in recent years (F. Ryan 2009, 93).

It has also been posited that viruses, which are intracellular parasites, have been agents in evolution from the earliest days of life on earth through various mechanisms, such as causing disease and eliminating susceptible genotypes or those carrying certain genes or by the insertion of viral material in host cells (Moelling and Broecker 2019). Thus viruses, of which each of us carries billions, are part and parcel of the grand scheme of the evolutionary nature of things. And even the harmful ones can be harnessed for human benefit, which is, of course, the principle of vaccines.

The word appears to be as tenacious as the entity. The more *virus* appears in multiple fields and disciplines, the more it stakes its claim as a noun. Although we can "avoid, kill, propagate or contract" a virus, the word itself has resisted the phenomenon of "verbing"—or, to use the technical term, *denomalization*—evidence, perhaps, of our insistence on its agency and mystery.

The entity, too, is surely showing its resistance, but the solution for humans may be to respond to viral tenacity with human flexibility. As the twenty-first century SARS-CoV-2 pandemic has shown, humans and viruses continue to coevolve. Humanity's attempts at prevention of viral contamination—from quarantine, isolation, hand washing, safe sex, social distancing, and healthy food preparations to vaccine and pharmaceutical developments—may be evolutionary responses. But since viruses evolve much more quickly than their human hosts, we are fortunate in having the ability to learn from experience. Or so we hope. SARS-CoV-2 in its many incarnations has shone a light on many of our social and geopolitical fault lines, from a changing climate and dwindling resources to the inequities of global poverty and structural racism. Our viruses will continue to teach us—or try to; the question is whether we are ready to learn.

65

Wound

Harris Solomon

The world was beginning to flower into wounds.

—J. G. Ballard, *Crash*

A wound is relational. The *Oxford English Dictionary* defines a wound as "a hurt caused by the laceration or separation of the tissues of the body by a hard or sharp instrument, a bullet, etc.; an external injury" (*OED Online* 2021, "wound"). Wounds are agentive materializations; it takes effort and action to make wounds happen. While *injury* may refer to a damaging and possibly wrongful act, a *wound* foregrounds the body as injury's primary object. One may follow the wound forward to consider what is entailed in recovery, and one may trace a wound backward to reflect on forensics. At stake in following wounds, then, are materialities of effect. Wounds are generative, giving rise to modes of critical attention both in ethnographic cases and in their different appearances in the health humanities. If the primacy of the concrete characterizes wounds, we might ask what wounds concretize in turn.

Wounds concretize medical specialties. For instance, the case of Phineas Gage, a railroad worker who survived an accident that drove a metal rod through his skull and brain, contributed to the development of psychology and neuroscience (Macmillan 2002). Relatedly, trauma surgery and emergency medicine each take wounds as their object, and both fields derive from historical and technological epochal shifts (Geroulanos and Meyers 2018; Cooter and Luckin 1997; Nurok 2003; Schlich 2006). There is an enduring tie between these

medical specialties and war: wounds are reminders of war-making both on and off the battlefield (Dewachi 2015; MacLeish 2013; Puar 2017; D. Nelson 1997; Serlin 2004), even as biomedicine both creates and disavows these attachments (Terry 2017; A. Young 1995). The triage of wounds spills into social rubrics, shaping moral economies of treatment deservingness and the ethics of rehabilitation (Linker 2011). In this light, as they make medicine, wounds connect healing to violence.

Wounds also constitute a unique object of inquiry for humanists and social scientists of medicine, an object both similar to and different from disease. Wounds mark specific forms of temporality, subjectivity, and visibility; they bridge the immanent and the chronic, the individuated and the collective, and the latent and the manifest. Like disease, wounds can spark questions of "What happened?" in the search for meaning amid scenes of suffering. Yet unlike disease, wounds from purposive action put the quest for healing in complex relation to questions about the intentionality and accountability of violence. The sick person's questions of "Why me?" have conventionally opened up space for health humanities analysis (Kleinman 1988). Yet the wounded person's questions of "Why me?" may also be understood as questions of "Why was this violence done to me?" (Das 2006). Agency figures here and can be the grounds for pursuits of compensation and justice (Jain 2006; Ralph 2020). Indeed, whether a bodily disruption can be visualized as a wound may be the deciding factor for legitimating or ignoring claims in law, especially in contexts where doubt clouds the truths of the body's evidence, such as sexual violence (Mulla 2014), disability (Ralph 2012; Wool 2015), and industrial disaster (K. Fortun 2001; Petryna 2002). Wounds also foreground pain as the grounds of political history (Wailoo 2014), ethics (L. Cohen 1999), and narrative itself (Scarry 1985).

To illustrate this problem of how wounds put credibility and accountability into tension, consider two cases from Mumbai, India, that speak to the social life of traumatic injury (Solomon 2022). One evening in the emergency department in one of the city's largest public hospitals, I sit with the casualty medical officer, or CMO. It is the CMO's job to triage the hundreds of cases that come to the hospital each day and to direct treatment for them. A man arrives with a leg fracture after being hit by a rickshaw while crossing the street. As the CMO assesses the fracture and takes notes in the examination sheet, the man insists that the doctor write the notes in such a way that the police will seek the most severe punishment for the rickshaw driver. In India, traffic accidents are considered medico-legal cases, meaning that a "case" consists of truths produced by both doctors and the police. These truths are active sites of social differentiation. Wounds, then, can bleed boundaries between authoritative institutions, such as the clinic, the police station, and the courtroom.

An additional challenge emerges in how wounds might be a conduit between blame and structural violence. One evening, a large group of shirtless teens, barefoot and drenched, bring in a young boy on a makeshift cloth stretcher. The teens were playing around the construction site, climbing and jumping, and the boy fell into a deep pool of water, which was filled with iron rods and concrete pylons. When he did not resurface, the others began looking for him. The dirty water clouded their ability to see beneath the surface, but they eventually found his body and brought him to the hospital. Now in the emergency room, the casualty medical officer says little, listens intently, and confers with the nurse who applies electrodes to the boy's body and reads the flatline on the EKG. The announcement of the boy's death sends waves of grief through the room, among the boy's family, among the friends who brought him,

and among the other people still waiting in line to be seen. The police arrive, and there are discussions about legal action against the builder who let the construction site remain unfinished. I watch the CMO fill out the paperwork and ask how he will account for the cause of death. Who or what is the agent of wounding here? Is it the iron rod? The standing water? The negligence of the builder or the real estate developer and the capitalist interests they represent? The CMO, with no easy answers, writes "iron rod" on the paper.

Whether structural explanations will bring relief or compensation to the boy's family is unclear, as the concreteness of wounds becomes fetishized at one scale of materiality to the exclusion of other possible scales. Still, this case points to ways that built environments might be examined as agents of wounding (Weizman 2017). Further, it points to questions scholars raise about how capitalism, colonialism, and technology are wounding forces, evinced in cases ranging from the expansion of the nineteenth-century railways (Schivelbusch 1986) to the lethality of the twenty-first-century United States / Mexico border (Jusionyte 2018; De León 2015). Mass injury may mark what has been termed *wound culture* in studies of how widespread traffic accidents in India (Sundaram 2009) and serial killers in the United States (Seltzer 1997) situate wounds in the everyday social fabric. Wound culture as a social form means that when medicine diagnoses and treats wounds, it is also diagnosing and treating the world.

Yet it is also crucial for health humanities scholars to confront how medicine *itself* is an agent of wounding. From chemotherapy to rehabilitative medicine, clinical pursuits call into question how much people can live with medicine's force as a *pharmakon* (Boyer 2019; Jain 2013). Also at stake is the challenge of tracing the histories of violence enacted on marginalized and often women's bodies in the name of making medical expertise, from obstetrics (Cooper Owens 2017) to reha-bilitative medicine (Kim 2017). Paradoxically and cru-elly, medicine's wounds may also ensnare patients in feedback loops where they must pursue *more* medicine after initial attempts at treatment fail, as the troubling instance of "failed back surgery syndrome" make clear (Crowley-Matoka 2020). As medicine marks bodies, of-ten indelibly, wounds may manifest medicine's very limits (Bosk 1979).

Finally, wounds concretize dilemmas of visibility. This matter comes into stark relief in Kevin Brockmei-er's novel *The Illumination* (2011). The book's premise is simple yet haunting: on a Friday evening, all around the world, people's wounds begin to shine. A woman's cut finger brightens a hospital room. She watches the TV and sees the phenomenon unfolding on the floor of the New York Stock Exchange, where "sparks ap-peared to swirl through the bodies of traders like the static on a broken television" (8). Newer wounds radi-ate; older ones twinkle. There is no explanation for The Illumination, just light. Brockmeier tracks how life adjusts to this new normal, including the life of medi-cine: "Doctors no longer had to rely on their patients to tell them how badly they were suffering," he writes (21). The Illumination also tilts everyday ethics. For one character in the novel, it is unclear how to regard the light of others. "Was it discourteous," he wonders, "to admit that you could see a person's sickness playing out on the surface of his body?" (140). To another character, the light of wounds seems to vary by setting: "People in the city exhibited the sickly luster of pollution rashes and the silver sparks of carpal tunnel syndrome, while in the country they wore the shimmering waves of home tattoo infections, the glowing white zippers of lig-ature abrasions" (148). And on gray days, another char-acter "would peer down the street and see nothing but a gleaming field of injuries, as if the traumas and diseases

from which people suffered had become so powerful, so hardy, that they no longer needed their bodies to sur-vive" (225). The capacity to see wounds, and for wounds to be seen, is the grounds of humanity itself.

This matter of visibility is perhaps what is most at stake in future studies of wounds. Such studies might ask these questions: What sets the terms of a wound's visibility and invisibility? What connections might there be between the revelation of a wound and medi-cine's response to it? And ultimately, what kinds of at-tachments will the health humanities have to tracing wounds, and to following what they concretize? Brock-meier writes, "The Illumination had overturned all the old categories of thought" (2011, 164). So too might the study of wounds continue to refresh modes of think-ing through an embodied politics of accountability.

References

AARP. "Better Together: Age-Friendly and Dementia-Friendly Communities." AARP Livable Communities. 2020. https://www.aarp.org.

Ablow, Rachel. "The Social Life of Pain." *Representations* 146, no. 1 (Spring 2019): 1–9.

Adams, Vincanne. "Against Global Health? Arbitrating Science, Non-science and Nonsense in Global Health." In *Against Health: How Health Became the New Morality*, edited by Jonathan M. Metzl and Anna Kirkland, 40–58. New York: New York University Press, 2010.

———. "Randomized Controlled Crime: Postcolonial Sciences in Alternative Medicine Research." *Social Studies of Science* 32, nos. 5–6 (2002): 659–90.

Adeola, Francis O. *Industrial Disasters, Toxic Waste, and Community Impact: The Health Effects and Environmental Justice Struggles around the Globe*. Lanham, MD: Rowman & Littlefield, 2012.

Adler-Milstein, Julia, and Ashish K. Jha. "HITECH Act Drove Large Gains in Hospital Electronic Health Record Adoption." *Health Affairs (Project Hope)* 36, no. 8 (2017): 1416–22. https://doi.org/10.1377/hlthaff.2016.1651.

Administration on Aging. *Profile of Older Americans*. Administration for Community Living, US Department of Health and Human Services, 2017. https://acl.gov.

———. "Who Will Provide Your Care?" US Department of Health and Human Services, 2020. https://longtermcare.acl.gov.

Agamben, Giorgio. *Homo Sacer: Sovereign Power and Bare Life*. Translated by Daniel Heller Roazen. Palo Alto, CA: Stanford University Press, 1998.

Ahmed, Aziza. "Medical Evidence and Expertise in Abortion Jurisprudence." *American Journal of Law & Medicine* 41, no. 1 (2015): 85–118.

Aiken, Linda H., Sean P. Clarke, Douglas M. Sloane, Julie Sochalski, and Jeffrey H. Silber. "Hospital Nurse Staffing and Patient Mortality, Nurse Burnout, and Job Dissatisfaction." *JAMA* 288, no. 16 (October 2002): 1987–93.

Akkermans, Rebecca. "Robert Heinrich Herman Koch." *Lancet Respiratory Medicine* 2, no. 4 (2014): 264–65.

Alaimo, Stacy. *Bodily Natures: Science, Environment, and the Material Self*. Bloomington: Indiana University Press, 2010.

Alaimo, Stacy, and Susan J. Hekman, eds. *Material Feminisms*. Bloomington: Indiana University Press, 2008.

Allen, Barbara L. *Uneasy Alchemy: Citizens and Experts in Louisiana's Chemical Corridor Disputes*. Cambridge, MA: MIT Press, 2003.

Allport, Gordon W. *The Nature of Prejudice*. Abbreviated ed. Garden City, NJ: Doubleday, 1958.

ALQahtani, Dalal A., Jerome I. Rotgans, Silvia Mamede, Ibrahim ALAlwan, Mohi Eldin M. Magzoub, Fatheya M. Altayeb, Manahil A. Mohamedani, and Henk G. Schmidt. "Does Time Pressure Have a Negative Effect on Diagnostic Accuracy?" *Academic Medicine* 91, no. 5 (2016): 710–16.

Alston, Vermonja. "Environment." In *Keywords for Environmental Studies*, edited by Joni Adamson, William A. Gleason, and David N. Pellow, 93–96. New York: New York University Press, 2016.

Altschuler, Sari. *The Medical Imagination: Literature and Health in the Early United States*. Philadelphia: University of Pennsylvania Press, 2018.

American Psychiatric Association DSM-5 Task Force. *Diagnostic and Statistical Manual of Mental Disorders*. 5th ed. Washington, DC: American Psychiatric Association, 2013.

Amin, Samir. *Class and Nation*. New York: Monthly Review Press, 1980.

———. "Crisis, Nationalism, and Socialism." In *Dynamics of Global Crisis*, edited by Samir Amin, Andre Gunder Frank, and Immanuel Wallerstein, 167–232. New York: Monthly Review Press, 1982.

———. *Unequal Development: An Essay on the Social Formations of Peripheral Capitalism*. New York: Monthly Review Press, 1976.

Amr, Samir S., and Abdulghani Tbakhi. "Abu Bakr Muhammad Ibn Zakariya Al Razi (Rhazes): Philosopher, Physician and Alchemist." *Annals of Saudi Medicine* 27, no. 4 (2007): 305–7. https://doi.org/10.5144/0256-4947.2007.305.

Amrith, S. Sunil. *Decolonizing International Health: India and Southeast Asia, 1930–1965*. Cambridge: Cambridge University Press, 2006.

Amutah, Christina, Kaliya Greenidge, Adjoa Mante, Michelle Munyikwa, Sanjna L. Surya, Eve Higginbotham, and David S. Jones. "Misrepresenting Race—the Role of Medical Schools in Propagating Physician Bias." *New England Journal of Medicine* 384, no. 9 (January 2021): 1–7.

Anagnost, Ann S. "Strange Circulations: The Blood Economy in Rural China." *Economy and Society* 34, no. 4 (2006): 509–29.

Anderson, Kyle. "Google's Larry Page and Sergey Brin Plan to Cure Aging with Biotech Venture." Money Morning. June 25, 2015.

Anderson, Misty. *Imagining Methodism in Eighteenth-Century Britain: Enthusiasm, Belief, and the Borders of the Self*. Baltimore: Johns Hopkins University Press, 2015.

Anderson, Warwick. *The Collectors of Lost Souls: Turning Kuru Scientists into Whitemen*. Baltimore: Johns Hopkins University Press, 2008.

———. *Colonial Pathologies: American Tropical Medicine, Race, and Hygiene in the Philippines*. Durham, NC: Duke University Press, 2006.

———. "Decolonizing Histories in Theory and Practice: An Introduction." *History and Theory* 59, no. 3 (September 2020): 369–75.

———. "Where Is the Postcolonial History of Medicine?" *Bulletin of the History of Medicine* 72, no. 3 (1998): 522–30.

Anderson Cooper 360. Season 6, Episode 8, "Finding Amanda." Aired April 2, 2008, on CNN.

Andrews, Billy F. "Sir William Osler's Emphasis on Physical Diagnosis and Listening to Symptoms." *Southern Medical Journal* 95, no. 10 (2002): 1173–78.

Antonetta, Susanne. *A Mind Apart: Travels in a Neurodiverse World*. New York: Tarcher, 2005.

Appelbaum, Paul S., and Joel I. Klein. "Therefore Choose Death?" *Commentary* 81, no. 4 (April 1986): 23–29.

Arendt, Hannah. *The Human Condition*. With an introduction by Margaret Canovan. 2nd ed. Chicago: University of Chicago Press, (1958) 1998.

Aristotle. "History of Animals." In *The Complete Works of Aristotle*, edited by Jonathan Barnes, 774–992. Vol. 1. Princeton, NJ: Princeton University Press, 1984a.

———. "On the Soul." In *The Complete Works of Aristotle*, edited by Jonathan Barnes, 641–92. Vol. 1. Princeton, NJ: Princeton University Press, 1984b.

———. "Parts of Animals." In *The Complete Works of Aristotle*, edited by Jonathan Barnes, 994–1086. Vol. 1. Princeton, NJ: Princeton University Press, 1984c.

———. "Physics." In *The Complete Works of Aristotle*, edited by Jonathan Barnes, 315–446. Vol. 1. Princeton, NJ: Princeton University Press, 1984d.

———. "Poetics." In *Poetics I*, translated by Richard Janko, 1–42. Indianapolis: Hackett, 1987.

Armelagos, George J., Peter J. Brow, and Bethany Turner. "Evolutionary, Historical and Political Economic Perspectives on Health and Disease." *Social Science & Medicine* 61, no. 4 (August 2005): 755–65.

Armiero, Marco, Thanos Andritsos, Stefania Barca, Rita Brás, Sergio Ruiz Cauyela, Çağdaş Dedeoğlu, Marica Di Pierri, et al. "Toxic Bios: Toxic Autobiographies—a Public Environmental Humanities Project." *Environmental Justice* 12, no. 1 (2019): 7–11.

Armstrong, David. "Embodiment and Ethics: Constructing Medicine's Two Bodies." *Sociology of Health & Illness* 28, no. 6 (2006): 866–81.

Arnold, David. *Colonizing the Body: State Medicine and Epidemic Disease in Nineteenth-Century India*. Berkeley: University of California Press, 1993.

Aronowitz, Robert A. *Risky Medicine: Our Quest to Cure Fear and Uncertainty*. Chicago: University of Chicago Press, 2015.

Aronson, Louise. *Elderhood: Redefining Aging, Transforming Medicine, Reimagining Life*. New York: Bloomsbury, 2019.

Arras, John D. *Bringing the Hospital Home: Ethical and Social Implications of High-Tech Home Care*. Baltimore: Johns Hopkins University Press, 1995.

———. *Methods in Bioethics: The Way We Reason Now*. New York: Oxford University Press, 2017.

Arvin, Maile. "Analytics of Indigeneity." In *Native Studies Keywords*, edited by Stephanie Nohelani Teves, Andrea Smith, and Michelle Raheja, 119–29. Tucson: University of Arizona Press, 2015.

Aschwanden, Christie. "The False Promise of Herd Immunity for COVID-19." *Nature* 587, no. 5 (November 2020): 26–28.

Askitopoulou, Helen. "Sleep and Dreams: From Myth to Medicine in Ancient Greece." *Journal of Anesthesia History* 1, no. 3 (2015): 70–75.

Atkinson, Sarah, Bethan Evans, Angela Woods, and Robin Kearns. "'The Medical' and 'Health' in Critical Medical Humanities." *Journal of Medical Humanities* 36, no. 1 (2015): 71–81.

Auerbach, Kelly, and Jay M. Baruch. "Beyond Comfort Zones: An Experiment in Medical and Art Education." *Journal for Learning through the Arts* 1, no. 8 (2012): 1–14.

Aulisio, Mark P., Robert M. Arnold, and Stuart J. Younger. "Health Care Ethics Consultation: Nature, Goals, and Competencies: A Position Paper from the Society for Health and Human Values—Society for Bioethics Consultation Task Force on Standards for Bioethics Consultation." *Annals of Internal Medicine* 133, no. 1 (2000): 59–69.

Ayalon, Liat, and Clemens Tesch-Römer. "Ageism—Concept and Origins." In *Contemporary Perspectives on Ageism*, edited by Liat Ayalon and Clemens Tesch-Römer, 1–10. Cham, Switzerland: Springer International, 2018.

Badiou, Alain. *The Century*. Malden, MA: Polity, 2007.

Baggs, Amanda. *Ballastexistenz*. WordPress, 2005. https://ballastexistenz.wordpress.com.

———. *In My Language*. YouTube channel, 2007. https://www.youtube.com/watch?v=JnylM1hI2jc.

Baker, Robert B. "The American Medical Association and Race." *AMA Journal of Ethics* 16, no. 6 (2014): 479–88.

Balasubramanian, Sai. "Anti-aging and Aesthetic Medicine: The Silent Rise of This Multibillion Dollar Industry." *Forbes*, January 28, 2020. https://www.forbes.com.

Baldwin, James. *Collected Essays*. Edited by Toni Morrison. New York: Library of America, 1998.

Ballard, J. G. *Crash*. New York: Picador, 2017.

Ballenger, Jesse. *Self, Senility and Alzheimer's Disease in Modern America*. Baltimore: Johns Hopkins University Press, 2006.

Bang, Megan, Ananda Marin, and Douglas Medin. "If Indigenous Peoples Stand with the Sciences, Will Scientists Stand with Us?" *Daedalus* 147, no. 2 (2018): 148–59.

Banner, Olivia. *Communicative Biocapitalism: The Voice of the Patient in Digital Health and the Health Humanities*. Ann Arbor: University of Michigan Press, 2017.

Barad, Karen. *Meeting the Universe Halfway: Quantum Physics and the Entanglement of Matter and Meaning*. Durham, NC: Duke University Press, 2007.

Barca, Stefania. "Telling the Right Story: Environmental Violence and Liberation Narratives." *Environment and History* 20, no. 4 (2014): 535–46.

Bardosh, Kevin, ed. *One Health: Science, Politics and Zoonotic Disease in Africa*. London: Routledge, 2016.

Barker, Pat. *Regeneration*. New York: Penguin, 1991.

Barnard, David. "Making a Place for the Humanities in Residency Education." *Academic Medicine* 69, no. 8 (August 1994): 628–30.

Barney, Richard, and Helen Schrek. "Introduction: Early and Modern Biospheres." *Journal for Early Modern Cultural Studies* 10, no. 2 (Fall/Winter 2010): 1–22.

Barocas, Solon, and Helen Nissenbaum. "Big Data's End Run Around Procedural Privacy Protections." *Communications of the ACM* 57, no. 11 (2014): 31–33.

———. "On Notice: The Trouble with Notice and Consent." Proceedings of the Engaging Data Forum: The First International Forum on the Application and Management of Personal Electronic Information. October 2009. https://nissenbaum.tech.cornell.edu.

Baron-Cohen, Simon. "The Concept of Neurodiversity Is Dividing the Autism Community." *Scientific American*, April 30, 2019. https://blogs.scientificamerican.com.

Barounis, Cynthia. *Vulnerable Constitutions: Queerness, Disability, and the Remaking of American Manhood*. Philadelphia: Temple University Press, 2019.

Barthes, Roland. "Introduction to the Structural Analysis of Narratives." In *The Semiotic Challenge*, translated by Richard Howard, 95–135. New York: Hill & Wang, 1988.

Baruch, Jay M. "Creative Writing as a Medical Instrument." *Journal of Medical Humanities* 34, no. 4 (2013): 459–69.

———. "Doctors as Makers." *Academic Medicine* 92, no. 1 (2017): 40–44.

Bashford, Alison, and Philippa Levine, eds. *The Oxford Handbook of the History of Eugenics*. Oxford: Oxford University Press, 2010.

Basting, Anne Davis. *Forget Memory: Creating Better Lives for People with Dementia*. Baltimore: Johns Hopkins University Press, 2009.

Baynton, Douglas C. *Defectives in the Land*. Chicago: University of Chicago Press, 2016.

Beam, Andrew, and Isaac Kohane. "Big Data and Machine Learning in Health Care." *JAMA* 319, no. 13 (2018): 1317–18.

Beard, George Miller. *American Nervousness: Its Causes and Consequences*. New York: G. P. Putnam's Sons, 1881.

Beauchamp, Tom L., and James Childress. *The Principles of Biomedical Ethics*. New York: Oxford University Press, 1979.

Beck, Ulrich. *Risk Society: Towards a New Modernity*. Translated by Mark Ritter. London: Sage, (1986) 1992.

Beecher, Henry K. "Ethics and Clinical Research." *New England Journal of Medicine* 274, no. 24 (1966): 1354–60.

Behbehani, Abbas M. "The Smallpox Story: Life and Death of an Old Disease." *Microbiological Reviews* 47, no. 4 (December 1983): 455–509.

Bell, Susan E. "Changing Ideas: The Medicalization of Menopause." *Social Science & Medicine* 24, no. 6 (1987): 535–42. https://doi.org/10.1016/0277-9536(87)90343-1.

Belling, Catherine. "Arts, Sciences, Humanities: Triangulating the Two Cultures." *Journal of Literature and Science* 10, no. 2 (2017): 19–25.

———. "Microbiography and Resistance in the Human Culture Medium." *Literature and Medicine* 22, no. 1 (2003): 84–101.

Benjamin, Ruha. "Assessing Risk, Automating Racism." *Science* 366, no. 6464 (2019a): 421–22.

———. *Race after Technology: Abolitionist Tools for the New Jim Code*. Medford, MA: Polity, 2019b.

Ben-Moshe, Liat, and Allison C. Carey. *Disability Incarcerated: Imprisonment and Disability in the United States and Canada*. New York: Palgrave Macmillan, 2014.

Bennett, Jane. *Vibrant Matter: A Political Ecology of Things*. Durham, NC: Duke University Press, 2010.

Benveniste, Emile. "La Doctrine Médicale des Indo-Européens." *Revue de l'Histoire des Religions* 130, no. 4 (1945): 5–12.

Berg, Jessica W., and Paul S. Appelbaum. *Informed Consent: Legal Theory and Clinical Practice*. New York: Oxford University Press, 2001.

Bergson, Henri. *Creative Evolution*. Translated by Arthur Mitchell. New York: Modern Library, 1944.

Berkeley, George. *Siris, or An Abstract of the Treatise on the Virtues of Tar-Water: With Additional Notes*. Dublin, 1744.

Berlant, Lauren, ed. *Compassion: The Culture and Politics of an Emotion*. New York: Routledge, 2004.

———. *Cruel Optimism*. Durham, NC: Duke University Press, 2011.

Bernard, Claude. *Introduction à l'étude de la médecine expérimentale*. Paris: Ballière, 1865.

———. *An Introduction to the Study of Experimental Medicine*. Translated by Henry Copley Greene. London: Macmillan, (1865) 1927.

———. *Principes de médecine expérimentale*. Paris: Presses Universitaires de France, (1867) 1947.

Best, John. *Hating Autism* (blog). 2006. Google now censors this blog.

Bettcher, Douglas, and Kelley Lee. "Globalisation and Public Health." *Journal of Epidemiology and Community Health* 56, no. 1 (2002): 8–17.

Bhattacharya, Sanjoy, Mark Harrison, and Michael Worboys. *Fractured States: Smallpox, Public Health and Vaccination Policy in British India 1800–1947*. Hyderabad, India: Orient Longman, 2005.

Binder, Douglas. "Re. [EXTERNAL][HealthHum] Who Teaches Humanities at Your Medical School?" Health Humanities (HealthHum) Listserv. Hiram College. Accessed September 5, 2020. https://archives.simplelists.com.

Birn, Anne-Emanuelle. *Marriage of Convenience: Rockefeller International Health and Revolutionary Mexico*. Rochester, NY: University of Rochester Press, 2006.

Bishop, Jeffrey P. "Rejecting Medical Humanism: Medical Humanities and the Metaphysics of Medicine." *Journal of Medical Humanities* 29, no. 1 (March 2008): 15–25.

Bivins, Roberta E. *Contagious Communities: Medicine, Migration, and the NHS in Post-war Britain*. Oxford: Oxford University Press, 2015.

Bivins, Roberta E., Stephanie Tierney, and Kate Seers. "Compassionate Care: Not Easy, Not Free, Not Only Nurses." *BMJ Quality and Safety* 26, no. 12 (2017): 1023–26.

Blackman, Lisa. *Hearing Voices: Embodiment and Experience.* London: Free Association Books, 2001.

Blanchflower, David G. "Is Happiness U-shaped Everywhere? Age and Subjective Well-Being in 132 Countries." National Bureau of Economic Research Working Papers, no. 26641 (2020): 1–63.

Blank, Hanne. *Straight: The Surprisingly Short History of Heterosexuality.* Boston: Beacon, 2012.

Bleakley, Alan. "Stories as Data, Data as Stories: Making Sense of Narrative Inquiry in Clinical Education." *Medical Education* 39, no. 5 (2005): 534–40.

———. "Towards a 'Critical Medical Humanities.'" In *Medicine, Health, and the Arts: Approaches to the Medical Humanities*, edited by Victoria Bates, Alan Bleakley, and Sam Goodman, 17–26. New York: Routledge, 2014.

Bleakley, Alan, Mike Wilson, and Jon Allard. "Story Telling." In *The Routledge Companion to Health Humanities*, edited by Paul Crawford, Brian Brown, and Andrea Charise, 341–45. New York: Routledge, 2020.

Blenkinsop, Sean. "Martin Buber: Educating for Relationship." *Ethics, Place and Environment* 8, no. 3 (2005): 285–307.

Block, Sharon. *Rape and Sexual Power in Early America.* Chapel Hill: University of North Carolina Press, 2006.

Bloom, Paul. *Against Empathy: The Case for Rational Compassion.* New York: HarperCollins, 2016.

Blume, H. "Neurodiversity." *Atlantic*, September 30, 1998. https://www.theatlantic.com.

Bock, Carl. *Das Buch von gesunden und kranken Menschen.* Leipzig, Germany: Ernst Keil, 1855.

Boesky, Amy, ed. *The Story Within: Personal Essays on Genetics and Identity.* Baltimore: Johns Hopkins University Press, 2013.

Boler, Megan. *Feeling Power: Emotions and Education.* New York: Routledge, 1999.

Bond, John. "The Medicalization of Dementia." *Journal of Aging Studies* 6, no. 4 (1992): 397–403.

Bond, Lucy, and Stef Craps. *Trauma.* Oxford: Routledge, 2020.

Bonnar, Deanne. "The Wages of Care: Change and Resistance in Support of Caregiving Work." *New Politics* 11, no. 1 (2006). https://archive.newpol.org.

Bonwitt, Jesse, Michael Dawson, Martin Kandeh, Rashid Ansumana, Foday Sahr, Hannah Brown and Ann H. Kelly. "Unintended Consequences of the 'Bushmeat Ban' in West Africa during the 2013–2016 Ebola Virus Disease Epidemic." *Social Science & Medicine* 200 (March 2018): 166–73.

Bookchin, Murray. *Our Synthetic Environment.* New York: Harper and Row, 1962.

Borgman, Albert. *Technology and the Character of Contemporary Life.* Chicago: University of Chicago Press, 1984.

Boris, Eileen, and Jennifer Klein. *Caring for America: Home Health Workers in the Shadow of the Welfare State.* New York: Oxford University Press, 2012.

Boris, Eileen, and Rhacel Salazar Parreñas, eds. *Intimate Labors: Cultures, Technologies, and the Politics of Care.* Palo Alto, CA: Stanford Social Sciences, 2010.

Bosk, Charles. *Forgive and Remember: Managing Medical Failure.* Chicago: University of Chicago Press, 1979.

Boudreau, Donald J., Eric J. Cassell, and Abraham Fuks. "Preparing Medical Students to Become Skilled at Clinical Observation." *Medical Teacher* 30, nos. 9–10 (2008): 857–62.

Bourgeois, Philippe. "Anthropology and Epidemiology on Drugs: The Challenges of Cross-Methodological and Theoretical Dialogue." *International Journal of Drug Policy* 13, no. 4 (October 2002): 259–69.

Bourke, Joanna. "Wartime." In *Medicine in the Twentieth Century*, edited by R. Cooter and J. Pickstone, 589–600. Amsterdam: Harwood, 2000.

Boyer, Anne. *The Undying: Pain, Vulnerability, Mortality, Medicine, Art, Time, Dreams, Data, Exhaustion, Cancer, and Care.* New York: Farrar, Straus and Giroux, 2019.

Braidotti, Rosi. "Four Theses on Posthuman Feminism." In *Anthropocene Feminism*, edited by Richard Grusin, 21–48. Minneapolis: University of Minnesota Press, 2017.

———. *Metamorphoses: Towards a Materialist Theory of Becoming.* Malden, MA: Polity, 2002.

Brandt, Allan M. *The Cigarette Century: The Rise, Fall, and Deadly Persistence of the Product That Defined America.* New York: Basic Books, 2007.

———. *No Magic Bullet. A Social History of Venereal Disease in the United States since 1880.* Oxford: Oxford University Press, 1985.

Braswell, Harold. *The Crisis of Us Hospice Care: Family and Freedom at the End of Life.* Baltimore: Johns Hopkins University Press, 2019.

Braun, Lundy, Anne Fausto-Sterling, Duana Fullwiley, Evelynn M. Hammonds, Alondra Nelson, William Quivers,

Susan M. Reverby, and Alexandra E. Sheilds. "Racial Categories in Medical Practice: How Useful Are They?" *PLoS Medicine* 4, no. 9 (2007): 1423–28.

Braveman, Paula. "Social Conditions, Health Equity, and Human Rights." *Health and Human Rights* 12, no. 2 (2010): 31–48.

Brian, Jenny Dyck, and Robert Cook-Deegan. "What's the Use? Disparate Purposes of U.S. Federal Bioethics Commissions." *Goals and Practice of Public Bioethics: Reflections on National Bioethics Commissions*, special report, *Hastings Center Report* 47, no. 3 (2017): S14–S16.

Bridges, Khiara M. *Reproducing Race: An Ethnography of Pregnancy as a Site of Racialization*. Berkeley: University of California Press, 2011.

Briggs, Charles L., and Clara Mantini-Briggs. *Tell Me Why My Children Died: Rabies, Indigenous Knowledge, and Communicative Justice*. Durham, NC: Duke University Press, 2016.

Briggs, Laura. *Reproducing Empire: Race, Sex, Science, and US Imperialism in Puerto Rico*. Berkeley: University of California Press, 2002.

Brock, Bastian, Vauclair Christin-Melanie, Steve Loughnan, Paul Bain, Ashwini Ashokkumar, Maja Becker, Michał Bilewicz, et al. "Explaining Illness with Evil: Pathogen Prevalence Fosters Moral Vitalism." *Proceedings of the Royal Society* 286, no. 1914 (2019): 1–10.

Brock, Dan W. "The Non-identity Problem and Genetic Harms—the Case of Wrongful Handicaps." *Bioethics* 9, no. 3 (1995): 269–75.

Brockmeier, Jens. *Beyond the Archive: Memory, Narrative, and the Autobiographical Process*. New York: Oxford University Press, 2015.

Brockmeier, Kevin. *The Illumination*. New York: Vintage, 2011.

Brooks, Cleanth. *The Well Wrought Urn*. New York: Harcourt, Brace, 1947.

Brown, Brené. "Brené Brown on Empathy vs. Sympathy." YouTube video, 2016. 2:53. https://www.youtube.com/watch?v=KZBTYViDPlQ.

Brown, Hannah, and Ann H. Kelly. "Material Proximities and Hotspots: Towards an Anthropology of Viral Haemorrhagic Fevers." *Medical Anthropology Quarterly* 28, no. 2 (2014): 280–303.

Brown, Hannah, and Alex M. Nading, eds. "Special Issue: Human Animal Health in Medical Anthropology." *Medical Anthropology Quarterly* 33, no. 1 (March 2019): 1–67.

Brown, Phil. "Naming and Framing: The Social Construction of Diagnosis and Illness." Extra issue, *Journal of Health and Social Behavior*, 1995, 34–52.

Brulle, J. Robert, and David N. Pellow. "Environmental Justice: Human Health and Environmental Inequalities." *Annual Review of Public Health* 27, no. 1 (April 2006): 103–24.

Bryan, Charles S., and Lawrence D. Longo. "Teaching and Mentoring the History of Medicine: An Oslerian Perspective." *Academic Medicine* 88, no. 1 (2013): 97–101.

Buckley, M. R. F. "Winds of Change." *Harvard Gazette*. Accessed September 23, 2020.

Buelens, Gert, Samuel Durrant, and Robert Eaglestone. *The Future of Trauma Theory: Contemporary Literary and Cultural Criticism*. New York: Routledge, 2014.

Buell, Lawrence. "Toxic Discourse." *Critical Inquiry* 24, no. 3 (1998): 639–65.

Bulkeley, Kelly. *Dreaming in the World's Religions: A Comparative History*. New York: New York University Press, 2008.

Bullard, Robert D. *Dumping in Dixie: Race, Class, and Environmental Quality*. Boulder, CO: Westview, (1990) 2000.

Bullard, Robert D., Paul Mohai, Robin Saha, and Beverly Wright. "Toxic Wastes and Race at Twenty: Why Race Still Matters after All These Years." *Environmental Law* 38, no. 2 (2008): 371–411.

Bullard, Robert D., and Beverly Wright. *The Wrong Complexion for Protection: How the Government Response to Disaster Endangers African American Communities*. New York: New York University Press, 2012.

Bulterijs, Sven, Raphaella S. Hull, Victor C. Björk, and Avi G. Roy. "It Is Time to Classify Biological Aging as a Disease." *Frontiers in Genetics* 6, no. 205 (2015): 1–5.

Burdick, Alan. "Monster or Machine? A Profile of the Coronavirus at 6 Months." *New York Times*, 2020. https://www.nytimes.com.

Burke, Peter. *Varieties of Cultural History*. Ithaca, NY: Cornell University Press, 1997.

Burke, Sarah. "These Artists Want Black People to Sleep." *Vice*. January 2019.

Butler, Judith. *Frames of War: When Is Life Grievable?* New York: Verso, 2009.

———. *Gender Trouble: Feminism and the Subversion of Identity*. New York: Routledge, 1990.

———. *Giving an Account of Oneself*. New York: Fordham University Press, 2005.

Büyüm, Ali Murad, Cordelia Kenney, Andrea Koris, Laura Mkumba, and Yadurshini Raveendran. "Decolonising Global Health: If Not Now, When?" *BMJ Global Health* 5, no. 8 (August 5, 2020): 1–4.

Bybee, Jay S. "Memorandum for Albert R. Gonzales, Counsel to the President Re: Standards of Conduct for Interrogation under 18 U.S.C. §§2340–2340A." Office of the Assistant Attorney General. August 1, 2002. https://nsarchive2.gwu.edu.

Bynum, William F. *Science and the Practice of Medicine in the Nineteenth Century*. Cambridge Studies in the History of Science. Cambridge: Cambridge University Press, 1994.

Cacchioni, Thea. "The Medicalization of Sexual Deviance, Reproduction, and Functioning." In *Handbook of the Sociology of Sexualities*, edited by John DeLamater and Rebeca F. Plante, 435–52. New York: Springer International, 2015.

Caduff, Carlo. *The Pandemic Perhaps: Dramatic Events in a Public Culture of Danger*. Berkeley: University of California Press, 2015.

Cajete, Gregory A. "Indigenous Science, Climate Change, and Indigenous Community Building: A Framework of Foundational Perspectives for Indigenous Community Resilience and Revitalization." *Sustainability* 12, no. 22 (2020): 1–11.

Callier, Shawneequa. "The Use of Racial Categories in Precision Medicine Research." *Ethnicity & Disease* 29, supplement 3 (2019): 651–58.

Cambridge English Dictionary, s.v. "drug." Cambridge University Press. Accessed October 20, 2022. https://dictionary.cambridge.org.

Campo, Rafael. "I Am Gula, Hear Me Roar: On Gender and Medicine." In *Health Humanities Reader*, edited by Therese Jones, Delese Wear, and Lester D. Friedman, 242–50. New Brunswick, NJ: Rutgers University Press, 2014.

———. "'The Medical Humanities,' for Lack of a Better Term." *JAMA* 294, no. 9 (September 2005): 1009–11.

Canguilhem, Georges. *Études d'histoire et de philosophie des sciences concernant les vivants et la vie*. Paris: Vrin, (1968) 1994.

———. *The Normal and the Pathological*. Translated by Carolyn Fawcett. New York: Zone, (1966) 1991.

Cantor, David, ed. *Reinventing Hippocrates*. Burlington, VT: Ashgate, 2002.

Cantor, David, and Edmund Ramsden, eds. *Stress, Shock, and Adaptation in the Twentieth Century*. Rochester, NY: University of Rochester Press, 2014.

Carey, Allison C. *On the Margins of Citizenship: Intellectual Disability and Civil Rights in Twentieth-Century America*. Philadelphia: Temple University Press, 2009.

Carlin, Claire L., ed. *Imagining Contagion in Early Modern Europe*. New York: Palgrave Macmillan, 2005.

Carlson, Licia. *The Faces of Intellectual Disability: Philosophical Reflections*. Bloomington: Indiana University Press, 2010.

Carmichael, Ann G. *Plague and the Poor in Renaissance Florence*. Cambridge: Cambridge University Press, 1986.

Carpenter, Morgan. "The Human Rights of Intersex People: Addressing Harmful Practices and Rhetoric of Change." *Reproductive Health Matters* 24, no. 47 (2016): 74–84.

———. *Unclaimed Experience: Trauma, Narrative and History*. Baltimore: Johns Hopkins University Press, 1996.

Carrigan, Anthony. "Towards a Postcolonial Disaster Studies." In *Global Ecologies and the Environmental Humanities: Postcolonial Approaches*, edited by Elizabeth DeLoughrey, Jill Didur, and Anthony Carrigan, 117–39. London: Routledge, 2015.

Carson, Rachel. *Silent Spring*. Boston: Houghton Mifflin Harcourt Trade & Reference, (1962) 2002.

Carstensen, Laura L., Monisha Pasupathi, Ulrich Mayr, and John R. Nesselroade. "Emotional Experience in Everyday Life across the Adult Life Span." *Journal of Personality and Social Psychology* 79, no. 4 (2000): 644–55.

Carter, Julian B. *The Heart of Whiteness: Normal Sexuality and Race in America, 1880–1940*. Durham, NC: Duke University Press, 2007.

Caruth, Cathy, ed. *Trauma: Explorations in Memory*. Baltimore: Johns Hopkins University Press, 1995.

Catanach, Ian. "Plague and the Tensions of Empire: India, 1896–1918." In *Imperial Medicine and Indigenous Societies*, edited by David Arnold, 149–71. Manchester: Manchester University Press, 1988.

Ceccarelli, Leah. *On the Frontier of Science: An American Rhetoric of Exploration and Exploitation*. East Lansing: Michigan State University Press, 2013.

Celermajer, Danielle, Sria Chatterji, Alasdair Cochrane, Stefanie Fishel, Astrida Neimanis, Anne O'Brien, Susan Reid, Krithika Srinivasan, David Schlosberg, and Anik Waldow. "Justice through a Multispecies Lens." *Contemporary Political Theory* 19, no. 3 (2020): 476–93.

Chadwick, J., W. N. Mann, and Geoffery Ernest Richard Lloyd. *Hippocratic Writings*. London: Penguin Classics, 1983.

Chakrabarti, Pratik. *Bacteriology in British India: Laboratory Medicine and the Tropics*. Rochester, NY: University of Rochester Press, 2012.

———. *Medicine and Empire, 1600–1960*. Basingstoke: Palgrave Macmillan, 2014.

Chambers, Tod. *The Fiction of Bioethics*. New York: Routledge, 1999.

Chan, Kit Yee, and Daniel D. Reidpath. "'Typhoid Mary' and 'HIV Jane': Responsibility, Agency and Disease Prevention." *Reproductive Health Matters* 11, no. 22 (2003): 40–50.

Chaney, Daniel W. "An Overview of the First Use of the Terms *Cognition* and *Behavior*." *Behavioral Sciences* 3, no. 1 (March 2013): 143–53.

Chang, E-Shien, Sneha Kannoth, Samantha Levy, Shi-Yi Wang, John E. Lee, and Becca R. Levy. "Global Reach of Ageism on Older Persons' Health: A Systematic Review." *PLoS One* 15, no. 1 (2020): 1–24. https://doi.org/10.1371/journal.pone.0220857.

Chaplin, Joyce. *Subject Matter Technology, the Body, and Science on the Anglo-American Frontier, 1500–1676*. Cambridge, MA: Harvard University Press, 2003.

Charise, Andrea. "'Let the Reader Think of the Burden': Old Age and the Crisis of Capacity." *Occasion: Interdisciplinary Studies in the Humanities* 4 (May 2012): 1–16. https://arcade.stanford.edu.

Charles, Dorothy, Kathryn Himmelstein, Keenan Walker, Nicolas Barcelo, and the White Coats for Black Lives National Working Group. "White Coats for Black Lives: Medical Students Responding to Racism and Police Brutality." *Journal of Urban Health* 92, no. 6 (December 2016): 1007–10.

Charlton, James I. *Nothing about Us without Us: Disability Oppression and Empowerment*. Berkeley: University of California Press, 2000.

Charon, Rita. "Literature and Medicine: Origins and Destinies." *Academic Medicine* 75, no. 1 (January 2000): 23–27.

———. "Narrative Medicine: A Model for Empathy, Reflection, Profession, and Trust." *JAMA* 286, no. 15 (2001): 1897–1902.

———. "Narrative Medicine: Attention, Representation, Affiliation." *Narrative* 13, no. 3 (2005): 261–70.

———. *Narrative Medicine: Honoring the Stories of Illness*. Oxford: Oxford University Press, 2006.

———. "Re. [EXTERNAL][HealthHum] Who Teaches Humanities at Your Medical School?" Health Humanities (HealthHum) Listserv. Hiram College. September 5, 2020. https://archives.simplelists.com.

———. "To Render the Lives of Patients." *Literature and Medicine* 5, no. 1 (1986): 58–74.

Charon, Rita, Sayantani DasGupta, Nellie Hermann, Craig Irvine, Eric R. Marcus, Edgar Rivera Colón, Danielle Spencer, and Maura Spiegel. *The Principles and Practice of Narrative Medicine*. New York: Oxford University Press, 2017.

Charon, Rita, Craig Irvine, Aaron Ngozi Oforlea, Edgar Rivera Colón, Cindy Smalletz, and Maura Spiegel. "Racial Justice in Medicine: Narrative Practices toward Equity." *Narrative* 29, no. 2 (2021): 160–77.

Charyn, Thelma. "The Etymology of Medicine." *Bulletin of the Medical Library Association* 39, no. 3 (July 1951): 216–21. https://www.ncbi.nlm.nih.gov.

Chase, Cheryl. "What Is the Agenda of the Intersex Patient Advocacy Movement?" *Endocrinologist* 13, no. 3 (2003): 240–42.

Chatzidakis, Andreas, Jamie Hakim, Jo Littler, Catherine Rottenberg, and Lynne Segal (the Care Collective). *The Care Manifesto: The Politics of Interdependence*. London: Verso, 2020.

Chekroud, Adam M., Hieronimus Loho, Martin Paulus, and John H. Krystal. "PTSD and the War of Words." *Chronic Stress* 2 (2018): 1–5. https://doi.org/10.1177/2470547018767387.

Chen, Mel Y. *Animacies: Biopolitics, Racial Mattering, and Queer Affect*. Durham, NC: Duke University Press, 2012.

Cheyne, George. *The Natural Method of Cureing the Diseases of the Body, and the Disorders of the Mind Depending on the Body*. London: Golden Ball, 1742.

Chigudu, Simukai. *The Political Life of an Epidemic: Cholera, Crisis and Citizenship in Zimbabwe*. Cambridge: Cambridge University Press, 2020.

Chilisa, Bagele. *Indigenous Research Methodologies*. Los Angeles: Sage, 2012.

Cho, Grace. *Haunting the Korean Diaspora: Shame, Secrecy, and the Forgotten War*. Minneapolis: University of Minnesota Press, 2008.

Cho, Mildred K., Sara L. Tobin, Henry T. Greely, Jennifer McCormick, Angie Boyce, and David Magnus. "Strangers at the Benchside: Research Ethics Consultation." *American Journal of Bioethics* 8, no. 3 (2008): 4–13.

Choi, Tina Young. *Anonymous Connections: The Body and Narratives of the Social in Victorian Britain*. Ann Arbor: University of Michigan Press, 2015.

Chowkwanyun, Merlin, Roland Bayer, and Sandro Galea. "'Precision' Public Health—between Novelty and Hype." *New England Journal of Medicine* 379, no. 15 (2018): 1398–1400.

Chown, Sheila, and K. F. Riegel, eds. *Psychological Functioning in the Normal Aging and Senile Aged*. Basel: Karger, 1968.

Chrisler, Joan C., Angela Barney, and Brigida Palatino. "Ageism Can Be Hazardous to Women's Health: Ageism, Sexism, and Stereotypes of Older Women in the Healthcare System." *Journal of Social Issues* 72, no. 1 (2016): 86–104. https://doi.org/10.1111/josi.12157.

Clapham, Christopher. "Decolonizing African Studies." *Journal of Modern African Studies* 58, no. 1 (2020): 137–53.

Clare, Eli. *Brilliant Imperfection: Grappling with Cure*. Durham, NC: Duke University Press, 2017.

Clark, Timothy. "Scale. Derangements of Scale." In *Telemorphosis: Theory in the Era of Climate Change*, vol. 1, edited by Tom Cohen, 148–66. London: Open Humanities, 2012.

Cleveland Clinic. "Empathy by Design." *Washington Post*, 2017. https://www.washingtonpost.com.

Cocchiara, Rosario Andrea, Margherita Peruzzo, Alice Mannocci, Livia Ottolenghi, Paolo Villari, Antonella Polimeni, Fabrizio Guerra et al. "The Use of Yoga to Manage Stress and Burnout in Healthcare Workers: A Systematic Review." *Journal of Clinical Medicine* 8, no. 3 (2019): 284. https://doi.org/10.3390/jcm8030284.

Cohen, Adam Seth. *Imbeciles: The Supreme Court, American Eugenics, and the Sterilization of Carrie Buck*. New York: Penguin, 2016.

Cohen, Deborah. *Family Secrets: Shame and Privacy in Modern Britain*. Oxford: Oxford University Press, 2013.

Cohen, Ed. *A Body Worth Defending: Immunity, Biopolitics, and the Apotheosis of the Modern Body*. Durham, NC: Duke University Press, 2009.

———. "Self, Not-Self, Not Not-Self but Not Self, or the Knotty Paradoxes of 'Autoimmunity': A Genealogical Rumination." *Parallax* 23, no. 1 (2017): 28–45.

Cohen, Glenn I., and Michelle M. Mello. "HIPAA and Protecting Health Information in the 21st Century." *JAMA* 320, no. 3 (2018): 231–32.

Cohen, Lawrence. *No Aging in India: Alzheimer's, the Bad Family, and Other Modern Things*. Berkeley: University of California Press, 1998.

———. "Where It Hurts: Indian Material for an Ethics of Organ Transplantation." *Daedalus* 128, no. 4 (1999): 135–65.

Colapinto, John. "Brain Games: The Marco Polo of Neuroscience." *New Yorker*, May 4, 2009. https://www.newyorker.com.

Coleman, William. "The Cognitive Basis of the Discipline: Claude Bernard on Physiology." *Isis* 76, no. 1 (1985): 49–70.

Coley, William B. "Contribution to the Knowledge of Sarcoma." *Annals of Surgery* 14, no. 3 (1891): 199–220.

Comfort, Nathaniel. "Can We Cure Genetic Diseases without Slipping into Eugenics?" In *Beyond Bioethics*, edited by Osagie K. Obasogie and Marcy Darnovsky, 175–85. Berkeley: University of California Press, 2018.

Condit, Celeste M. "How the Public Understands Genetics: Non-deterministic and Non-discriminatory Interpretations of the 'Blueprint' Metaphor." *Public Understanding of Science* 8, no. 3 (1999): 169–80.

Conrad, Peter. *The Medicalization of Society: On the Transformation of Human Conditions into Treatable Disorders*. Baltimore: Johns Hopkins University Press, 2007.

Conrad, Peter, and Deborah Potter. "From Hyperactive Children to ADHD Adults: Observations on the Expansion of Medical Categories." *Social Problems* 47, no. 4 (2000): 559–82.

"Constitution of the World Health Organization." *American Journal of Public Health* 36, no. 11 (November 1, 1946): 1315–23.

Cook, Gordon Charles. "Thomas Southwood Smith FRCP (1788–1861): Leading Exponent of Diseases of Poverty and Pioneer of Sanitary Reform in the Mid-nineteenth Century." *Journal of Medical Biography* 10, no. 4 (2002): 194–205.

Cooke, Anne, ed. *Understanding Psychosis: Why People Sometimes Hear Voices, Believe Things That Others Find Strange, or Appear Out of Touch with Reality, and What Can Help*. London: British Psychological Society, 2017.

Coole, Diana, and Samantha Frost, eds. *New Materialisms: Ontology, Agency, and Politics*. Durham, NC: Duke University Press, 2010.

Cooper, Claudia, Paul Bebbington, and Gill Livingston. "Cognitive Impairment and Happiness in Old People in Low and Middle Income Countries: Results from the 10/66 Study." *Journal of Affective Disorders* 130, nos. 1–2 (2011): 198–204. https://doi.org/10.1016/j.jad.2010.09.017.

Cooper, Melinda. *Life as Surplus: Biotechnology and Capitalism in the Neoliberal Era*. Seattle: University of Washington Press, 2008.

Cooper Owens, Dierdre. *Medical Bondage: Race, Gender, and the Origins of American Gynecology*. Athens: University of Georgia Press, 2017.

Cooter, Roger. "'Framing' the End of the Social History of Medicine." In *Locating Medical History: The Stories and Their Meanings*, edited by Frank Huisman and John Harley Warner, 309–37. Baltimore: Johns Hopkins University Press, 2004.

Cooter, Roger, and Bill Luckin. *Accidents in History: Injuries, Fatalities and Social Relations*. Amsterdam: Rodopi, 1997.

Cooter, Roger, Mark Harrison, and Steven Sturdy, eds. *War, Medicine, and Modernity*. Stroud, UK: Sutton, 1998.

Corbin, Alain. *The Foul and the Fragrant: Odor and the French Social Imagination*. Cambridge, MA: Harvard University Press, 1986.

Corrigan, Patrick. *The Stigma Effect: Unintended Consequences of Mental Health Campaigns*. New York: Columbia University Press, 2019.

Corrigan, Patrick, Amy Watson, Mark Heyrman, Amy Warpinski, Gabriela Gracia, Natalie Slopen, and Laura Hall. "Structural Stigma in State Legislation." *Psychiatric Services* 56, no. 5 (2005): 557–63.

Costandi, Moheb. "Against Neurodiversity." *Aeon*, 2019. https://aeon.co.

Cottingham, John. "Descartes on 'Thought.'" *Philosophical Quarterly* 28, no. 112 (1978): 208–14.

Coulton, C. G. *The Black Death*. London: Benn's Six Penny Library, 1929.

Couser, Thomas G. "What Disability Studies Has to Offer Medical Education." *Journal of Medical Humanities* 32, no. 1 (2011): 21–30.

Cowdry, E. V., ed. *Problems of Ageing: Biological and Medical Aspects*. London: Bailliere, Tindall & Cox, 1939.

Crafts, Lydia. "Ivermectin Experiments in Arkansas Jail Recall Long History of Medical Abuse." *Washington Post*, September 15, 2021. https://www.washingtonpost.com.

Cram, Sharon. "Living in Dose: Nuclear Work and the Politics of Permissible Exposure." *Public Culture* 28, no. 3 (2016): 519–39.

Crary, Jonathan. *24/7: Late Capitalism and the Ends of Sleep*. London: Verso, 2013.

Crawford, Paul, Brian Brown, Charlotte Baker, Victoria Tischler, and Brian Abrams. *Health Humanities*. London: Palgrave Macmillan, 2015.

Crawford, Paul, Brian Brown, and Andrea Charise, eds. *The Routledge Companion to Health Humanities*. London: Routledge, 2020.

Crawford, Paul, Brian Brown, Victoria Tischler, and Charlotte Baker. "Health Humanities: The Future of Medical Humanities?" *Mental Health Review Journal* 15, no. 3 (2010): 4–10.

Creighton, Charles. *A History of Epidemics in Britain from A.D. 664 to the Extinction of Plague*. 2 vols. Cambridge: Cambridge University Press, 1891.

Crimp, Douglas, ed. *AIDS: Cultural Analysis/Cultural Activism*. Cambridge, MA: MIT Press, 1988.

———. *Melancholia and Moralism: Essays on AIDS and Queer Politics*. Cambridge, MA: MIT Press, 2002.

———. "Mourning and Militancy." *October* 51 (1989): 3–18.

Crocq, Marc-Antoine. "The History of Generalized Anxiety Disorder as a Diagnostic Category." *Dialogues in Clinical Neuroscience* 19, no. 2 (2017): 107–16.

Cronon, William. "A Place for Stories: Nature, History, and Narrative." *Journal of American History* 78, no. 4 (March 1992): 1347–76.

Crosby, Alfred. "Virgin Soil Epidemics as a Factor in the Aboriginal Depopulation in America." *William and Mary Quarterly* 33, no. 2 (1976): 289–99.

Croskerry, Pat. "Cognitive Forcing Strategies in Clinical Decision Making." *Annals of Emergency Medicine* 41, no. 1 (2003): 110–20.

Cross-Call, Jesse, and Matt Broadus. "States That Have Expanded Medicaid Are Better Positioned to Address COVID-19 and Recession." Center on Budget and Policy Priorities. July 14, 2020. https://www.cbpp.org.

Crossman, Ashley. "Understanding Poverty and Its Various Types." ThoughtCo. July 18, 2019. https://www.thoughtco.com.

Crowley-Matoka, Megan. "Operating (for) Legitimacy: Pain, Surgical Seriality, and 'Failed Back Surgery Syndrome' in US Biomedicine." *American Ethnologist* 47, no. 1 (2020): 58–71.

Cryle, Peter, and Elizabeth Stephens. *Normality: A Critical Genealogy*. Chicago: University of Chicago Press, 2017.

Cueto, Marcos. *The Return of Epidemics: Health and Society in Peru during the Twentieth Century*. London: Routledge, 2001.

Cunningham, Andrew, and Perry Williams, eds. *The Laboratory Revolution in Medicine*. Cambridge: Cambridge University Press, 1992.

Cvetkovich, Ann. *An Archive of Feelings: Trauma, Sexuality, and Lesbian Public Cultures*. Durham, NC: Duke University Press, 2003.

Daniel, Michelle, Sorabh Khandelwal, Sally A. Santen, Matthew Malone, and Pat Croskerry. "Cognitive Debiasing Strategies for the Emergency Department." *Academic Emergency Medicine Education and Training* 1, no. 1 (January 19, 2017): 41–42.

Darwin, Charles. *On the Origin of Species*. New York: Norton, 2002.

Das, Veena. *Life and Words: Violence and the Descent into the Ordinary*. Berkeley: University of California Press, 2006.

DasGupta, Sayantani. "Medicalization." In *Keywords for Disability Studies*, edited by Rachel Adams, Benjamin Reiss, and David Serlin, 120–21. New York: New York University Press, 2015.

———. "Narrative Humility." *Lancet* 371, no. 9617 (March 2008): 980–81. https://doi.org/10.1016/S0140-6736(08)60440-7.

Daston, Lorraine, and Peter Galison. "The Image of Objectivity." *Representations* 40 (1992): 81–128.

Dauber, Michele Landis. *The Sympathetic State: Disaster Relief and the Origins of the American Welfare State*. Chicago: University of Chicago Press, 2013.

Davis, Dena S. *Genetic Dilemmas: Reproductive Technology, Parental Choices, and Children's Futures*. New York: Oxford University Press, 2010.

Davis, Kathy. *Dubious Equalities and Embodied Differences: Cultural Studies on Cosmetic Surgeries*. Lanham, MD: Rowman & Littlefield, 2003.

Davis, Lennard J., ed. *Disability Studies Reader*. 5th ed. New York: Routledge, 2016.

———. *Enforcing Normalcy: Disability, Deafness, and the Body*. London: Verso, 1995.

Davis, Mark H. *Empathy: A Social Psychological Approach*. New York: Routledge, 2018.

Davis, Natalie Zemon. "Decentering History: Local Stories and Cultural Crossings in a Global World." *History and Theory* 50, no. 2 (May 2011): 188–202.

Deaton, Angus, and Anne Case. *Deaths of Despair and the Future of Capitalism*. Princeton, NJ: Princeton University Press, 2020.

de Certeau, Michel. *The Practice of Everyday Life*. Translated by Steven Rendall. Berkeley: University of California Press, 1984.

"A Definition of Irreversible Coma: Report of the Ad Hoc Committee of the Harvard Medical School to Examine the Definition of Brain Death." *JAMA* 205, no. 6 (August 5, 1968): 337–40.

Degler, Carl N. *In Search of Human Nature: The Decline and Revival of Darwinism in American Social Thought*. Oxford: Oxford University Press, 1991.

De Grandis, Giovanni, and Vidar Halgunset. "Conceptual and Terminological Confusion around Personalised Medicine: A Coping Strategy." *BMC Medical Ethics* 17, no. 43 (2016): 1–12.

De Kruif, Paul. *Microbe Hunters*. New York: Blue Ribbon, 1926.

Delaporte, François. *Disease and Civilization. The Cholera in Paris, 1832*. Translated by Arthur Goldhammer. Cambridge, MA: MIT Press, 1986.

De León, Jason. *The Land of Open Graves: Living and Dying on the Migrant Trail*. Berkeley: University of California Press, 2015.

Deleuze, Gilles, and Felix Guattari. *Anti-Oedipus Capitalism and Schizophrenia*. Translated by Robert Hurley, Mark Seem, and Helen R. Lane. New York: Viking, 1977.

Demaitre, Luke. "The Description and Diagnosis of Leprosy by Fourteenth-Century Physicians." *Bulletin of the History of Medicine* 59, no. 3 (1985): 327–44.

De Melo-Martin, Inmaculada. "The Ethics of Sex Selection." In *Ethics and Emerging Technologies*, edited by Ronald Sandler, 90–103. Basingstoke: Palgrave, 2014.

Depraz, Natalie, and Thomas Desmidt. "Cardiophenomenology: A Refinement of Neurophenomenology." *Phenomenology and the Cognitive Sciences* 18 (2019): 493–507.

Derickson, Alan. *Black Lung: Anatomy of a Public Health Disaster*. Ithaca, NY: Cornell University Press, 2014a.

———. *Dangerously Sleepy: Overworked Americans and the Cult of Manly Wakefulness*. Philadelphia: University of Pennsylvania Press, 2014b.

Derrida, Jacques. *The Beast & the Sovereign*. Vol. 1. Translated by Geoffrey Bennington. Chicago: University of Chicago Press, 2009.

———. *Dissemination*. Translated by Barbara Johnson. Chicago: University of Chicago Press, 1981.

Desmarais, Michele M., and Regina E. Robbins. "From the Ground Up: Indigenizing Medical Humanities and Narrative Medicine." *Survive & Thrive: A Journal for Medical Humanities and Narrative as Medicine* 4, no. 1 (2019). https://repository.stcloudstate.edu.

D'Esposito, Mark, and Bradley R. Postle. "The Cognitive Neuroscience of Working Memory." *Annual Review of Psychology* 66 (2015): 115–42.

Dewachi, Omar. "When Wounds Travel." *Medicine Anthropology Theory* 2, no. 3 (2015): 61–82.

Di Chiro, Giovanna. "Local Actions, Global Visions: Remaking Environmental Expertise." *Frontiers* 18, no. 2 (1997): 203–31.

Diedrich, Lisa. "Against Compassion: Attending to Histories and Methods in Medical Humanities; or, Doing Critical Medical Studies." *Narrative Matters in Medical Contexts across Disciplines* 41, no. 1 (2015): 167–82.

Digby, Anne, and Helen Sweet. "Social Medicine and Medical Pluralism: The Valley Trust and Botha's Hill Health Centre, South Africa, 1940s to 2000s." *Social History of Medicine* 25, no. 2 (May 2012): 425–45.

Dingwall, Robert, Lily M. Hoffman, and Karen Staniland. "Introduction: Why a Sociology of Pandemics?" *Sociology of Health & Illness* 35, no. 2 (2013): 167–73.

Donaldson, Molla S., Janet M. Corrigan, and Linda T. Kohn. *To Err Is Human: Building a Safer Health System*. Vol. 6. Washington, DC: National Academies Press, 2000.

Donnelly, Jack. *Universal Human Rights in Theory and Practice*. Ithaca, NY: Cornell University Press, 2013.

Doty, Mark. "In Favor of Uncertainty." In *Views from the Loft: A Portable Writer's Workshop*, edited by Daniel Slager, 68–72. Minneapolis: Milkweed, 2010.

Downs, Jim. *Sick from Freedom: African-American Illness and Suffering during the Civil War and Reconstruction*. New York: Oxford University Press, 2012.

Doz, François, Patrice Marvanne, and Anne Fagot-Largeault. "The Person in Personalised Medicine." *European Journal of Cancer* 49, no. 5 (2013): 1159–60.

Dreger, Alice Domurat. *Hermaphrodites and the Medical Invention of Sex*. 3rd ed. Cambridge, MA: Harvard University Press, 2000.

———. *One of Us: Conjoined Twins and the Future of Normal*. Cambridge, MA: Harvard University Press, 2004.

Dubal, Sam. *Against Humanity: Lessons from the Lord's Resistance Army*. Oakland: University of California Press, 2018.

Dubois, W. E. B. *Black Reconstruction in America 1860–1880*. New York: Free Press, 1998.

Duffield, Mark R. *Development, Security and Unending War: Governing the World of Peoples*. Cambridge: Polity, 2007.

Duffin, Jacalyn. *To See with a Better Eye: A Life of R. T. H. Laennec*. Princeton, NJ: Princeton University Press, 1998.

Dumes, Abigail. "Lyme Disease and the Epistemic Tensions of 'Medically Unexplained Illnesses.'" *Medical Anthropology* 39, no. 6 (2020): 441–56.

Dumit, Joseph. *Drugs for Life: How Pharmaceutical Companies Define Our Health*. Durham, NC: Duke University Press, 2012.

———. *Picturing Personhood: Brain Scans and Biomedical Identity*. Raleigh, NC: Duke University Press, 2004.

Dunglison, Robley. *History of Medicine from the Earliest Ages to the Commencement of the Nineteenth Century*. Philadelphia: Lindsay and Blakiston, 1872.

Dunn, Jennifer L. "'Victims' and 'Survivors': Emerging Vocabularies of Motive for 'Battered Women Who Stay.'" *Sociological Inquiry* 75, no. 1 (2004): 1–30.

Dupré, John. "Understanding Contemporary Genomics." *Perspectives on Science* 12, no. 3 (2004): 320–38.

During, Simon. "What Were the Humanities, Anyway?" *Chronicle of Higher Education* 31. August 2020. https://www.chronicle.com.

Dusenbery, Maya. *Doing Harm: The Truth about How Bad Medicine and Lazy Science Leave Women Dismissed, Misdiagnosed, and Sick*. New York: HarperCollins, 2017.

Dutta, Prafulla C. *Rural Health and Medical Care in India*. Ambala Cantt, India: Army Educational Press, 1955.

Dwork, Cynthia, Frank McSherry, Kobbi Nissim, and Adam Smith. "Calibrating Noise to Sensitivity in Private Data Analysis." In *Proceedings of the Third Conference on Theory of Cryptography (TCC'06)*, edited by Shai Halevi and Tal Rabin, 265–84. Berlin: Springer-Verlag, 2006.

Ebbinghaus, Hermann. *Memory: A Contribution to Experimental Psychology*. Translated by Clara Bussenius and Henry Ruger. New York: Columbia University Press, (1885) 1913.

Ebeling, Mary F. E. *Healthcare and Big Data: Digital Specters and Phantom Objects*. New York: Palgrave, 2016.

Echenberg, Myron. *Plague Ports: The Global Urban Impact of Bubonic Plague 1894–1901*. New York: New York University Press, 2007.

Eckhert, Erik. "A Case for the Demedicalization of Queer Bodies." *Yale Journal of Biology and Medicine* 89, no. 2 (2016): 239–46.

Eddy, David M. "Practice Policies: Guidelines for Methods." *JAMA* 263, no. 13 (1990): 1839–41.

Edelman, Lee. "The Plague of Discourse: Politics, Literary Theory and AIDS." In *The Postmodern Turn: New Perspectives on Social Theory*, edited by Steven Seidman, 299–312. Cambridge: Cambridge University Press, 1994.

Ehrenreich, Barbara. *Witches, Midwives and Nurses: A History of Women Healers*. New York: Feminist Press at the City University of New York, 1972.

Ehrenreich, Barbara, and John Ehrenreich. *The American Health Empire: Power, Profits, and Politics*. New York: Vintage, 1971.

Ehrenreich, Barbara, and Deirdre English. *Complaints and Disorders: The Sexual Politics of Sickness*. New York: Feminist Press at the City University of New York, (1973) 2011.

Ehrenreich, Barbara, and Arlie Russell Hochschild, eds. *Global Woman: Nannies, Maids, and Sex Workers in the New Economy*. New York: Metropolitan Books, 2003.

Eichbaum, Quentin G. "Thinking about Thinking and Emotion: The Metacognitive Approach to the Medical Humanities That Integrates the Humanities with the Basic and Clinical Sciences." *Permanente Journal* 18, no. 4 (2014): 64–75.

Ekirch, Roger A. "The Modernization of Western Sleep, or Does Insomnia Have a History?" *Past & Present* 226, no. 1 (2015): 149–92. https://doi.org/10.1093/pastj/gtu040.

———. "Sleep We Have Lost: Pre-industrial Slumber in the British Isles." *American Historical Review* 106, no. 2 (2001): 343–86. https://doi.org/10.2307/2651611.

Elbe, Stefan. *Security and Global Health*. Cambridge: Polity, 2010.

Elliott, Carl. "Pharmaceutical Propaganda." In *Against Health: How Health Became the New Morality*, edited by Jonathan M. Metzl and Anna Kirkland, 93–104. New York: New York University Press, 2010.

Elliot, Denielle, and Timothy K. Thomas. "Lost in Translation? On Collaboration between Anthropology and Epidemiology." *Medicine Anthropology Theory* 4, no. 2 (2017): 1–17.

Ellman, Nora. "State Actions Undermining Abortion Rights in 2020." Center for American Progress. August 27, 2020. https://www.americanprogress.org.

Emanuel, Linda L., and Leigh B. Bienen. "Physician Participation in Executions: Time to Eliminate Anonymity Provisions and Protest the Practice." *Annals of Internal Medicine* 135, no. 10 (2001): 922–24.

Eng, David, Judith Halberstam, and José Esteban Muñoz. "Introduction: What's Queer about Queer Studies." *Social Text* 23, nos. 3–4 (2005): 1–17.

Epstein, Steven. *Impure Science: AIDS, Activism, and the Politics of Knowledge*. Vol. 7. Berkeley: University of California Press, 1996.

Erikson, Kai T. *Everything in Its Path: Destruction of Community in the Buffalo Creek Flood*. New York: Simon & Schuster, 1976.

———. *A New Species of Trouble: Explorations of Disaster, Trauma, and Community*. New York: Norton, 1994.

Escobar, Arturo. *Encountering Development*. Princeton, NJ: Princeton University Press, 2012.

Evans, Howard Martin, and David Alan Greaves. "Ten Years of Medical Humanities: A Decade in the Life of a Journal and a Discipline." *Medical Humanities* 36, no. 2 (December 2010): 66–68. https://www.ncbi.nlm.nih.gov.

Evans, Richard J. *Death in Hamburg: Society and Politics in the Cholera Years 1830–1910*. Oxford: Clarendon, 1987.

Eyerman, Ron. *Cultural Trauma: Slavery and the Formation of African American Identity*. Cambridge: Cambridge University Press, 2002.

Fadiman, Anne. *The Spirit Catches You and You Fall Down: A Hmong Child, Her American Doctors, and the Collision of Two Cultures*. New York: Farrar, Straus and Giroux, 1997.

Fagan, Brian, and Nadia Durrani. *What We Did in Bed: A Horizontal History*. New Haven, CT: Yale University Press, 2019.

Fairhead, James. "Technology, Inclusivity and the Rogue: Bats and the War against the 'Invisible Enemy.'" *Conservation and Society* 16, no. 2 (2018): 170–80.

Fang, Fang. *Wuhan Diary: Dispatches from a Quarantined City*. Translated by Michael Berry. New York: HarperCollins, 2020.

Fanon, Frantz, and Jacques Azoulay. "Daily Life in the Douars." In *Alienation and Freedom: Frantz Fanon*, edited by Jean Khalfa and J. C. Young, 373–84. London: Bloomsbury Academic, 2015a.

———. "Social Therapy in a Ward of Muslim Men: Methodological Difficulties." In *Alienation and Freedom: Frantz Fanon*, edited by Jean Khalfa and J. C. Young, 353–71. London: Bloomsbury Academic, 2015b.

Farmer, Paul. *Infections and Inequalities: The Modern Plagues*. Berkeley: University of California Press, 1999a.

———. "Pathologies of Power: Rethinking Health and Human Rights." *American Journal of Public Health* 89, no. 10 (1999b): 1486–96.

Farrell, Amy Erdman. *Fat Shame*. New York: New York University Press, 2011.

Fassin, Didier, and Richard Rechtman. *The Empire of Trauma: An Inquiry into the Condition of Victimhood*. Princeton, NJ: Princeton University Press, 2009.

Faulkner, Alison. "Survivor Research and Mad Studies: The Role and Value of Experiential Knowledge in Mental Health Research." *Disability & Society* 32, no. 4 (2017): 500–520.

Faust, Drew Gilpin. *This Republic of Suffering: Death and the American Civil War*. New York: Alfred A. Knopf, 2008.

Fausto-Sterling, Anne. *Sexing the Body: Gender Politics and the Construction of Sexuality*. Revised ed. New York: Basic Books, 2000.

Fawcett, Jonathan M., and Justin C. Hulbert. "The Many Faces of Forgetting: Toward a Constructive View of Forgetting in Everyday Life." *Journal of Applied Research in Memory and Cognition* 9 (2020): 1–18.

Fearnley, Lyle. *Virulent Zones. Animal Disease and Global Health at China's Pandemic Epicenter*. Durham, NC: Duke University Press, 2020.

Featherstone, Katie, and Paul Atkinson. *Creating Conditions: The Making and Remaking of Genetic Medicine*. New York: Taylor & Francis, 2013.

Feierman, Steven. "Struggles for Control: The Social Roots of Health and Healing in Modern Africa." *African Studies Review* 28, no. 2/3 (1985): 73–147.

Feinberg, Joel. "Wrongful Life and the Counterfactual Element in Harming." *Social Philosophy and Policy* 4, no. 1 (1986): 145–78.

Feinstein, Alvan R. *Clinical Judgment*. Baltimore: Williams & Wilkins, 1967.

Fenner, Frank, Donald A. Henderson, Isao Arita, Zdenek Jezek, and Ivan Danilovich Ladnyi. *Smallpox and Its Eradication*. Geneva: World Health Organization, 1988.

Ferguson, James. *Global Shadows: Africa in the Neocolonial World Order*. Durham, NC: Duke University Press, 2006.

Fett, Sharla M. *Working Cures: Healing, Health, and Power on Southern Slave Plantations*. Chapel Hill: University of North Carolina Press, 2002.

Feudtner, John Christopher. *Bittersweet: Diabetes, Insulin, and the Transformation of Illness*. Chapel Hill: University of North Carolina Press, 2003.

Fiedler, Leslie A. *Tyranny of the Normal: Essays on Bioethics, Theology & Myth*. Boston: D. R. Godine, 1996.

Filipe, Angela M. "Making ADHD Evident." *Medical Anthropology* 35, no. 5 (2015): 390–403.

Fineman, Martha. *The Autonomy Myth: A Theory of Dependency*. New York: New Press, 2004.

Fink, Marty. "Choir Boy: Trans Vocal Performance and the Depathologization of Transition." *Journal of Medical Humanities* 40, no. 1 (2019): 21–31.

Finkelstein, Avram. *After Silence: A History of AIDS through Its Images*. Berkeley: University of California Press, 2020.

Finney, Carolyn. *Black Faces, White Spaces: Reimagining the Relationship of African Americans to the Great Outdoors*. Chapel Hill: University of North Carolina Press, 2014.

Fischer, David Hackett. *Growing Old in America*. New York: Oxford University Press, 1977.

Fisher, Mark. *Capitalist Realism: Is There No Alternative?* London: Zer0 Books, 2009.

Fitzgerald, Des, and Felicity Callard. "Entangling the Medical Humanities." In *The Edinburgh Companion to the Critical Medical Humanities*, edited by Anne Whitehead, Angela Woods, Sarah Atkinson, Jane MacNaughton, and Jennifer Richards, 35–36. Edinburgh: Edinburgh University Press, 2016.

Fleck, Ludwik. *Genesis and Development of a Scientific Fact*. Chicago: University of Chicago Press, 1979.

Flexner, Abraham. *Medical Education: A Comparative Study*. New York: Macmillan, 1925.

———. *Medical Education in the United States and Canada*. New York: Carnegie Foundation, 1910.

Fortun, Kim. *Advocacy after Bhopal Environmentalism, Disaster, New Global Orders*. Chicago: University of Chicago Press, 2001.

Fortun, Mike. *Promising Genomics: Iceland and deCODE Genetics in a World of Speculation*. Berkeley: University of California Press, 2008.

Foucault, Michel. *The Birth of the Clinic: An Archaeology of Medical Perception*. Translated by A. M. Sheridan Smith. New York: Vintage, (1963) 1975.

———. *The History of Sexuality Volume 1: An Introduction*. Translated by Robert Hurley. New York: Vintage, (1976) 1990.

———. *Madness and Civilization*. London: Tavistock, (1961) 2001.

———. *The Order of Things: An Archaeology of the Human Sciences*. New York: Vintage, (1966) 1994.

———. *"Society Must Be Defended": Lectures at the Collège de France, 1975–1976*. Translated by David Macey. New York: Picador, 2003.

Fox, Renée. "Cultural Competence and the Culture of Medicine." *New England Journal of Medicine* 353, no. 13 (2005): 1316–19.

Frank, Arthur W. "Being a Good Story: The Humanities as Therapeutic Practice." In *Health Humanities Reader*, edited by Therese Jones, Delese Wear, and Lester D. Friedman, 13–25. New Brunswick, NJ: Rutgers University Press, 2014.

———. *The Wounded Storyteller: Body, Illness, and Ethics*. Chicago: University of Chicago Press, 1995.

Fraser, Nancy, and Linda Gordon. "A Genealogy of Dependency: Tracing a Keyword of the U.S. Welfare State." *Signs: Journal of Women in Culture and Society* 19, no. 2 (1994): 309–36.

Freud, Sigmund. *Three Contributions to the Sexual Theory*. Translated by A. A. Brill. New York: Journal of Nervous and Mental Disease, 1910.

Friedlander, Henry. *The Origins of Nazi Genocide: From Euthanasia to the Final Solution*. Chapel Hill: University of North Carolina Press, 2000.

Fuller, Thomas. *The Historie of the Holy Warre*. Cambridge: T. Buck, 1639.

Gale, Henry. "Psychosis Is Nothing like a Badger." YouTube video, 2013. https://www.youtube.com/watch?v=z50ILDXkA0w.

Galtung, Johan. "Violence, Peace, and Peace Research." *Journal of Peace Research* 6, no. 3 (1969): 167–91.

Gamble, Vanessa Northington. *Making a Place for Ourselves: The Black Hospital Movement, 1920–1945*. Oxford: Oxford University Press, 1995.

Gammeltoft, Tine. *Haunting Images: A Cultural Account of Selective Reproduction in Vietnam*. Oakland: University of California Press, 2014.

Garber, Marjorie. "Compassion." In *Compassion: The Culture and Politics of an Emotion*, edited by Lauren Berlant, 15–27. New York: Routledge, 2004.

Garden, Rebecca Elizabeth. "Critical Healing: Queering Diagnosis and Public Health through the Health Humanities." *Journal of Medical Humanities* 40, no. 1 (2019): 1–5.

———. "The Problem of Empathy: Medicine and the Humanities." *New Literary History* 38, no. 3 (2007): 551–67. https://doi.org/10.1353/nlh.2007.0037.

Gardner, Hunter H. *Pestilence and the Body Politic in Latin Literature*. Oxford: Oxford University Press, 2019.

Garland-Thomson, Rosemarie. "The Case for Conserving Disability." *Journal of Bioethical Inquiry* 9, no. 3 (2012): 339–55.

———. "Disability Bioethics: From Theory to Practice." *Kennedy Institute of Ethics Journal* 27, no. 2 (2017): 323–39.

———. *Extraordinary Bodies: Figuring Physical Disability in American Culture and Literature*. New York: Columbia University Press, 1996.

———. "Feminist Disability Studies." *Signs: Journal of Women in Culture and Society* 30, no. 2 (2005): 1557–87.

———. "How We Got to CRISPR: The Dilemma of Being Human." *Perspectives in Biology and Medicine* 63, no. 1 (2020): 28–43.

Garland-Thomson, Rosemarie, and Lisa I. Iezzoni. "Disability Cultural Competence for All as a Model." *American Journal of Bioethics* 21, no. 9 (2021): 26–28.

Garment, Ann, Susan Lederer, Naomi Rogers, and Lisa Boult. "Let the Dead Teach the Living: The Rise of Body Bequeathal in 20th-Century America." *Academic Medicine* 82, no. 10 (October 2007): 1000–1005.

Gasquet, Francis Aidan. *The Great Pestilence (A.D. 1348–9) Now Commonly Known as the Black Death*. London: Simpkin Marshall, Hamilton, Kent, 1893.

Gavrilov, Leonid A., and Natalia S. Gavrilova. "Is Aging a Disease? Biodemographers' Point of View." *Advances in Gerontology* 30, no. 6 (2017): 841–42.

Gawande, Atul. *Being Mortal: Medicine and What Matters in the End*. New York: Metropolitan Books, 2014.

———. *The Checklist Manifesto: How to Get Things Right*. London: Picador, 2011.

———. "On Washing Hands." *New England Journal of Medicine* 350, no. 13 (2004): 1283–86.

Genette, Gérard. *Narrative Discourse: An Essay in Method*. Translated by Jane E. Lewin. Ithaca, NY: Cornell University Press, 1980.

"Germ-ane." *Phrenological Journal & Science of Health* 79, no. 2 (August 1884): 110; Reprint, *Scientific American* 51, no. 6 (August 9, 1884): 83.

Gernsbacher, Morton Ann. "Autistics Need Acceptance, Not Cure." *Wisconsin State Journal*, May 24, 2004, A6. https://www.madison.com.

Geroulanos, Stefanos, and Todd Meyers. *The Human Body in the Age of Catastrophe*. Chicago: University of Chicago Press, 2018.

Getz, Faye Marie. "Black Death and the Silver Lining: Meaning, Continuity, and Revolutionary Change in Histories of Medieval Plague." *Journal of the History of Biology* 24, no. 2 (1991): 265–89.

Geuss, Raymond. *Who Needs a World View?* Cambridge, MA: Harvard University Press, 2020.

Gevitz, Norman. "'The Devil Hath Laughed at the Physicians': Witchcraft and Medical Practice in Seventeenth-Century New England." *Journal of the History of Medicine and Allied Sciences* 55, no. 1 (2000): 5–36.

Gibson, Alexandra Farren, Christina Lee, and Shona Crabb. "'If You Grow Them, Know Them': Discursive Constructions of the Pink Ribbon Culture of Breast Cancer in the Australian Context." *Feminism & Psychology* 24, no. 4 (2014): 521–41.

Giddens, Anthony. *The Consequences of Modernity*. Palo Alto, CA: Stanford University Press, 1990.

———. *Modernity and Self-Identity*. Palo Alto, CA: Stanford University Press, 1991.

Gigante, Denise. *Life: Organic Form and Romanticism*. New Haven, CT: Yale University Press, 2009.

Gilbert, Daniel. *Stumbling on Happiness*. New York: Vintage Canada, 2009.

Gilbert, Melody, dir. *Whole*. London: Frozen Feet Films, 2003.

Gilbert, Sandra M. *Death's Door: Modern Dying and the Ways We Grieve*. New York: W. W. Norton, 2006.

Gilbert, Sandra M., and Susan Gubar. *The Madwoman in the Attic: The Woman Writer and the Nineteenth-Century Literary Imagination*. New Haven, CT: Yale University Press, 1979.

Gilbreth, Lillian, and Edna Yost. *Normal Lives for the Disabled*. New York: Macmillan, 1944.

Gilligan, Carol. "The Listening Guide Method of Psychological Inquiry." *Qualitative Psychology* 2, no. 1 (2015): 69–77.

Gillon, Raanan. "'Primum Non Nocere' and the Principle of Non-maleficence." *British Medical Journal* 291, no. 6488 (1985): 130–31.

Gilman, Sander L. "AIDS and Syphilis: The Iconography of Disease." *October* 43 (1987): 87–107.

———. *Difference and Pathology: Stereotypes of Sexuality, Race, and Madness*. Ithaca, NY: Cornell University Press, 1985.

Gitelman, Lisa. "'Raw Data' Is an Oxymoron." In *New Media, Old Media: A History and Theory Reader*, edited by Wendy Hui Kyong Chun, Anna Watkins Fisher, and Thomas Keenan, 167–76. 2nd ed. New York: Routledge, 2015.

Glenn, Evelyn Nakano. *Forced to Care: Coercion and Caregiving in America*. Cambridge, MA: Harvard University Press, 2010.

Goffman, Erving. *Stigma: Notes on the Management of Spoiled Identity*. Englewood Cliffs, NJ: Prentice-Hall, 1963.

Goldberg, Daniel S. "Pain and the Human Condition." *Medical Humanities* 44, no. 2 (2018): 72–73.

Golinski, Jan. *British Weather and the Climate of the Enlightenment*. Chicago: University of Chicago Press, 2007.

Gómez, Pablo. *The Experiential Caribbean: Creating Knowledge and Healing in the Early Modern Atlantic*. Chapel Hill: University of North Carolina Press, 2017.

Goodwin, James. "Akira Kurosawa and the Atomic Age." In *Hibakusha Cinema*, edited by Mick Broderick, 190–214. New York: Routledge, 2013.

Goodwin, Michele. *Policing the Womb: Invisible Women and the Criminalization of Motherhood*. New York: Cambridge University Press, 2020.

Google Books. "Bioethics, Medical Ethics." Ngram Viewer, 2021. https://books.google.com/ngrams.

Gordon, Deborah. "Tenacious Assumptions in Western Medicine." In *Biomedicine Examined*, edited by Margaret Lock and Deborah Gordon, 19–56. Dordrecht, Netherlands: Kluwer Academic, 1988.

Gostin, Lawrence O. "Public Health, Ethics, and Human Rights: A Tribute to the Late Jonathan Mann." *Journal of Law, Medicine & Ethics* 29, no. 2 (2001): 121–30.

Goudsmit, Jaap. *Viral Fitness: The Next SARS and West Nile in the Making*. New York: Oxford University Press, 2004.

Graboyes, Melisa. *The Experiment Must Continue: Medical Research and Ethics in East Africa, 1940–2014*. Athens: Ohio University Press, 2014.

Gradmann, Christoph. "Robert Koch and the Invention of the Carrier State: Tropical Medicine, Veterinary Infections and Epidemiology around 1900." *Studies in History and Philosophy of Science Part C: Studies in History and Philosophy of Biological and Biomedical Sciences* 41, no. 3 (2010): 232–40.

Graff, Gerald. *Professing Literature: An Institutional History*. Chicago: University of Chicago Press, 1987.

Grafton, Anthony. *Defenders of the Text: The Tradition of Scholarship in an Age of Science 1450–1800*. Cambridge, MA: Harvard University Press, 1991.

Grafton, Anthony, and Lisa Jardine. *From Humanism to the Humanities: Education and the Liberal Arts in Fifteenth- and Sixteenth-Century Europe*. Cambridge, MA: Harvard University Press, 1986.

Greene, Jeremy A. *Prescribing by Numbers: Drugs and the Definition of Disease*. Baltimore: Johns Hopkins University Press, 2007.

Greene, Jeremy A., and David S. Jones. "The Shared Goals and Distinct Strengths of the Medical Humanities: Can the Sum of the Parts Be Greater Than the Whole?" *Academic Medicine* 92, no. 12 (December 2017): 1661–64.

Greenhalgh, Tricia. "The Limits of Evidence-Based Medicine." *Respiratory Care* 46, no. 12 (December 2001): 1435–40. PMID 11728302.

Greenwall Foundation. "About Us." Greenwall Foundation. Accessed October 20, 2022. https://greenwall.org.

Greenwood, Anna, and Harshad Topiwala. *Indian Doctors in Kenya, 1890–1940: The Forgotten History*. Basingstoke: Palgrave Macmillan, 2015.

Gross, Cary P., and Kent A. Sepkowitz. "The Myth of the Medical Breakthrough: Smallpox, Vaccination, and Jenner Reconsidered." *International Journal of Infectious Diseases* 3, no. 1 (July–September 1998): 54–60.

Grosz, Elizabeth. *Becoming Undone: Darwinian Reflections on Life, Politics, and Art*. Durham, NC: Duke University Press, 2011.

Guha, Ramachandra. "Radical American Environmentalism and Wilderness Preservation: A Third World Critique." *Environmental Ethics* 11, no. 1 (1989): 71–83.

———. *The Ramachandra Guha Omnibus*. New Delhi: Oxford University Press, (2000) 2005.

Gullette, Margaret Morganroth. *Aged by Culture*. Chicago: University of Chicago Press, 2011.

Gutierrez, Kevin J., and Sayantani DasGupta. "The Space That Difference Makes: On Marginality, Social Justice and the Future of the Health Humanities." *Journal of Medical Humanities* 37, no. 4 (2016): 435–48.

Gutmann, Amy, and Dennis Thompson. "Deliberating about Bioethics." *Hastings Center Report* 27, no. 3 (1997): 38–41.

Guyatt, Gordon, John Cairns, David Churchill, Deborah Cook, Brian Haynes, Jack Hirsh, Jan Irvine, et al. "Evidence-Based Medicine: A New Approach to Teaching the Practice of Medicine." *JAMA* 268, no. 17 (1992): 2420–25. https://doi.org/10.1001/jama.1992.03490170092032.

Hacking, Ian. "Dreams in Place." *Historical Ontology* 59, no. 3 (2002): 227–54.

———. "Making Up People." *London Review of Books* 28, nos. 16–17 (2006): 23–26.

———. *Rewriting the Soul: Multiple Personality and the Sciences of Memory*. Princeton, NJ: Princeton University Press, 1995.

———. *The Social Construction of What?* Cambridge, MA: Harvard University Press, 1999.

———. *The Taming of Chance*. Cambridge: Cambridge University Press, 1990.

Hafner, Marco, Martin Stepanek, Jirca Taylor, Wendy M. Troxel, and Christian van Stolk. *Why Sleep Matters—Quantifying the Economic Costs of Insufficient Sleep: A Cross-Country Comparative Analysis*. Santa Monica, CA: Rand Corporation, 2016. https://www.rand.org.

Halbwachs, Maurice. *On Collective Memory*. Translated by L. Coser. Chicago: University of Chicago Press, (1941) 1992.

Halliwell, Martin. *American Health Crisis: One Hundred Years of Panic, Planning, and Politics*. Berkeley: University of California Press, 2021.

Halpern, Jodi. *From Detached Concern to Empathy: Humanizing Medical Practice*. Oxford: Oxford University Press, 2011.

Hammill, Gary. "Miracles and Plagues: Plague Discourse as Political Thought." *Journal for Early Modern Cultural Studies* 10, no. 2 (Fall/Winter 2010): 85–104.

Hamraie, Aimi. *Building Access: Universal Design and the Politics of Disability*. Minneapolis: University of Minnesota Press, 2017.

Hancock, Jason, and Karen Mattick. "Tolerance of Ambiguity and Psychological Well-Being in Medical Training: A Systematic Review." *Medical Education* 54, no. 2 (2020): 125–37.

Handley, Sasha. *Sleep in Early Modern England*. New Haven, CT: Yale University Press, 2016.

Hanemaayer, Arianne. "Evidence-Based Medicine: A Genealogy of the Dominant Science of Medical Education." *Journal of Medical Humanities* 37, no. 4 (2016): 449–73. https://doi.org/10.1007/s10912-016-9398-0.

Hansen, Helena. "Assisted Technologies of Social Reproduction: Pharmaceutical Prosthesis for Gender, Race, and Class in the White Opioid 'Crisis.'" *Contemporary Drug Problems* 44, no. 4 (2017): 321–38.

Hansen, Helena, and Samuel K. Roberts. "Two Tiers of Biomedicalization: Methadone, Buprenorphine, and the Racial Politics of Addiction Treatment." *Critical Perspectives on Addiction* 14 (2012): 79–102.

Hanson, Marta E. *Speaking of Epidemics in Chinese Medicine: Disease and the Geographic Imagination in Late Imperial China*. London: Routledge, 2011.

Haraway, Donna. "Anthropocene, Capitalocene, Plantationocene, Chthulucene: Making Kin." *Environmental Humanities* 6, no. 1 (2015): 159–65.

———. *Simians, Cyborgs, and Women. The Reinvention of Nature*. London: Routledge, (1990) 1991.

———. "Situated Knowledges: The Science Question in Feminism and the Privilege of Partial Perspective." *Feminist Studies* 14, no. 3 (1988): 575–99. https://doi.org/10.2307/3178066.

Harden, Blaine. "The Moral Superiority of Lying." *Washington Post Magazine*, May 2, 1982. https://www.washingtonpost.com.

Harding, Sandra G. *Is Science Multicultural? Postcolonialisms, Feminisms, and Epistemologies*. Bloomington: Indiana University Press, 1998.

Hardon, Anita, and Emilia Sanabria. "Fluid Drugs: Revisiting the Anthropology of Pharmaceuticals." *Annual Review of Anthropology* 46 (2017): 117–32.

Harjo-Sapulpa, Joy. "Three Generations of Native American Women's Birth Experience." In *Imagine What It's Like*, edited by Victoria Bonebakker, 126–30. Manoa: University of Hawai'i Press, 2008.

Harmon, Amy. "Neurodiversity Forever: The Disability Movement Turns to Brains." *New York Times*, May 2004.

Harper, Lynn Casteel. *On Vanishing: Mortality, Dementia, and What It Means to Disappear*. New York: Catapult, 2020.

Harrington, Anne. *The Cure Within: A History of Mind/Body Medicine*. New York: W. W. Norton, 2009.

Harris, La Donna, and Jacqueline Wasilewski. "Indigeneity, an Alternative Worldview: Four R's (Relationship, Responsibility, Reciprocity, Redistribution) vs. Two P's (Power and Profit). Sharing the Journey Towards Conscious Evolution." *Systems Research and Behavioral Science: The Official Journal of the International Federation for Systems Research* 21, no. 5 (2004): 489–503.

Harrison, Mark. *Climates and Constitutions: Health, Race, Environment and British Imperialism in India, 1600–1850*. Oxford: Oxford University Press, 1999.

———. *Contagion: How Commerce Has Spread Disease*. New Haven, CT: Yale University Press, 2013.

———. "Pandemic." In *The Routledge History of Disease*, edited by Mark Jackson, 129–46. London: Routledge, 2017.

Hart, Michael A. "Indigenous Worldviews, Knowledge, and Research: The Development of an Indigenous Research Paradigm." *Journal of Indigenous Voices in Social Work* 1, no. 1 (2010): 1–16.

Hartman, Chester, and Gregory D. Squires, ed. *There Is No Such Thing as a Natural Disaster: Race, Class, and Hurricane Katrina*. New York: Routledge, 2006.

Hartman, Saidiya. *Lose Your Mother: A Journey along the Atlantic Slave Route*. New York: Farrar, Straus and Giroux, 2008.

Hartmann, Betsy. *Reproductive Rights and Wrongs: The Global Politics of Population Control*. Chicago: Haymarket, 2016.

Hatch, Anthony Ryan. *Silent Cells: The Secret Drugging of Captive America*. Minneapolis: University of Minnesota Press, 2019.

Hawkins, Anne Hunsaker, James O. Ballard, and David J. Hufford. "Humanities Education at Pennsylvania State University College of Medicine, Hershey, Pennsylvania." *Academic Medicine* 78, no. 10 (2003): 1001–5.

Hawkins, Mike. *Social Darwinism in European and American Thought, 1860–1945: Nature as Model and Nature as Threat*. Cambridge: Cambridge University Press, 1997.

Haynes, Todd, dir. *Safe*. Culver City, CA: Columbia TriStar Entertainment, 1995. 1 hr., 35 min.

Hays, J. N. *The Burdens of Disease: Epidemics and Human Response in Western History*. New Brunswick, NJ: Rutgers University Press, 1998.

Healy, David. *Pharmageddon*. Berkeley: University of California Press, 2012.

Healy, Margaret. "Defoe's *Journal* and the English Plague Writing Tradition." *Literature and Medicine* 22, no. 1 (2003): 25–44.

Heath, Deborah, Rayna Rapp, and Karen-Sue Taussig. "Genetic Citizenship." In *A Companion to the Anthropology of Politics*, edited by David Nugent and Joan Vincent, 152–67. Malden, MA: Blackwell, 2004.

Hecker, I. F. C. *The Black Death in the Fourteenth Century*. Translated by B. G. Babington. London: A. Schloss, 1833.

Hedgecoe, Adam. *The Politics of Personalised Medicine: Pharmacogenetics in the Clinic*. Cambridge: Cambridge University Press, 2004.

Heise, Ursula K. "Toxins, Drugs, and Global Systems: Risk and Narrative in the Contemporary Novel." *American Literature* 74, no. 4 (2002): 747–78.

Helmich, Esther, Laura Diachun, Radha Joseph, Kori LaDonna, Nelleke Noeverman-Poel, Lorelei Lingard, and Sayra Cristancho. "'Oh My God, I Can't Handle This!': Trainees' Emotional Responses to Complex Situations." *Medical Education* 52, no. 2 (2018): 206–15.

Hemsley, Jeff. "Virality: Developing a Rigorous and Useful Definition of an Information Diffusion Process." Syracuse University, School of Information Studies, April 15, 2011. https://ssrn.com.

Henne, Kate, and Bridget Livingstone. "More Than Unnatural Masculinity: Gendered and Queer Perspectives on Human Enhancement Drugs." In *Human Enhancement Drugs*, edited by Katinka van de Ven, Kyle J. D. Mulrooney, and Jim McVeigh, 13–26. London: Routledge, 2019.

Herek, Gregory M. "Confronting Sexual Stigma and Prejudice: Theory and Practice." *Journal of Social Issues* 63, no. 4 (2007): 905–25.

Heritage, John. "Revisiting Authority in Physician-Patient Interaction." In *Diagnosis as Cultural Practice*, edited by Judith Felson Duchan and Dana Kovarsky, 83–102. New York: Mouton de Gruyter, 2005.

Herman, Judith. *Trauma and Recovery: The Aftermath of Violence—from Domestic Abuse to Political Terror*. New York: Basic Books, 1992.

Hernández, Robb. *Archiving an Epidemic: Art, AIDS, and the Queer Chicanx Avant-Garde*. Berkeley: University of California Press, 2019.

Herndl, Diane Price. "Reconstructing the Posthuman Feminist Body Twenty Years after Audre Lorde's Cancer Journals." In *Disability Studies: Enabling the Humanities*, edited by Sharon L. Snyder, Brenda Jo Brueggemann, and Rosemarie Garland-Thomson, 144–55. New York: Modern Language Association of America, 2002.

Herrera, Salvador. "Already Quarantined: Yes, the 'Spanish' Flu Was Racist Too." *Synapsis: A Health Humanities Journal*, July 3, 2020. https://medicalhealthhumanities.com.

Herring, Ann D., and Alan C. Swedlund, eds. *Plagues and Epidemics: Infected Spaces Past and Present*. Oxford: Berg, 2010.

Hershatter, Gail. *The Gender of Memory: Rural Women and China's Collective Past*. Berkeley: University of California Press, 2011.

Herzberg, David. *White Market Drugs: Big Pharma and the Hidden History of Addiction in America*. Chicago: University of Chicago Press, 2020.

Herzog, Dagmar. *Cold War Freud: Psychoanalysis in an Age of Catastrophes*. Cambridge: Cambridge University Press, 2017.

———. *Unlearning Eugenics: Sexuality, Reproduction, and Disability in Post-Nazi Europe*. Madison: University of Wisconsin Press, 2018.

Heymann, David L., and G. R. Rodier. "Global Surveillance of Communicable Diseases." *Emerging Infectious Diseases* 4, no. 3 (1998): 362–65.

Higgins, Jenny A., Susie Hoffman, and Shari L. Dworkin. "Rethinking Gender, Heterosexual Men, and Women's Vulnerability to HIV/AIDS." *American Journal of Public Health* 100, no. 3 (2010): 435–45.

Highmore, Ben, ed. *The Everyday Life Reader*. London and New York: Routledge, 2002.

Hill, Kristina. "Shifting Sites." In *Site Matters: Design Concepts, Histories, and Strategies*, edited by Carol Burns and Andrea Kahn, 131–56. New York: Routledge, 2005.

Hinchliffe, Steven, Nick Bingham, John Allen, and Simon Carter. *Pathological Lives: Disease, Space and Biopolitics*. West Sussex, UK: Wiley-Blackwell, 2016.

Hinshaw, Stephen P. *The Mark of Shame: Stigma of Mental Illness and an Agenda for Change*. Oxford and New York: Oxford University Press, 2007.

Hinton, Devon E., and Byron J. Good. *Culture and PTSD: Trauma in Global and Historical Perspective*. Philadelphia: University of Pennsylvania Press, 2015.

Hippocrates. *The Genuine Works of Hippocrates*. Translated by Francis Adams. London: Sydenham Society, 1849.

———. *On Airs, Waters, and Places*. London: Wyman & Sons, 1881.

Hirschberger, Gilad. "Collective Trauma and the Social Construction of Meaning." *Frontiers in Psychology* 9 (2018): 1–14.

Hirst, Fabian L. *The Conquest of Plague. A Study of the Evolution of Epidemiology*. Oxford: Clarendon, 1953.

Hirst, William, and Alin Coman. "Building a Collective Memory: The Case for Collective Forgetting." *Current Opinion in Psychology* 23 (2018): 88–92.

Hirst, William, Jeremy Yamashiro, and Alin Coman. "Collective Memory from a Psychological Perspective." *Trends in Cognitive Sciences* 22 (2018): 438–51.

Hochschild, Arlie. *The Managed Heart: Commercialization of Human Feeling*. Berkeley: University of California Press, 1983.

Hoffman, Kelly M., Sophie Trawalter, Jordan R. Axt, and M. Norman Oliver. "Racial Bias in Pain Assessment and Treatment Recommendations, and False Beliefs about Biological Differences between Blacks and Whites." *Proceedings of the National Academy of Sciences of the United States of America* 113, no. 16 (2016): 4296–301.

Hofstadter, Richard. *Social Darwinism in American Thought*. Boston: Beacon, 1955.

Hogarth, Rana A. *Medicalizing Blackness: Making Racial Difference in the Atlantic World, 1780–1840*. Chapel Hill: University of North Carolina Press, 2017.

Holloway, Karla F. C. *Private Bodies, Public Texts: Race, Gender, and a Cultural Bioethics*. Durham, NC: Duke University Press, 2011.

Holmes, Brooke. *The Symptom and the Subject: The Emergence of the Physical Body in Ancient Greece*. Princeton, NJ: Princeton University Press, 2010.

Hond, Paul. "US Poet Laureate Tracy K. Smith '97SOA Gives Wings to Words." *Columbia Magazine*, spring/summer 2018. https://magazine.columbia.edu.

Honigsbaum, Mark. "'Tipping the Balance': Karl Friedrich Meyer, Latent Infections, and the Birth of Modern Ideas of Disease Ecology." *Journal of the History of Biology* 49, no. 2 (2016): 261–309.

hooks, bell. *Representing Whiteness in the Black Imagination*. New York: Routledge, 1992.

Hooton, Earnest Albert. *Young Man, You Are Normal*. New York: G. P. Putnam's Sons, 1945.

Horden, Peregrine. "What's Wrong with Early Medieval Medicine?" *Social History of Medicine* 24, no. 1 (2011): 5–25.

Horton, Richard. "The Myth of 'Decolonising Global Health.'" *Lancet* 398, no. 10312 (November 2021): 1673.

Horwitz, Allan. *Creating Mental Illness*. Chicago: University of Chicago Press, 2002.

Horwitz, Allan, and Jerome C. Wakefield. *All We Have to Fear: Psychiatry's Transformation of Natural Anxieties into Mental Disorders*. New York: Oxford University Press, 2012.

Houser, Heather. *Ecosickness in Contemporary U.S. Fiction: Environment and Affect*. New York: Columbia University Press, 2014.

———. *Infowhelm: Environmental Art and Literature in an Age of Data*. New York: Columbia University Press, 2020.

Houston, Donna. "Environmental Justice Storytelling: Angels and Isotopes at Yucca Mountain, Nevada." *Antipode* 45, no. 2 (2013): 417–35.

Howes, David. *Sensual Relations: Engaging the Senses in Culture and Social Theory*. Ann Arbor: University of Michigan Press, 2003.

Hsu, Hsuan L. "Naturalist Smellscapes and Environmental Justice." *American Literature* 88, no. 4 (2016): 787–814.

Hsu, Stephanie. "Fanon and the New Paraphilias: Towards a Trans of Color Critique of the DSM-V." *Journal of Medical Humanities* 40, no. 1 (2019): 53–68. https://doi.org/10.1007/s10912-018-9531-3.

Huber, Valeska. *Channelling Mobilities: Migration and Globalisation in the Suez Canal Region and Beyond, 1869–1914*. Cambridge: Cambridge University Press, 2013.

Huisman, Frank, and John Harley Warner. "Medical Histories." In *Locating Medical History: The Stories and Their Meanings*, edited by Frank Huisman and John Harley Warner, 1–30. Baltimore: Johns Hopkins University Press, 2004.

Hulkower, Raphael. "From Sacrilege to Privilege: The Tale of Body Procurement for Anatomical Dissection in the United States." *Einstein Journal of Biology and Medicine* 27, no. 1 (2011): 23–26.

Human Rights Watch and InterACT Advocates for Intersex Youth. "'I Want to Be like Nature Made Me': Medically Unnecessary Surgeries in Intersex Children in the US." Human Rights Watch. 2017. https://www.hrw.org.

Hume, David. *An Enquiry concerning the Principles of Morals*. Edited by Tom L. Beauchamp. England, 1751; Reprint, Oxford: Oxford University Press, 1998.

———. *A Treatise of Human Nature*. England, 1739; Project Gutenberg, 2002. https://www.gutenberg.org.

Hunt, Lynn. *Inventing Human Rights: A History*. New York: W. W. Norton, 2007.

Hurford, Christianna Elrene Thomas. "'In His Arm the Scar': Medicine, Race, and the Social Implications of the 1721 Inoculation Controversy on Boston." PhD Diss., Ohio State University, 2010.

Hurwitz, Brian. "Medical Humanities: Lineage, Excursionary Sketch and Rationale." *Journal of Medical Ethics* 39, no. 11 (2013): 672–74.

Hutchings, Rich. "Understanding of and Vision for the Environmental Humanities." *Environmental Humanities* 4, no. 1 (2014): 213–20.

Idoate, Regina, Michele Marie Desmarais, Brittany Strong, Anne Steinhoff, Lilly Tamayo, Gretchen Carroll, Chaulette DeCora, Cassie Rhoads-Carroll, Nicole Tamayo-Bergman, and Camille Voorhees. "An Indigenist Theory of Health Advocacy." *Great Plains Research* 30, no. 1 (2020): 35–48.

Igea, Juan Manuel. "From the Old Immunitas to the Modern Immunity: Do We Need a New Name for the Immune System?" *Current Immunology Reviews* 11, no. 1 (2015): 55–65.

Imperato, Pascal J., and Gavin H. Imperato. "Smallpox Inoculation (Variolation) in East Africa with Special Reference to the Practice among the Boran and Gabra of Northern Kenya." *Journal of Community Health* 39, no. 6 (December 2014): 1053–62.

Imperfect Cognitions Network (website). Accessed November 30, 2021. https://imperfectcognitions.blogspot.com.

Inhorn, Marcia C. "Medical Anthropology and Epidemiology: Divergences or Convergences?" *Social Science & Medicine* 40, no. 3 (1995): 285–90.

Inhorn, Marcia C., and Peter J. Brown. "The Anthropology of Infectious Disease." *Annual Review of Anthropology* 19 (1990): 89–117.

"Instructions for Authors." *Journal of the American Medical Association*. https://jamanetwork.com.

International Association for the Study of Pain. "Pain." IASP Terminology. Last updated 2017. https://www.iasp-pain.org.

"The International Health Organization of the League of Nations: The Work of the Cancer Commission, 1923 to 1927." *British Medical Journal* 1, no. 3302 (1924): 672–75. https://www.ncbi.nlm.nih.gov.

Itzen, Peter, and Simone Muller. "Risk as a Category of Analysis for a Social History of the Twentieth Century: An Introduction." *Historical Social Research* 41, no. 1 (2016): 7–29.

Iwai, Yoshiko, Zahra Khan, and Sayantani DasGupta. "Abolition Medicine." *Lancet* 396, no. 10245 (July 2020): 158–59.

Jabr, Ferris. "The Earth Is Just as Alive as You Are." *New York Times*, April 2019. https://www.nytimes.com.

Jackson, Mark. *The Age of Stress: Science and the Search for Stability*. Oxford: Oxford University Press, 2013.

Jackson, Zakiyyah Iman. *Becoming Human: Matter and Meaning in an Antiblack World*. New York: New York University Press, 2020.

Jaggar, Alison M. "Love and Emotion in Feminist Epistemology." In *Gender / Body / Knowledge: Feminist Reconstructions of Being and Knowing*, edited by Alison M. Jaggar and Susan R. Bordo, 145–71. New Brunswick, NJ: Rutgers University Press, 1989.

Jain, Lochlann S. *Injury: The Politics of Product Design and Safety Law in the United States*. Princeton, NJ: Princeton University Press, 2006.

———. *Malignant: How Cancer Becomes Us*. Berkeley: University of California Press, 2013.

———. "The WetNet: What the Oral Polio Vaccine Hypothesis Exposes about Globalized Interspecies Fluid Bonds." *Medical Anthropology Quarterly* 34, no. 4 (2020): 504–24.

James, Henry. *The Art of the Novel: Critical Prefaces by Henry James*. Boston: Northeastern University Press, 1984.

Jameson, Fredric. *Postmodernism or the Cultural Logic of Late Capitalism*. London: Verso, 1991.

Jamison, Kay Redfield. *An Unquiet Mind: A Memoir of Moods and Madness*. New York: Random House, 1996.

Janković, Vladimir. *Confronting the Climate: British Airs and the Making of Environmental Medicine*. New York: Palgrave Macmillan, 2010.

Jasanoff, Sheila. "Future Imperfect: Science, Technology, and the Imaginations of Modernity." In *Dreamscapes of Modernity: Sociotechnical Imaginaries and the Fabrication of Power*, edited by Sheila Jasanoff and Sang Hyun-Kim, 1–33. Chicago: University of Chicago Press, 2015.

Jaudon, Toni Wall. "Obeah's Sensations: Rethinking Religion at the Transnational Turn." *American Literature* 84, no. 4 (2012): 715–41.

Jauhar, Sandeep. "What Is Death?" *New York Times*, February 16, 2019.

Jenkins, Janice Hunter. "The State Construction of Affect: Political Ethos and Mental Health among Salvadoran Refugees." *Culture, Medicine, and Psychiatry* 15, no. 2 (1991): 139–65.

Jenner, Mark, and Patrick Wallis, eds. *Medicine and the Market in England and Its Colonies, c.1450–c.1850*. Basingstoke: Palgrave, 2007.

Jenson, Deborah, and Marco Iacoboni. "Literary Bio-Mimesis: Mirror Neurons and the Ontological Priority of Representation." *California Italian Studies* 2 (2011): 1–18.

Jewson, Norman. "The Disappearance of the Sick Man in Medical Cosmology." *Sociology* 10, no. 2 (1976): 225–44.

Jobson, Ryan Cecil. "The Case for Letting Anthropology Burn: Sociocultural Anthropology in 2019." *American Anthropologist* 122, no. 2 (2020): 259–71.

Johannsen, Wilhelm. "The Genotype Conception of Heredity." *American Naturalist* 45, no. 531 (1911): 129–59.

Jones, Anne Hudson. "Narrative in Medical Ethics." *BMJ* 318, no. 7178 (1999): 253–56.

———. "Reading Patients—Cautions and Concerns." *Literature and Medicine* 13, no. 2 (1994): 190–200.

Jones, David S. *Rationalizing Epidemics: Meanings and Uses of American Indian Mortality since 1600*. Cambridge, MA: Harvard University Press, 2004.

Jones, David S., Jeremy A. Greene, Jaclyn Duffin, and John Harley Warner. "Making the Case for History in Medical Education." *Journal of the History of Medicine and Allied Sciences* 70, no. 4 (October 2015): 623–52.

Jones, Donna V. *The Racial Discourses of Life Philosophy: Négritude, Vitalism, and Modernity*. New York: Columbia University Press, 2010.

Jones, James H. *Bad Blood: The Tuskegee Syphilis Experiment*. New York: Free Press, 1993.

Jones, Therese. "'Oh, the Humanit(ies)!': Dissent, Democracy, and Danger." In *Medicine, Health, and the Arts: Approaches to the Medical Humanities*, edited by Victoria Bates, Alan Bleakley, and Sam Goodman, 27–38. New York: Routledge, 2014.

Jones, Therese, Michael Blackie, Rebecca Garden, and Delese Wear. "The Almost Right Word: The Move from Medical to Health Humanities." *Academic Medicine* 92, no. 7 (2017): 932–35.

Jones, Therese, Delese Wear, and Lester D. Friedman, eds. *Health Humanities Reader*. New Brunswick, NJ: Rutgers University Press, 2014.

Jones, W. H. S. *Hippocrates II*. Loeb Classical Library. Cambridge, MA: Harvard University Press, 1931.

Jongsma, Karin R., and Bredenoord, Annelien L. "Ethics Parallel Research: An Approach for (Early) Ethical Guidance of Biomedical Innovation." *BMC Medical Ethics* 21, no. 81 (2020): 1–9. https://doi.org/10.1186/s12910-020-00524-z.

Jonsen, Albert R. *The Birth of Bioethics*. New York: Oxford University Press, 1998.

———. "Do No Harm." *Annals of Internal Medicine* 88, no. 6 (1978): 827–32.

Jopp, Daniela, and Christoph Rott. "Adaptation in Very Old Age: Exploring the Role of Resources, Beliefs, and Attitudes for Centenarians' Happiness." *Psychology and Aging* 21, no. 2 (2006): 266–80.

Jordanova, L. J. "Earth Science and Environmental Medicine: The Synthesis of Late Enlightenment." In *Images of the Earth: Essays in the History of the Environmental Sciences*, edited by L. J. Jordanova and Roy S. Porter, 119–46. London: British Society for the History of Science Monographs, 1978.

Jordan-Young, Rebecca M. *Brain Storm: The Flaws in the Science of Sex Differences*. Cambridge, MA: Harvard University Press, 2011.

Jurecic, Ann. "Empathy and the Critic." *College English* 74, no. 1 (September 2011): 10–27.

———. *Illness as Narrative*. Pittsburgh: University of Pittsburgh Press, 2012.

Jusionyte, Ieva. *Threshold: Emergency Responders on the US-Mexico Border*. Berkeley: University of California Press, 2018.

Jutel, Annemarie. *Putting a Name to It: Diagnosis in Contemporary Society*. Baltimore: Johns Hopkins University Press, 2011.

Kafer, Alison. *Feminist, Queer, Crip*. Bloomington: Indiana University Press, 2013.

Kahneman, Daniel. *Thinking, Fast and Slow*. New York: Macmillan, 2011.

Kalathil, Jayasree, and Nev Jones. "Unsettling Disciplines: Madness, Identity, Research, Knowledge." *Philosophy, Psychiatry & Psychology* 23, no. 3/4 (2016): 183–88.

Kall, Lisa Folkmarson, ed. *Dimensions of Pain: Humanities and Social Science Perspectives*. New York: Routledge, 2013.

Karamanou, Marianna, George Panayiotakopoulos, Gregory Tsoucalas, Antonis A. Kousoulis, and George Androutsos. "From Miasmas to Germs: A Historical Approach to Theories of Infectious Disease Transmission." *Infez Med* 20, no. 1 (2012): 58–62.

Karkazis, Katrina. *Fixing Sex: Intersex, Medical Authority, and Lived Experience*. Durham, NC: Duke University Press, 2008.

Karkazis, Katrina, Rebecca Jordan-Young, Georgiann Davis, and Silvia Camporesi. "Out of Bounds? A Critique of the New Policies on Hyperandrogenism in Elite Female Athletes." *American Journal of Bioethics* 12, no. 7 (2012): 3–16.

Karpin, Isabel, and Roxanne Mykitiuk. "Reimagining Disability: The Screening of Donor Gametes and Embryos in IVF." *Journal of Law and the Biosciences* 8, no. 2 (2020): 1–24.

Kassirer, Jerome P. "Our Stubborn Quest for Diagnostic Certainty." *New England Journal of Medicine* 320, no. 22 (1989): 1489–91.

Katz, Jonathan Ned. *The Invention of Heterosexuality*. Chicago: University of Chicago Press, 1995.

Kaufman, Sharon. *And a Time to Die: How American Hospitals Shape End of Life Care*. New York: Scribner, 2005.

Keck, Frédéric. *Avian Reservoirs: Virus Hunters and Birdwatchers in Chinese Sentinel Posts*. Durham, NC: Duke University Press, 2019.

Keck, Frédéric, and Christos Lynteris, eds. "The Anthropology of Zoonosis." *Medicine Anthropology Theory* 5, no. 3 (June 2018): 21–34.

Kelly, Ann H., Frédéric Keck, and Christos Lynteris, eds. *The Anthropology of Epidemics*. London: Routledge, 2019.

Kelly, Christine. *Disability Politics and Care: The Challenge of Direct Funding*. Vancouver: UBC Press, 2016.

Kelton, Paul. *Cherokee Medicine, Colonial Germs: An Indigenous Nation's Fight against Smallpox, 1518–1824*. Norman: University of Oklahoma Press, 2015.

Kendall-Taylor, Nat, Aly Neumann, and Julie Schoen. "Advocating for Age in an Age of Uncertainty." *Stanford Social Innovation Review*, May 28, 2020. https://ssir.org.

Kendi, Ibram X. "Post-traumatic Slave Syndrome Is a Racist Idea." *Black Perspectives* (blog), June 21, 2016. https://www.aaihs.org.

Kendrick, Karen. "Is This What Sociology Is For?" Medium. Accessed November 11, 2020. https://medium.com.

Kennedy, Helen, Thomas Poell, and Jose van Dijck. "Data and Agency." *Big Data & Society*, December 2015. https://doi.org/10.1177/2053951715621569.

Kenney, Martha, and Laura Mamo. "The Imaginary of Precision Public Health." *Medical Humanities* 46, no. 3 (September 2020): 192–203.

Kessler, Ronald C., Sandro Galea, Russell T. Jones, and Holly A. Parker. "Mental Illness and Suicidality after Hurricane Katrina." *Bulletin of the World Health Organization* 84, no. 12 (December 2006): 930–39.

Kevles, Daniel J. *In the Name of Eugenics: Genetics and the Uses of Human Heredity*. Cambridge, MA: Harvard University Press, 1995.

Kickett, Marion. *Examination of How a Culturally-Appropriate Definition of Resilience Affects the Physical and Mental Health of Aboriginal People*. PhD diss., University of Western Australia, 2011.

Killingsworth, Ben, Renata Kokanovic, Huong Tran, and Chris Dowrick. "A Care-Full Diagnosis: Three Vietnamese Australian Women and Their Accounts of Becoming 'Mentally Ill.'" *Medicine Anthropology Quarterly* 24, no. 1 (2010): 108–23. https://doi.org/10.1111/j.1548-1387.2010.01087.x.

Kim, Eunjung. *Curative Violence: Rehabilitating Disability, Gender, and Sexuality in Modern Korea*. Durham, NC: Duke University Press, 2017.

King, Lester S. "Commentary." In *Education in the History of Medicine*, edited by. John B. Blake, 28–31. New York: Hafner, 1968.

King, Nicholas B. "The Scale Politics of Emerging Diseases." *Osiris* 19 (2004): 62–76.

King, Thomas. *The Truth about Stories: A Native Narrative*. Minneapolis: University of Minnesota Press, 2003.

Kirby, Vicki. Foreword to *What If Culture Was Nature All Along?*, edited by Vicki Kirby, viii–xii. Edinburgh: Edinburgh University Press, 2017.

Kirkness, Verna J., and Ray Barnhardt. "First Nations and Higher Education: The Four R's—Respect, Relevance, Reciprocity, Responsibility." *Journal of American Indian Education* 30, no. 3 (1991): 1–15.

Kirksey, Eben S., and Stefan Helmreich. "The Emergence of Multispecies Ethnography." *Cultural Anthropology* 25, no. 4 (2010): 545–76.

Kittay, Eva Feder. "Dependency, Difference, and the Global Ethic of Long-Term Care." *Journal of Political Philosophy* 13, no. 4 (2005): 441–69.

———. *Love's Labor: Essays on Women, Equality, and Dependency*. New York: Routledge, 1999.

Klar, Estée. *The Joy of Autism* (blog). 2005. Now defunct.

Klawiter, Maren. *The Biopolitics of Breast Cancer: Changing Cultures of Disease and Activism*. Minneapolis: University of Minnesota Press, 2008.

Kleider-Offutt, Heather M., Alesha D. Bond, and Shanna E. A. Hegerty. "Black Stereotypical Features: When a Face Type Can Get You in Trouble." *Current Directions in Psychological Science* 26, no. 1 (2017): 28–33.

Klein, Richard. "What Is Health and How Do You Get It?" In *Against Health: How Health Became the New Morality*, edited by Jonathan M. Metzl and Anna Kirkland, 15–25. New York: New York University Press, 2010.

Kleinman, Arthur. *The Illness Narratives: Suffering, Healing, and the Human Condition*. New York: Basic Books, 1988.

———. *Social Origins of Distress and Disease: Depression, Neurasthenia and Pain in Modern China*. New Haven, CT: Yale University Press, 1986.

Kleinman, Arthur, Veena Das, and Margaret Lock, eds. *Social Suffering*. Berkeley: University of California Press, 1997.

Kleinman, Arthur, L. Eisenberg, and Byron Good. "Culture, Illness, and Care: Clinical Lessons from Anthropologic and Cross-Cultural Research." *Annals of Internal Medicine* 88, no. 2 (1978): 251–58.

Kline, Wendy. *Bodies of Knowledge: Sexuality, Reproduction, and Women's Health in the Second Wave*. Chicago: University of Chicago Press, 2010.

Klugman, Craig M. "Who Teaches Humanities at Your Medical School?" Health Humanities Listserv. Hiram College. September 2020. https://archives.simplelists.com.

Klugman, Craig M., and Erin Gentry Lamb. *Research Methods in Health Humanities*. Oxford: Oxford University Press, 2019.

Knadler, Stephen. *Vitality Politics: Health, Debility, and the Limits of Black Emancipation*. Ann Arbor: University of Michigan Press, 2019.

Knott, Sarah. *Sensibility and the American Revolution*. Chapel Hill: University of North Carolina Press, 2009.

Kohn, Eduardo. *How Forests Think: Toward an Anthropology beyond the Human*. Berkeley: University of California Press, 2013.

Kolata, Gina. "'Partly Alive': Scientists Revive Cells in Brains from Dead Pigs." *New York Times*, April 17, 2019. https://www.nytimes.com.

Koslofsky, Craig. "Knowing Skin in Early Modern Europe." *History Compass* 12, no. 10 (2014): 794–806.

Kottow, Miguel H. "Should Medical Ethics Justify Violence?" *Journal of Medical Ethics* 32, no. 8 (2006): 464–67.

Kovach, Margaret. *Indigenous Methodologies: Characteristics, Conversations, and Contexts*. Toronto: University of Toronto Press, 2009.

Koven, Suzanne (@SuzanneKovenMD). "A whole issue of @JAMA_current devoted to narratives. . . . Who knew interest in storytelling and #medhum [medical humanities] would surge during a pandemic? (We knew)." Twitter, May 6, 2020, 8:46 a.m. https://twitter.com/SuzanneKovenMD/status/1258015218787135491?s=20&t=r97FbYFoF2hAbAi1u8cnSg.

Kraut, Alan M. *Silent Travelers: Germs, Genes, and the "Immigrant Menace."* Baltimore: Johns Hopkins University Press, 1994.

Kreiswirth, Martin. "Trusting the Tale: The Narrativist Turn in the Human Sciences." *New Literary History* 23 (1992): 629–57.

Krisberg, Kim. "Humanities Programs Help Medical Students See Life through a Patient's Eyes." *AAMC Reporter*, May 2014. https://www.aamc.org.

Kristeller, Paul Oskar. "'Creativity' and 'Tradition.'" *Journal of the History of Ideas* 44, no. 1 (1983): 105–13.

Kristeva, Julia, Marie Rose Moro, John Ødemark, and Eivind Engebretsen. "Cultural Crossings of Care: An Appeal to the Medical Humanities." *Medical Humanities* 44, no. 1 (March 2018): 55–58.

Kroker, Kenton. *The Sleep of Others and the Transformation of Sleep Research.* Toronto: University of Toronto Press, 2007.

Kroll-Smith, Steven, Phil Brown, and Valerie J. Gunter, eds. *Illness and the Environment: A Reader in Contested Medicine.* New York: New York University Press, 2000.

Kroll-Smith, Steven, and H. Hugh Floyd. *Bodies in Protest: Environmental Illness and the Struggle over Medical Knowledge.* New York: New York University Press, 1997.

Kruger, Steven F. *AIDS Narratives: Gender and Sexuality, Fiction and Science.* New York: Routledge, 1996.

Krznaric, Roman. *Empathy: Why It Matters and How to Get It.* New York: Penguin Random House, 2014.

Kujit, Ian. "The Regeneration of Life Neolithic Structures of Symbolic Remembering and Forgetting." *Current Anthropology* 49, no. 2 (April 2008): 171–97.

Kumagai, Arno K., and Monica L. Lypson. "Beyond Cultural Competence: Critical Consciousness, Social Justice, and Multicultural Education." *Academic Medicine* 84, no. 6 (2009): 782–87.

Kumagai, Arno K., and Thirusha Naidu. "The Cutting Edge: Health Humanities for Equity and Social Change." In *Routledge Handbook of the Medical Humanities*, edited by Alan Bleakley, 83–96. London: Routledge, 2019.

Kumagai, Arno K., and Delese Wear. "'Making Strange': A Role for the Humanities in Medical Education." *Academic Medicine* 89, no. 7 (2014): 973–77.

LaCapra, Dominick. *Writing History, Writing Trauma.* Baltimore: Johns Hopkins University Press, 2001.

Ladurie, Emmanuel Le Roy. "Un concept: L'unification microbienne du monde (XIVe–XVIIe siecles)." *Schweizerische Zeitschrift für Geschichte* 23, no. 4 (1973): 627–94.

Lakoff, Andrew. *Pharmaceutical Reason: Knowledge and Value in Global Psychiatry.* New York: Cambridge University Press, 2005.

———. *Unprepared: Global Health in a Time of Emergency.* Berkeley: University of California Press, 2017.

Lally, John, and Peter Cantillon. "Uncertainty and Ambiguity and Their Association with Psychological Distress in Medical Students." *Academic Psychiatry* 38, no. 3 (2014): 339–44.

Lane, Christopher. *Shyness: How Normal Became a Sickness.* New Haven, CT: Yale University Press, 2008.

Langfelder, Elinor J., and Eric T. Juengst. "Ethical, Legal, and Social Implications (ELSI) Program National Center for Human Genome Research, National Institutes of Health." *Politics and the Life Sciences* 12, no. 2 (1993): 273–75.

Langston, Nancy. *Toxic Bodies: Hormone Disruptors and the Legacy of DES.* New Haven, CT: Yale University Press, 2010.

Lanser, Susan S., and Shlomith Rimmon-Kenan. "Narratology at the Checkpoint: The Politics and Poetics of Entanglement." *Narrative* 27, no. 3 (2019): 245–69.

Lanzarotta, Tess. "Ethics in Retrospect: Biomedical Research, Colonial Violence, and Iñupiat Sovereignty in the Alaskan Arctic." *Social Studies of Science* 50, no. 5 (2020): 778–801.

Larkin, Marilyn. "The 'Medicalization' of Aging: What It Is, How It Harms, and What to Do about It." *Journal on Active Aging* 28 (January/February 2011): 28–36.

Latour, Bruno. *The Pasteurization of France.* Translated by Alan Sheridan. Cambridge, MA: Harvard University Press, 1988.

Lau, Travis Chi Wing. "Defoe before Immunity: A Prophylactic. *Journal of the Plague Year.*" *Digital Defoe: Studies in Defoe & His Contemporaries* 8, no. 1 (2016): 23–39.

Lawrence, Christopher, and George Weisz. *Greater Than the Parts: Holism in Biomedicine, 1920–1950.* New York: Oxford University Press, 1998.

Lawrence, Jane. "The Indian Health Service and the Sterilization of Native American Women." *American Indian Quarterly* 24, no. 3 (2000): 400–419.

Leach, Melissa. "Epidemics and Anthropologists." *Anthropology Today* 35, no. 6 (December 2019): 1–2.

Leavitt, Judith Walzer. *Typhoid Mary: Captive to the Public's Health*. Boston: Beacon, 1997.

Lederberg, Joshua. "Infectious History." *Science* 288, no. 5464 (2000): 287–93.

———. "Viruses and Humankind: Intracellular Symbiosis and Evolutionary Competition." In *Emerging Viruses*, edited by Stephen S. Morse, 3–9. Oxford: Oxford University Press, 1996.

Lederer, Susan. *Subjected to Science: Human Experimentation in America before the Second World War*. Baltimore: Johns Hopkins University Press, 1998.

Lee, Lisa M. "A Bridge Back to the Future: Public Health Ethics, Bioethics, and Environmental Ethics." *American Journal of Bioethics* 17, no. 9 (2017): 5–12.

Lee, Lisa M., and Frances A. McCarty. "Emergence of a Discipline? Growth in U.S. Postsecondary Bioethics Degrees." *Hastings Center Report* 46, no. 2 (2016): 19–21.

Lee, Sandra Soo-Jin. "Waiting on the Promise of Prescribing Precision: Race in the Era of Pharmacogenomics." In *Genetics and the Unsettled Past*, edited by K. A. Wailoo, A. Nelson, and C. Lee, 164–80. New Brunswick, NJ: Rutgers University Press, 2011.

Lee, Stephanie M. "Want to Cure Aging? Calico Is Now Hiring." SF Gate. December 1, 2014. https://blog.sfgate.com.

Lees, Lynn Hoollen. *The Solidarities of Strangers: The English Poor Laws and the People, 1770–1948*. Cambridge: Cambridge University Press, 1998.

Leitch, Kevin. *Left Brain / Right Brain*. Accessed September 1, 2020. https://leftbrainrightbrain.co.uk.

Lema, Mark J. "Taking the 'Non' out of 'Primum Non Nocere.'" *Regional Anesthesia* 18, no. 4 (1993): 205–6.

Lemoine, Maël. "Neither from Words, nor from Visions: Understanding P-Medicine from Innovative Treatments." *Lato Sensu: Revue de la société de philosophie des sciences* 4, no. 2 (2017): 12–23.

Leopold, Aldo. *For the Health of the Land: Previously Unpublished Essays and Other Writings*, edited by J. Baird Callicott and Eric T. Freyfogle. Washington, DC: Island Press, (1949) 2014.

———. *A Sand County Almanac: And Sketches Here*. Oxford: Oxford University Press, 1949.

Lerner, Paul. *Hysterical Men: War, Psychiatry, and the Politics of Trauma in Germany, 1890–1930*. Ithaca, NY: Cornell University Press, 2009.

Lerner, Steve. *Sacrifice Zones: The Front Lines of Toxic Chemical Exposure in the United States*. Cambridge, MA: MIT Press, 2010.

Leski, Kyna. *The Storm of Creativity*. Cambridge, MA: MIT Press, 2015.

Leung, Angela Ki Che, and Qizi Liang. *Leprosy in China: A History*. New York: Columbia University Press, 2009.

Levina, Marina. "Googling Your Genes: Personal Genomics and the Discourse of Citizen Bioscience in the Network Age." *Journal of Science Communication* 9, no. 1 (2010): 1–8.

Levinas, Emmanuel. *Totality and Infinity*. Translated by Alphonso Lingis. Boston: M. Nijhoff, 1979.

Levy, Becca R. "Stereotype Embodiment: A Psychosocial Approach to Aging." *Current Directions in Psychological Science* 18, no. 6 (2009): 332–36.

Levy, Becca R., and Lindsey M. Myers. "Preventive Health Behaviors Influenced by Self-Perceptions of Aging." *Preventive Medicine* 39, no. 3 (2004): 625–29.

Levy, Becca R., Martin D. Slade, E-Shien Chang, Sneha Kannoth, and Shi-Yi Wang. "Ageism Amplifies Cost and Prevalence of Health Conditions." *Gerontologist* 60, no. 1 (2020): 174–81.

Levy, Becca R., Martin D. Slade, Suzanne R. Kunkel, and Stanislav V. Kasl. "Longevity Increased by Positive Self-Perceptions of Aging." *Journal of Personality and Social Psychology* 83, no. 2 (2002): 261–70.

Levy, Becca R., Martin D. Slade, Robert H. Pietrzak, and Luigi Ferrucci. "Positive Age Beliefs Protect against Dementia Even among Elders with High-Risk Gene." *PLoS One* 13, no. 2 (2018): 1–8.

Levy, Becca R., Alan B. Zonderman, Martin D. Slade, and Luigi Ferrucci. "Age Stereotypes Held Earlier in Life Predict Cardiovascular Events in Later Life." *Psychological Science* 20, no. 3 (2009): 296–98.

Levy, Nicholas, J. Sturgess, and Pam Mills. "'Pain as the Fifth Vital Sign' and Dependence on the 'Numerical Pain Scale' Is Being Abandoned in the US: Why?" *British Journal of Anaesthesia* 120, no. 3 (2018): 435–38. https://bjanaesthesia.org.

Lewis, Abram J. "'We Are Certain of Our Own Insanity': Antipsychiatry and the Gay Liberation Movement, 1968–1980." *Journal of the History of Sexuality* 25, no. 1 (2016): 83–113.

Lewis, Arthur W. "The Dual Economy Revisited." *Manchester School* 47, no. 3 (1979): 211–29.

———. "The Industrialization of the British West Indies." *Caribbean Economic Review* 2 (1950): 1–53.

Leys, Ruth. *Trauma: A Genealogy*. Chicago: University of Chicago Press, 2000.

Link, Bruce G., and Jo Phelan. "Conceptualizing Stigma." *Annual Review of Sociology* 27, no. 1 (2001): 363–85.

———. "Stigma Power." *Social Science & Medicine* 103 (2014): 24–32.

Linker, Beth. "On the Borderland of Medical and Disability History: A Survey of the Fields." *Bulletin of the History of Medicine* 87, no. 4 (2013): 499–535.

———. *War's Waste: Rehabilitation in World War I America*. Chicago: University of Chicago Press, 2011.

Liou, Kevin T., Daniel S. Jamorabo, Richard H. Dollase, Luba Dumenco, Fred J. Schiffman, and Jay M. Baruch. "Playing in the 'Gutter': Cultivating Creativity in Medical Education and Practice." *Academic Medicine* 91, no. 3 (2016): 322–27.

Lipson, Ephraim. *The Economic History of England*. Vol. 1. *The Middle Ages*. London: A. & C. Black, 1929.

Lira, Natalie, and Alexandra Minna Stern. "Mexican Americans and Eugenic Sterilization: Resisting Reproductive Injustice in California, 1920–1950." *Aztlán: A Journal of Chicano Studies* 39, no. 2 (2014): 9–34.

Liu, Jenny X., Yevgeniy Goryakin, Akiko Maeda, Tim Bruckner, and Richard Scheffler. "Global Health Workforce Labor Market Projections for 2030." *Human Resources for Health* 15, no. 11 (2017): 1–12.

Livingston, James. "Mental Illness-Related Structural Stigma: The Downward Spiral of Systemic Exclusion Final Report." Mental Health Commission of Canada. October 31, 2013.

Livingston, Julie. *Debility and the Moral Imagination in Botswana*. Bloomington: Indiana University Press, 2005.

———. *Improvising Medicine: An African Oncology Ward in an Emerging Cancer Epidemic*. Durham, NC: Duke University Press, 2012.

Lock, Margaret. *Encounters with Aging: Mythologies of Menopause in Japan and North America*. Berkeley: University of California Press, 1993.

Logan, Peter Melville. *Nerves and Narratives: A Cultural History of Hysteria in Nineteenth-Century British Prose*. Berkeley: University of California Press, 1997.

Lombardo, Paul A. "Eugenics Laws Restricting Immigration." *Chesterton Review* 43, no. 1/2 (2017): 174–77.

———. *Three Generations, No Imbeciles: Eugenics, the Supreme Court, and Buck v. Bell*. Baltimore: Johns Hopkins University Press, 2002.

London School of Hygiene & Tropical Medicine. "Decolonising Global Health LSHTM." Accessed October 30, 2022. https://www.lshtm.ac.uk.

Long, Edward. *The History of Jamaica: Reflections on Its Situation, Settlements, Inhabitants, Climate, Products, Commerce, Laws, and Government*. Vol. 2. London: T. Lowndes, 1774.

Lorde, Audre. *A Burst of Light: Essays*. Ithaca, NY: Firebrand, 1988.

———. *The Cancer Journals*. San Francisco: Aunt Lute, 1980.

Lovejoy, Arthur O. *The Great Chain of Being: A Study of the History of an Idea*. Cambridge, MA: Harvard University Press, 1976.

Lovelock, James. *Gaia: A New Look at Life on Earth*. Revised ed. Oxford: Oxford University Press, 2016.

Löwy, Ilana, ed. *The Polish School of Philosophy of Medicine: From Tytus Chalubinski (1820–1889) to Ludwik Fleck (1896–1961)*. Vol. 37. Berlin: Springer Science & Business Media, 2012.

Ludmerer, Kenneth M. "Genetics, Eugenics, and the Immigration Restriction Act of 1924." *Bulletin of the History of Medicine* 46, no. 1 (1972): 59–81.

Luhrmann, Tanya. *Of Two Minds: An Anthropologist Looks at American Psychiatry*. New York: Vintage, 2001.

———. *When God Talks Back: Understanding the American Evangelical Relationship with God*. New York: Vintage, 2012.

Lupton, Deborah. *Medicine as Culture: Illness, Disease and the Body*. London: Sage, 2012.

———. "Quantifying the Body: Monitoring and Measuring Health in the Age of MHealth Technologies." *Critical Public Health* 23, no. 4 (2013): 393–403. https://doi.org/10.1080/09581596.2013.794931.

Lurie, Peter, Percy Hintzen, and Robert Lowe. "Socioeconomic Obstacles to HIV Prevention and Treatment in Developing Countries: The Roles of the International Monetary Fund and the World Bank." *AIDS* 9, no. 6 (1995): 539–46.

Luther, Vera P., and Sonia J. Crandall. "Commentary: Ambiguity and Uncertainty: Neglected Elements of Medical Education Curricula?" *Academic Medicine* 86, no. 7 (2011): 799–800.

Lwanda, John. "The [In]visibility of HIV/AIDS in the Malawi Public Sphere." *African Journal of AIDS Research* 2, no. 2 (2003): 113–26.

Lynch, Lisa. "The Neo/Bio/Colonial Hot Zone: African Viruses, American Fairytales." *International Journal of Cultural Studies* 1, no. 2 (1998): 233–52.

Lynteris, Christos, ed. *Framing Animals as Epidemic Villains: Histories of Non-human Disease Vectors.* London: Palgrave Macmillan, 2019a.

———. *Human Extinction and the Pandemic Imaginary.* London: Routledge, 2019b.

Lyons, Maryinez. *The Colonial Disease: A Social History of Sleeping Sickness in Northern Zaire, 1900–1940.* Cambridge: Cambridge University Press, 1992.

MacLeish, Kenneth T. *Making War at Fort Hood: Life and Uncertainty in a Military Community.* Princeton, NJ: Princeton University Press, 2013.

Macmillan, Malcolm. *An Odd Kind of Fame: Stories of Phineas Gage.* Cambridge, MA: MIT Press, 2002.

MacRae, Donald Gunn. "Thomas Malthus." *Encyclopedia Britannica*, December 2019. https://www.britannica.com.

Madness and Literature Network (website). Accessed November 5, 2021. http://www.madnessandliterature.org.

Magi, Jill, Nev Jones, and Timothy Kelly. "How Are/Our Work: 'What, If Anything, Is the Use of Any of This?'" In *The Edinburgh Companion to the Critical Medical Humanities*, edited by Anne Whitehead and Angela Woods, 136–52. Edinburgh: Edinburgh University Press, 2016.

Major, Brenda, John F. Dovidio, and Bruce G. Link. *The Oxford Handbook of Stigma, Discrimination, and Health.* New York: Oxford University Press, 2018.

Mäkelä, Maria, Samuli Björninen, Laura Karttunen, Matias Nurminen, Juha Raipola, and Tytti Rantanen. "Dangers of Narrative: A Critical Approach to Narratives of Personal Experience in Contemporary Story Economy." *Narrative* 29, no. 2 (2021): 139–59.

Malabou, Catherine. *The Ontology of the Accident: An Essay on Destructive Plasticity.* Translated by Carolyn Shread. Malden, MA: Polity, (2009) 2012.

———. *What Should We Do with Our Brain.* Translated by Sebastian Rand. New York: Fordham University Press, 2008.

Malafouris, Lambros. "Beads for a Plastic Mind: The 'Blind Man's Stick' (BMS) Hypothesis and the Active Nature of Material Culture." *Cambridge Archeological Journal* 18, no. 3 (2008): 401–14.

———. *How Things Shape the Mind: A Theory of Material Engagement.* Cambridge, MA: MIT Press, 2013.

Maldonado-Torres, Nelson. "Interrogating Systemic Racism and the White Academic Field." Foundation Frantz Fanon. 2020. https://fondation-frantzfanon.com.

Malthus, Thomas Robert. *An Essay on the Principle of Population and Other Writings.* London: Penguin Classics, (1798) 2015.

Mamo, Laura, and Jennifer R. Fishman. "Potency in All the Right Places: Viagra as a Technology of the Gendered Body." *Body & Society* 7, no. 4 (2001): 13–35.

Mangione, Salvatore, Chayan Chakraborti, Giuseppe Staltari, Rebecca Harrison, Allan R. Tunkel, Kevin T. Liou, Elizabeth Cerceo et al. "Medical Students' Exposure to the Humanities Correlates with Positive Personal Qualities and Reduced Burnout: A Multi-institutional U.S. Survey." *Journal of General Internal Medicine* 33, no. 5 (2018): 628–34.

Mann, Annika. *Reading Contagion: The Hazards of Reading in the Age of Print.* Charlottesville: University of Virginia Press, 2018.

Mann, Jonathan M. "Health and Human Rights." *British Medical Journal* 312, no. 7036 (1996): 924–25.

Marini, Maria Giulia. *Language of Care in Narrative Medicine: Words, Space and Time in the Health Care Ecosystem.* Berlin: Springer, 2019.

———. *Narrative Medicine: Bridging the Gap between Evidence-Based Care and Medical Humanities.* Berlin: Springer, 2016.

Markley, Robert. "'A Putridness in the Air': Monsoons and Mortality in Seventeenth-Century Bombay." *Journal for Early Modern Cultural Studies* 10, no. 2 (Fall/Winter 2010): 105–25.

Marsland, Rebecca. "The Modern Traditional Healer: Locating 'Hybridity' in Modern Traditional Medicine, Southern Tanzania." *Journal of Southern African Studies* 33, no. 4 (December 2007): 751–65.

Martenson, Robert. "The History of Bioethics: An Essay Review." *Journal of the History of Medicine and Allied Sciences* 56, no. 2 (April 2001): 168–75.

Martin, Emily. *Bipolar Expeditions: Mania and Depression in American Culture.* Princeton, NJ: Princeton University Press, 2007.

——. *Flexible Bodies: Tracking Immunity in American Culture from the Days of Polio to the Age of AIDS*. Boston: Beacon, 1995.

——. "The Pharmaceutical Person." *BioSocieties* 1, no. 3 (2006): 273–87.

Massumi, Brian. *The Politics of Affect*. Malden, MA: Polity, 2015.

Matthew, Dayna Bowen. *Just Medicine: A Cure for Racial Inequality in Health Care*. New York: New York University Press, 2015.

——. "Two Threats to Precision Medicine Equity." *Ethnicity & Disease* 29, no. 3 (2019): 629–40.

Maturana, Humberto, and Francisco J. Varela. *Autopoiesis and Cognition: The Realization of the Living*. Berlin: Springer Dordrecht, 1980.

Mavhunga, Clapperton Chak. *The Mobile Workshop: The Tsetse Fly and African Knowledge Production*. Cambridge, MA: MIT Press, 2018.

May, Jacques M. *The Ecology of Human Disease* New York: MD Publications, 1958.

Mayer-Schönberger, Viktor, and Kenneth Cukier. *Big Data: A Revolution That Will Transform How We Live, Work, and Think*. New York: Houghton Mifflin Harcourt, 2013.

Mayr, Ernst. *The Growth of Biological Thought: Diversity, Evolution, and Inheritance*. Cambridge: Belknap, 1982.

Mbali, Mandisa. "AIDS Discourses and the South African State: Government Denialism and Post-apartheid AIDS Policy-Making." *Transformation: Critical Perspectives on Southern Africa* 54, no. 1 (2004): 104–22.

Mbembe, Achille. "Necropolitics." Translated by Libby Meintjes. In *Biopolitics: A Reader*, edited by Timothy Campbell and Adam Sitze, 161–92. Durham, NC: Duke University Press, 2013.

McCarthy, Anna. "From the Ordinary to the Concrete: Cultural Studies and the Politics of Scale." In *Questions of Method in Cultural Studies*, edited by Mimi White and James Schwoch, 17–53. Malden, MA: Blackwell, 2006.

McCrudden, Christopher. "Institutional Discrimination." *Oxford Journal of Legal Studies* 2, no. 3 (1982): 303–67.

McDonald, Kathryn M., Hector P. Rodriguez, and Stephen M. Shortell. "Organizational Influences on Time Pressure Stressors and Potential Patient Consequences in Primary Care." *Medical Care* 56, no. 10 (2018): 822.

McDowell, Paula. *The Women of Grub Street: Press, Politics, and Gender in the London Literary Marketplace, 1678–1730*. Oxford: Oxford University Press, 1998.

McGee, Glenn, Arthur L. Caplan, Joshua P. Spanogle, and David A. Asch. "A National Study of Ethics Committees." *American Journal of Bioethics* 1, no. 4 (2001): 60–64.

McGuire, Danielle L. *At the Dark End of the Street*. New York: Penguin Random House, 2011.

McKeown, Thomas. *The Role of Medicine: Dream, Mirage or Nemesis?* Nuffield Provincial Hospitals Trust, 1976; Reprint, Princeton, NJ: Princeton University Press, 1980.

McNeill, William H. *Plagues and Peoples*. New York: Anchor, 1976; Reprint, New York: Knopf, 2010.

McRuer, Robert. *Crip Theory: Cultural Signs of Queerness and Disability*. New York: New York University Press, 2006.

Mendelsohn, J. Andrew. "'Like All That Lives': Biology, Medicine and Bacteria in the Age of Pasteur and Koch." *History and Philosophy of the Life Sciences* 24, no. 1 (2002): 3–36.

Merton, Robert K. "The Self-Fulfilling Prophecy." *Antioch Review* 8, no. 2 (1948): 193–210.

Metzl, Jonathan M. *Dying of Whiteness: How the Politics of Racial Resentment Is Killing America's Heartland*. New York: Basic Books, 2019.

——. *The Protest Psychosis: How Schizophrenia Became a Black Disease*. Boston: Beacon, 2009.

——. "Selling Sanity through Gender: The Psychodynamics of Psychotropic Advertising." *Journal of Medical Humanities* 24, no. 1/2 (2003): 79–103.

Metzl, Jonathan M., and Helena Hansen. "Structural Competency: Theorizing a New Medical Engagement with Stigma and Inequality." *Social Science & Medicine* 103 (2014): 126–33.

Metzl, Jonathan M., and Rebecca M. Herzig. "Medicalisation in the 21st Century: Introduction." *Lancet* 369, no. 9562 (February 2007): 697–98.

Metzl, Jonathan M., and Anna Kirkland. *Against Health: How Health Became the New Morality*. New York: New York University Press, 2010.

Meyerowitz, Joanne. *How Sex Changed: A History of Transsexuality in the United States*. Cambridge, MA: Harvard University Press, 2002.

Micale, Mark S. "On the 'Disappearance' of Hysteria: A Study in the Clinical Deconstruction of a Diagnosis." *Isis* 84, no. 3 (1993): 496–526. https://doi.org/10.1086/356549.

Micale, Mark S., and Paul Lerner. *Traumatic Pasts: History, Psychiatry, and Trauma in the Modern Age, 1870–1930*. Cambridge: Cambridge University Press, 2001.

Micale, Mark S., and Hans Pols. *Traumatic Pasts in Asia: History, Psychiatry, and Trauma from the 1930s to the Present*. New York: Berghahn, 2021.

Mignolo, Walter D., and Catherine E. Walsh. *On Decoloniality: Concepts, Analytics, Praxis*. Durham, NC: Duke University Press, 2018.

Miller, J. Hillis. *The Ethics of Reading: Kant, de Man, Eliot, Trollope, James, and Benjamin*. New York: Columbia University Press, 1987.

Miner, Dylan A. T. "Stories as *Mshkiki*: Reflections on the Healing and Migratory Practices of Minwaajimo." In *Centering Anishinaabeg Studies: Understanding the World through Stories*, edited by Jill Doerfler, Niigaanwewidam James Sinclair, and Heidi Kiiwetinepinesiik Stark, 317–39. East Lansing: Michigan State University Press, 2013.

Mintz, Susannah B. *Hurt and Pain: Literature and the Suffering Body*. London: Bloomsbury, 2013.

Mitchell, David, and Sharon L. Snyder. *The Biopolitics of Disability: Neoliberalism, Ablenationalism, and Peripheral Embodiment*. Ann Arbor: University of Michigan Press, 2015.

Mitchell, Peta. *Contagious Metaphor*. London: Bloomsbury Academic, 2012.

Mitchell, Robert. *Experimental Life: Vitalism in Romantic Science and Literature*. Baltimore: Johns Hopkins University Press, 2013.

Moeller, Susan. *Compassion Fatigue: How the Media Sell Disease, Famine, War, and Death*. New York: Routledge, 1999.

Moelling, Karin, and Felix Broecker. "Viruses and Evolution—Viruses First? A Personal Perspective." *Frontiers in Microbiology* 10, no. 523 (2019): 1–13. https://doi.org/10.3389/fmicb.2019.00523.

Mol, Annemarie. *The Body Multiple: Ontology in Medical Practice*. Raleigh, NC: Duke University Press, 2005.

Moore, Andrew. "What's the Point of Paracetamol?" Conversation. October 2016. https://theconversation.com.

Morales, Laurel. "The Navajo Nation, Uranium Mining's Deadly Legacy Lingers." NPR. April 2016. https://www.npr.org.

Moran, J. A. "Primum non nocere." *CMAJ: Canadian Medical Association Journal* 146, no. 10 (1992): 1700.

Moran, Joe. *Reading the Everyday*. London: Taylor & Francis, 2005.

Morantz-Sanchez, Regina Markell. *Sympathy & Science: Women Physicians in American Medicine*. New York: Oxford University Press, 1985.

Moreton-Robinson, Aileen. "I Still Call Australia Home: Indigenous Belonging and Place in a White Postcolonizing Society." In *Uprootings/Regroundings Questions of Home and Migration*, edited by Sara Ahmed, Claudia Castada, Anne-Marie Fortier, and Mimi Sheller, 1–23. New York: Routledge, 2020.

Moriyama, Iwao, Ruth M. Loy, and Alastair H. T. Robb-Smith. *History of the Statistical Classification of Diseases and Causes of Death*. Hyattsville, MD: National Center for Health Statistics, 2011.

Morris, David B. *The Culture of Pain*. Berkeley: University of California Press, 1991.

Morrison, Kerrianne E., Kilee M. DeBrabander, Desiree R. Jones, Daniel J. Faso, Robert A. Ackerman, and Noah J. Sasson. "Outcomes of Real-World Social Interaction for Autistic Adults Paired with Autistic Compared with Typically Developing Partners." *Autism* 24, no. 5 (2019): 1067–80.

Morrison, Toni. *The Origin of Others (The Charles Eliot Norton Lectures 2016)*. Cambridge, MA: Harvard University Press, 2017.

Morse, Stephen S. "Examining the Origins of Emerging Viruses." In *Emerging Viruses*, edited by Stephen S. Morse, 10–28. New York: Oxford University Press, 1996.

Moser, Benjamin. *Sontag: Her Life and Work*. New York: Ecco, 2019.

Moss, Lenny. *What Genes Can't Do*. Cambridge, MA: MIT Press, 2004.

Motola, Jacob. "When and How Did the Metaphor of the Computer 'Virus' Arise?" *Scientific American*, September 1997. https://www.scientificamerican.com.

Moulton, Carol-Anne E., Glenn Regehr, Maria Mylopoulos, and Helen M. MacRae. "Slowing Down When You Should: A New Model of Expert Judgment." *Academic Medicine* 82, no. 10 (2007): S109–S116.

Muir, John. *My First Summer in the Sierra*. Boston: Houghton Mifflin, 1911.

Mukharji, Projit B. *Doctoring Traditions: Ayurveda, Small Technologies, and Braided Sciences*. Chicago: University of Chicago Press, 2016.

Mukherjee, Pablo. "'Tomorrow There Will Be More of Us': Toxic Postcoloniality in *Animal's People*." In *Postcolonial Ecologies: Literatures of the Environment*, edited by Elizabeth DeLoughrey and George B. Handley, 216–31. New York: Oxford University Press, 2011.

Mulla, Sameena. *The Violence of Care: Rape Victims, Forensic Nurses, and Sexual Assault Victims*. New York: New York University Press, 2014.

Muller, Lorraine. *A Theory for Indigenous Australian Health and Human Service Work: Connecting Indigenous Knowledge and Practice*. New York: Routledge, 2020.

Murison, Justine. *The Politics of Anxiety in Nineteenth-Century American Literature*. Cambridge: Cambridge University Press, 2011.

Muskie. "Institute for the Study of the Neurologically Typical" (website), 1998. Now defunct.

Naimark, Norman. *Genocide: A World History*. Oxford: Oxford University Press, 2016.

Nancy, Jean Luc. *The Fall of Sleep*. Translated by Charlotte Mandell. New York: Fordham University Press, 2009.

Narat, Victor, Lys Alcayna-Stevens, Stephanie Rupp, and Tamara Giles-Vernick. "Rethinking Human-Nonhuman Primate Contact and Pathogenic Disease Spillover." *EcoHealth* 14, no. 4 (2017): 840–50. https://doi.org/10.1007/s10393-017-1283-4.

Nash, Linda Lorraine. *Inescapable Ecologies: A History of Environment, Disease, and Knowledge*. Berkeley: University of California Press, 2006.

National Institute for Health and Care Excellence. "Psychosis and Schizophrenia in Adults: Prevention and Management [Clinical Guideline CG178]." 2014. https://www.nice.org.uk.

National Research Council. National Science Education Standards. National Committee on Science Education Standards and Assessment, 1996. https://www.csun.edu.

Needham, Joseph. *Science and Civilization in China*. Vol. 6. Cambridge: Cambridge University Press, 2000.

Ne'eman, Ari. "The Future (and the Past) of Autism Advocacy, or Why the ASA's Magazine, *The Advocate*, Wouldn't Publish This Piece." *Disability Studies Quarterly* 30, no. 1 (2010). https://dsq-sds.org.

Neff, Gina, and Dawn Nafus. *Self-Tracking*. Cambridge, MA: MIT Press, 2016.

Nelkin, Dorothy. "Molecular Metaphors: The Gene in Popular Discourse." *Nature Reviews Genetics* 2, no. 7 (2001): 555–59.

Nelson, Alondra. *Body and Soul: The Black Panther Party and the Fight against Medical Discrimination*. New York: New York University Press, 2011.

Nelson, Diane. *A Finger in the Wound: Body Politics in Quincentennial Guatemala*. Berkeley: University of California Press, 1997.

Nelson, Jennifer. *More Than Medicine: A History of the Women's Health Movement*. New York: New York University Press, 2015.

Nerlich, Brigitte, Robert Dingwall, and David D. Clarke. "The Book of Life: How the Completion of the Human Genome Project Was Revealed to the Public." *Health* 6, no. 4 (2002): 445–69.

Neuberger, Julia, and Raymond Tallis. "Do We Need a New Word for Patients?" *BMJ* 318, no. 7200 (1999): 1756–58.

Neuhaus, Carolyn P. "Does Solidarity Require 'All of Us' to Participate in Genomics Research?" *Hastings Center Report* 50, no. 1 (2020): S62–S69.

Newen, Albert, Leon de Bruin, and Shaun Gallagher. *The Oxford Handbook of 4E Cognition*. Oxford: Oxford University Press, 2018.

Nguyen, Vinh-Kim, and Karine Peschard. "Anthropology, Inequality, and Disease: A Review." *Annual Review of Anthropology* 32 (2003): 447–74.

Ngwira, Emmanuel. "'Daughters of Eve': Portrayal of the Female Body in Selected HIV/AIDS Songs in Malawi." *Journal of Humanities* 25, no. 1 (2017): 94–111.

Nicolaidis, Christina. "What Can Physicians Learn from the Neurodiversity Movement?" *American Medical Association Journal of Ethics* 14, no. 6 (2012): 503–10.

Nissenbaum, Helen. "A Contextual Approach to Privacy Online." *Daedalus* 140, no. 4 (Fall 2011): 32–48.

Nixon, Kari. *Kept from All Contagion: Germ Theory, Disease, and the Dilemma of Human Contact in Late Nineteenth-Century Literature*. Albany: SUNY Press, 2020.

Nixon, Kari, and Lorenzo Servitje, eds. *Endemic: Essays in Contagion Theory*. New York: Palgrave Macmillan, 2016.

Nixon, Rob. *Slow Violence and the Environmentalism of the Poor*. Cambridge, MA: Harvard University Press, 2011.

Noddings, Nel. *Caring, a Feminine Approach to Ethics & Moral Education*. Berkeley: University of California Press, 1984.

Noel, Maxine. "My Grandmother's Eyes." In *Me Artsy*, edited by Drew Hayden Taylor, 41–57. Madeira Park, BC: Douglas & McIntyre, 2015.

Norris, Philip. *A History of Disease in Ancient Times*. London: Palgrave, 2016.

Nozick, Robert. *Anarchy, State, and Utopia*. New York: Basic Books, 1974.

Nudelman, Franny. *Fighting Sleep: The War for the Mind and the US Military*. London: Verso, 2019.

Nuffield Council on Bioethics. "Genome Editing: An Ethical Review." Nuffield Council on Bioethics. September 2016. https://www.nuffieldbioethics.org.

Núñez Noriega, Guillermo, and Claudia Esthela Espinoza Cid. "Drug-Trafficking as a Dispositif of Sex-Gender Power: Organized Crime, Masculinity and Queer Theory." *Revista interdisciplinaria de estudios de género de El Colegio de México* 3, no. 5 (2017): 90–128.

"Nuremberg Code (1947)." *British Medical Journal* 313, no. 7070 (1996): 1448.

Nurok, Michael. "Elements of the Medical Emergency's Epistemological Alignment: 18–20th-Century Perspectives." *Social Studies of Science* 33, no. 4 (2003): 563–79.

Nutton, Vivian. "Did the Greeks Have a Word for It? Contagion and Contagion Theory in Classical Antiquity." In *Contagion: Perspectives from Pre-modern Societies*, edited by L. I. Conrad and D. Wajastyk, 137–62. Aldershot, UK: Ashgate, 2000.

———. *Galen: A Thinking Doctor in Imperial Rome*. London: Routledge, 2020.

Obermeyer, Ziad, Brian Powers, Christine Vogeli, and Sendhil Mullainathan. "Dissecting Racial Bias in an Algorithm Used to Manage the Health of Populations." *Science* 366, no. 6464 (2019): 447–53. https://doi.org/10.1126/science.aax2342.

O'Brien, Susan M. "Spirit Discipline: Gender, Islam, and Hierarchies of Treatment in Postcolonial Northern Nigeria." *Interventions* 3, no. 2 (January 2001): 222–41.

O'Connor, Erin. *Raw Material: Producing Pathology in Victorian Culture*. Durham, NC: Duke University Press, 2000.

OED Online, s.v. "access." Oxford University Press, December 2021. https://www.oed.com.

———, s.v. "accuracy." Oxford University Press, May 2021. https://www.oed.com.

———, s.v. "anxiety." Oxford University Press, December 2021. https://www.oed.com.

———, s.v. "colonialism." Oxford University Press, September 2022. https://www.oed.com.

———, s.v. "colony." Oxford University Press, September 2022. https://www.oed.com.

———, s.v. "compassion." Oxford University Press, December 2021. https://www.oed.com.

———, s.v. "creativity." Oxford University Press, December 2021. https://www.oed.com.

———, s.v. "data." Oxford University Press, December 2021. https://www.oed.com.

———, s.v. "datum." Oxford University Press, December 2021. https://www.oed.com.

———, s.v. "death." Oxford University Press, September 2022. https://www.oed.com.

———, s.v. "diagnosis." Oxford University Press, December 2021. https://www.oed.com.

———, s.v. "germ." Oxford University Press, September 2020. https://www.oed.com.

———, s.v. "history." Oxford University Press, December 2020. https://www.oed.com.

———, s.v. "humanism." Oxford University Press, September 2020. https://www.oed.com.

———, s.v. "humanities." Oxford University Press, September 2020. https://www.oed.com.

———, s.v. "humanity." Oxford University Press, September 2020. https://www.oed.com.

———, s.v. "microbe." Oxford University Press, September 2020. https://www.oed.com.

———, s.v. "observation." Oxford University Press, May 2021. https://www.oed.com.

———, s.v. "pathological." Oxford University Press, May 2021. https://www.oed.com.

———, s.v. "patient." Oxford University Press, May 2021. https://www.oed.com.

———, s.v. "physician." Oxford University Press, May 2021. https://www.oed.com.

———, s.v. "pollution." Oxford University Press, December 2021. https://www.oed.com.

———, s.v. "psychosis." Oxford University Press, December 2021. https://www.oed.com.

————, s.v. "reproduction." Oxford University Press, December 2021. https://www.oed.com.

————, s.v. "sense." Oxford University Press, December 2021. https://www.oed.com.

————, s.v. "toxic." Oxford University Press, December 2021. https://www.oed.com.

————, s.v. "trauma." Oxford University Press, December 2021. https://www.oed.com.

————, s.v. "virus." Oxford University Press, September 2022. https://www.oed.com.

————, s.v. "wound." Oxford University Press, December 2021. https://www.oed.com.

Office of the High Commissioner for Human Rights. "A Human Rights-Based Approach to Health." Accessed September 22, 2022. https://www.ohchr.org.

Ogden, Emily. "*Edgar Huntly* and the Regulation of the Senses." *American Literature* 85, no. 3 (2013): 419–45.

Oliver, Mary. *Upstream: Selected Essays*. New York: Penguin, 2019.

Olopade, Dyo. *The Bright Continent: Breaking Rules & Making Change in Modern Africa*. Boston: Houghton Mifflin Harcourt, 2014.

Ong, Aihwa. "Ecologies of Expertise: Assembling Flows, Managing Citizenship." In *Global Assemblages: Technology, Politics, and Ethics as Anthropological Problems*, edited by Aihwa Ong and Stephen J. Collier, 337–53. Malden, MA: Blackwell, 2005.

————. *Neoliberalism as Exception: Mutations in Citizenship and Sovereignty*. Durham, NC: Duke University Press, 2006.

Orwin, Clifford. "Stasis and Plague: Thucydides on the Dissolution of Society." *Journal of Politics* 50, no. 4 (November 1988): 831–47.

Osborne, Thomas. "The Ordinariness of the Archive." *History of Human Sciences* 12, no. 2 (1999): 51–64.

Osler, William. "A Note on the Teaching of the History of Medicine." *British Medical Journal* 2, no. 2167 (1902): 93.

————. "The Old Humanities and the New Science: The Presidential Address Delivered before the Classical Association at Oxford." *British Medical Journal* 2, no. 3053 (May 1919): 1–7.

Osseo-Asare, Abena Dove Agyepoma. *Bitter Roots: The Search for Healing Plants in Africa*. Chicago: University of Chicago Press, 2014.

Osteen, Mark. Review of *See It Feelingly: Classic Novels, Autistic Readers, and the Schooling of a No-Good English Professor. ALH Online Review* 20, no. 1 (2019): 273 https://static.primary.prod.gcms.the-infra.com/static/site/alh/document/ALH_Online_Review_Series_20/20Mark_Osteen.pdf?node=a903aec794bb840033fc&version=324070:9582e2319425555edaac&preview=true.

Ostherr, Kirsten. "Artificial Intelligence and Medical Humanities." *Journal of Medical Humanities* 43 (July 2020a): 211–32. https://doi.org/10.1007/s10912-020-09636-4.

————. *Cinematic Prophylaxis: Globalization and Contagion in the Discourse of World Health*. Durham, NC: Duke University Press, 2005.

————. "Risk Media in Medicine: The Rise of the Metaclinical Health App Ecosystem." In *The Routledge Companion to Media and Risk*, edited by Bishnupriya Gosh and Bhaskar Sarkar, 107–17. New York: Routledge, 2020b. https://doi.org/10.4324/9781315637501-6.

Ostherr, Kirsten, Svetlana Borodina, Rachel Conrad Bracken, Charles Lotterman, Eliot Storer, and Brandon Williams. "Trust and Privacy in the Context of User-Generated Health Data." *Big Data & Society* 4, no. 1 (2017): 1–11. https://doi.org/10.1177/2053951717704673.

Otis, Laura. *Membranes: Metaphors of Invasion in Nineteenth-Century Literature, Science, and Politics*. Baltimore: Johns Hopkins University Press, 1999.

Ouellette, Alicia. *Bioethics and Disability: Toward a Disability-Conscious Bioethics*. Cambridge: Cambridge University Press, 2011.

————. "Hearing the Deaf: Cochlear Implants, the Deaf Community, and Bioethical Analysis." *Valparaiso University Law Review* 45, no. 3 (2010): 1247–70.

Packard, Randall M. *A History of Global Health: Interventions into the Lives of Other Peoples*. Baltimore: Johns Hopkins University Press, 2016.

————. *The Making of a Tropical Disease: A Short History of Malaria*. Baltimore: Johns Hopkins University Press, 2007.

————. "Post-colonial Medicine." In *Companion to Medicine in the Twentieth Century*, edited by Roger Cooter and John V. Pickstone, 97–112. London: Routledge, 2004.

————. *White Plague, Black Labor: Tuberculosis and the Political Economy of Health and Disease in South Africa*. Berkeley: University of California Press, 1989.

Packard, Randall M., and Paul Epstein. "Epidemiologists, Social Scientists, and the Structure of Medical Research on AIDS in Africa." *Social Science & Medicine* 33, no. 7 (1991): 771–94.

Painter, Nell. *The History of White People*. New York: W. W. Norton, 2010.

Palmer, Steven. "Migrant Clinics and Hookworm Science: Peripheral Origins of Int'l Health, 1840–1920." *Bulletin of the History of Medicine* 83, no. 4 (2009): 676–709.

Panda, S. C. "Medicine: Science or Art?" *Mens Sana Monographs* 4, no. 1 (2006): 127–38.

Paradiz, Valerie. *Elijah's Cup: A Family's Journey into the Community and Culture of High Functioning Autism and Asperger's Syndrome*. New York: Free Press, 2002.

Parens, Erik. "Is Better Always Good? The Enhancement Project." *Hastings Center Report* 28, no. 1 (1998): S1–S15.

Parens, Erik, and Adrienne Ash. "The Disability Rights Critique of Prenatal Testing." In *Prenatal Testing and Disability Rights*, edited by Erik Parens and Adrienne Ash, 3–43. Washington, DC: Georgetown University Press, 2000.

Parks, Lisa, and Nicole Starosielski, eds. *Signal Traffic: Critical Studies of Media Infrastructures*. Champaign: University of Illinois Press, 2015.

Parreñas, Rhacel Salazar. *The Force of Domesticity: Filipina Migrants and Globalization*. New York: New York University Press, 2008.

———. "Mothering from a Distance: Emotions, Gender, and Intergenerational Relations in Filipino Transnational Families." Feminist Studies 27, no. 2 (2001): 361–90.

———, ed. *Servants of Globalization: Migration and Domestic Work*. 2nd ed. Palo Alto, CA: Stanford University Press, 2015.

Parsons, Talcott. *The Social System*. New York: Free Press, 1964.

Parzen, Micah David. "Toward a Culture-Bound Syndrome-Based Insanity Defense?" *Culture, Medicine, and Psychiatry* 27, no. 2 (2003): 131–55.

Pasupathi, Monisha, and Corinna E. Löckenhoff. "Ageist Behavior." In *Ageism: Stereotyping and Prejudice against Older Persons*, edited by Todd D. Nelson, 201–46. Cambridge, MA: MIT Press, 2002.

Patel, Rikinkumar S., Ramya Bachu, Archana Adikey, Meryem Malik, and Mansi Shah. "Factors Related to Physician Burnout and Its Consequences: A Review." *Behavioral*

Sciences 8, no. 11 (October 2018): 1–7. https://doi.org/10.3390/bs8110098.

Paul, Diane B., and James Moore. "The Darwinian Context: Evolution and Inheritance." In *The Oxford Handbook of the History of Eugenics*, edited by Alison Bashford and Philippa Levine, 27–42. Oxford: Oxford University Press, 2010.

Paxson, Heather, and Stefan Helmreich. "The Perils and Promise of Microbial Abundance: Novel Natures and Model Ecosystems." *Social Studies of Science* 44, no. 2 (2014): 165–93.

Peckham, Robert. *Epidemics in Modern Asia*. Cambridge: Cambridge University Press, 2016.

Peckham, Robert, and Ria Sinha. "Satellites and the New War on Infection: Tracking Ebola in West Africa." *Geoforum* 80 (2017): 24–38.

Pellegrino, Edmund D. "Prescribing and Drug Ingestion Symbols and Substances." *Drug Intelligence & Clinical Pharmacy* 10, no. 11 (November 1976): 624–30. https://doi.org/10.1177/106002807601001101.

Pelling, Margaret. "The Meaning of Contagion: Reproduction, Medicine, and Metaphor." In *Contagion: Historical and Cultural Studies*, edited by Alison Bashford and Claire Hooker, 15–38. London: Routledge, 2001.

Perrot, Michelle. *The Bedroom: An Intimate History*. Translated by Lauren Elkin. New Haven, CT: Yale University Press, 2018.

Persaud, Nav, Heather Butts, and Philip Berger. "William Osler: Saint in a 'White Man's Dominion.'" *Canadian Medical Association Journal* 192, no. 45 (November 2020): E1414–16. https://doi.org/10.1503/cmaj.201567.

Persson, Asha. "Incorporating Pharmakon: HIV, Medicine, and Body Shape Change." *Body & Society* 10, no. 4 (2004): 45–67.

Pescosolido, A. Bernice, and Jack K. Martin. "The Stigma Complex." *Annual Review of Sociology* 41, no. 1 (2015): 87–116.

Petryna, Adriana. *Life Exposed: Biological Citizens after Chernobyl*. Princeton, NJ: Princeton University Press, 2002.

———. *When Experiments Travel: Clinical Trials and the Global Search for Human Subjects*. Princeton, NJ: Princeton University Press, 2009.

Pew Research Center. "Attitudes about Aging: A Global Perspective." January 2014. https://www.pewresearch.org.

Phelan, James. *Narrative as Rhetoric: Techniques, Audiences, Ethics, Ideology*. Columbus: Ohio State University Press, 2010.

Pickersgill, Martyn, and Linda Hogle. "Enhancement, Ethics and Society: Towards an Empirical Research Agenda for the Medical Humanities and Social Sciences." *Medical Humanities* 41 (2015): 136–42.

Pierce, Andrew J. "Whose Lives Matter? The Black Lives Matter Movement and the Contested Legacy of Philosophical Humanism." *Journal of Social Philosophy* 51, no. 2 (2020): 261–82.

Pine, Adrienne. "From Healing to Witchcraft: On Ritual Speech and Roboticization in the Hospital." *Culture, Medicine, and Psychiatry* 35, no. 2 (2011): 262–84.

Pitts-Taylor, Victoria. "Mattering: Feminism, Science, and Corporeal Politics." In *Mattering: Feminism, Science, and Materialism*, edited by Pitts-Taylor, 1–20. New York: New York University Press, 2016.

Politi, Mary C., and France Légaré. "Physicians' Reactions to Uncertainty in the Context of Shared Decision Making." *Patient Education and Counseling* 80, no. 2 (2010): 155–57.

Pollock, Anne. *Medicating Race: Heart Disease and Durable Preoccupations with Difference*. Durham, NC: Duke University Press, 2012.

——. "Queering Endocrine Disruption." In *Object Oriented Feminism*, edited by Katherine Behar, 183–99. Minneapolis: University of Minnesota Press, 2016.

Porter, Natalie. *Viral Economies: Bird Flu Experiments in Vietnam*. Chicago: University of Chicago Press, 2019.

Porter, Roy. *Doctor of Society: Thomas Beddoes and the Sick Trade in Late-Enlightenment England*. New York: Routledge, 1992.

——. *The Greatest Benefit to Mankind: A Medical History of Humanity*. New York: W. W. Norton, 1999.

——. *Medicine in the Enlightenment*. Atlanta: Rodopi, 1995.

——. "The Patient's View: Doing Medical History from Below." *Theory and Society* 14, no. 2 (1985): 175–98.

Porter, Roy, and Dorothy Porter. "The Rise of the English Drugs Industry: The Role of Thomas Corbyn." *Medical History* 33, no. 3 (1989): 277–95.

Potter, Van Rensellaer. *Bioethics: Bridge to the Future*. Englewood Cliffs, NJ: Prentice-Hall, 1971.

Povinelli, Elizabeth A. *Economies of Abandonment: Social Belonging and Endurance in Late Liberalism*. Durham, NC: Duke University Press, 2011.

Powers, Richard. *Gain*. New York: Farrar, Straus and Giroux, 1998.

Preciado, Paul B. *Testo Junkie: Sex, Drugs, and Biopolitics in the Pharmacopornographic Era*. Translated by Bruce Benderson. New York: Feminist Press, 2013.

Presidential Commission for the Study of Bioethical Issues. *Bioethics for Every Generation: Deliberation and Education in Health, Science, and Technology*. Washington, DC: Presidential Commission for the Study of Bioethical Issues, 2016.

President's Council on Bioethics. *Beyond Therapy: Biotechnology and the Pursuit of Happiness*. Washington, DC: President's Council on Bioethics, 2003.

Price, Janet, and Margrit Shildrick. "Bodies Together: Touch, Ethics and Disability." In *Disability/Postmodernity: Embodying Disability Theory*, edited by Mairian Corker and Tom Shakespeare, 62–75. London: Bloomsbury, 2002.

Price, W. Nicholson, II, and I. Glenn Cohen. "Privacy in the Age of Medical Big Data." *Nature Medicine* 25, no. 1 (2019): 37–43.

Price, W. Nicholson, II, Margot E. Kaminski, Timo Minssen, and Kayte Spector-Bagdady. "Shadow Health Records Meet New Data Privacy Laws." *Science* 363, no. 6426 (2019): 448–50.

Proctor, Robert. *Racial Hygiene: Medicine under the Nazis*. Cambridge, MA: Harvard University Press, 1988.

Propp, Vladimir. *Morphology of the Folk Tale*. Translated by Laurence Scott and Svatava Pirkova-Jakobson. Austin: University of Texas Press, (1928) 1968.

Puar, Jasbir K. "Prognosis Time: Towards a Geopolitics of Affect, Debility, and Capacity." *Women and Performance: A Journal of Feminist Theory* 19, no. 2 (2009): 161–72.

——. *The Right to Maim: Debility, Capacity, Disability*. Durham, NC: Duke University Press, 2017.

Puig de la Bellacasa, María. *Matters of Care: Speculative Ethics in More Than Human Worlds*. Minneapolis: University of Minnesota Press, 2017.

Purswani, Juhi M., Adam P. Dicker, Colin E. Champ, Matt Cantor, and Nitin Ohri. "Big Data from Small Devices: The Future of Smartphones in Oncology." *Seminars in Radiation Oncology* 29, no. 4 (2019): 338–47.

Putnam, Hilary. *Ethics without Ontology*. Cambridge, MA: Harvard University Press, 2004.

Quarantelli, E. L., ed. *What Is a Disaster? Perspectives on the Question*. London: Routledge, 1998.

Quigley, William P. "Five Hundred Years of English Poor Laws, 1349–1834: Regulating the Working and Non-working Poor." *Akron Law Review* 30, no. 1 (1996): 73–128.

Rabinbach, Anson. *The Human Motor: Energy, Fatigue, and the Origins of Modernity*. Berkeley: University of California Press, 1990.

Race, Kane. *Pleasure Consuming Medicine: The Queer Politics of Drugs*. Durham, NC: Duke University Press, 2009.

Radden, Jennifer. "Is This Dame Melancholy? Equating Today's Depression and Past Melancholia." *Philosophy, Psychiatry & Psychology* 10, no. 1 (2003): 37–52.

Radin, Joanna. "Collecting Human Subjects." *Curator: The Museum Journal* 57, no. 2 (2014): 249–58.

Rae, Philip A., Vivian Zhang, and Yelena S. Baras. "Ivermectin and River Blindness." *American Scientist* 98 (2010): 294–303.

Raffle Angela E., and J. A. Muir Gray. *Screening: Evidence and Practice*. Oxford: Oxford University Press, 2007.

Raley, Rita. "Dataveillance and Countervailance." In *"Raw Data" Is an Oxymoron*, edited by Lisa Gitelman, 121–46. Cambridge, MA: MIT Press, 2013.

Ralph, Laurence. *The Torture Letters: Reckoning with Police Violence*. Chicago: University of Chicago Press, 2020.

———. "What Wounds Enable: The Politics of Disability and Violence in Chicago." *Disability Studies Quarterly* 32, no. 3 (2012): 1–27.

Ramey, Sarah. *The Lady's Handbook for Her Mysterious Illness*. New York: Doubleday, 2020.

Ramos, Kimberly G., Ian Christopher N. Rocha, Trisha Denise Cedeño, Ana Carla dos Santos Costa, Shoaib Ahmad, Mohammad Yasir Essar, and Christos Tsagkaris. "Suez Canal Blockage and Its Global Impact on Healthcare amidst the COVID-19 Pandemic." *International Maritime Health* 72, no. 2 (2021): 145–46.

Ramos, Marco, Tess Lanzarotta, and Iris Chandler. "COVID-19 Is Changing What It Means to Be a Doctor." *Boston Review*, July 2020. https://bostonreview.net.

Rankin, William W., Sean Brennan, Ellen Schell, Jones Laviwa, and Sally H. Rankin. "The Stigma of Being HIV-Positive in Africa." *PLoS Medicine* 2, no. 8 (2005): e247.

Rapp, Rayna. "Moral Pioneers: Women, Men and Fetuses on a Frontier of Reproductive Technology." *Women & Health* 13, nos. 1–2 (1988): 101–17.

———. *Testing Women, Testing the Fetus: The Social Impact of Amniocentesis in America*. New York: Routledge, 1999.

Ray, Keisha Shantel. "It's Time for a Black Bioethics." *American Journal of Bioethics* 21, no. 2 (2021): 38–40.

Ray, Sarah Jaquette. *The Ecological Other: Environmental Exclusion in American Culture*. Tucson: University of Arizona Press, 2013.

Redman, Peter. "Invasion of the Monstrous Others: Heterosexual Masculinities, the 'AIDS Carrier' and the Horror Genre." In *Border Patrols: Policing the Boundaries of Heterosexuality*, edited by Deborah Lynn Steinberg, Debbie Epstein, and Richard Johnson, 98–116. London: Cassell, 1997.

Reich, Warren Thomas. "The Word 'Bioethics': The Struggle over Its Earliest Meanings." *Kennedy Institute of Ethics Journal* 5, no. 1 (March 1995): 19–34.

Reid, Fiona. *Broken Men: Shell Shock, Treatment and Recovery in Britain, 1914–1930*. London: Continuum, 2014.

Reiss, Benjamin. "African Americans Don't Sleep as Well as Whites, an Inequality Stretching Back to Slavery." *Los Angeles Times*, April 2017a. https://www.latimes.com.

———. *Wild Nights: How Taming Sleep Created Our Restless World*. New York: Basic Books, 2017b.

Reiss, Elizabeth. *Bodies in Doubt: An American History of Intersex*. Baltimore: Johns Hopkins University Press, 2009.

Reiss, Elizabeth, and Matthew W. McCarthy. "What Hospitalists Should Know about Intersex Adults." *Perspectives in Biology and Medicine* 59, no. 3 (2016): 391–98.

Remein, Christy DiFrances, Ellen Childs, John Carlo Pasco, Ludovic Trinquart, David B. Flynn, Sarah L. Wingerter, Robina M. Bhasin, Lindsay B. Demers, and Emelia J. Benjamin. "Content and Outcomes of Narrative Medicine Programmes: A Systematic Review of the Literature through 2019." *BMJ Open* 10, no. 1 (2020): e031568. https://doi.org/10.1136/bmjopen-2019-031568.

Reverby, Susan M. *Examining Tuskegee: The Infamous Syphilis Study and Its Legacy*. Chapel Hill: University of North Carolina Press, 2009.

———. *Ordered to Care: The Dilemma of American Nursing, 1850–1945*. Cambridge: Cambridge University Press, 1987.

Reynolds, Joel Michael. "Toward a Critical Theory of Harm: Ableism, Normativity, and Transability." *American Philosophical Association Newsletter on Philosophy and Medicine* 16, no. 1 (2016): 37–46.

Rich, Adrienne. "Compulsory Heterosexuality and Lesbian Existence." *Signs: Journal of Women in Culture and Society* 5, no. 4 (1980): 631–60.

Richards, Paul. *Ebola: How a People's Science Helped End an Epidemic*. London: Zed Books, 2016.

Richards, Robert J. *The Romantic Conception of Life: Science and Philosophy in the Age of Goethe*. Chicago: University of Chicago Press, 2002.

Richardson, Eugene. *Epidemic Illusions: On the Coloniality of Global Public Health*. Cambridge, MA: MIT Press, 2020.

Richmond, Chantelle, Vanessa Ambtman-Smith, Carrie Bourassa, Chenoa Cassidy-Mathews, Karine R. Duhamel, Miranda Keewatin, Malcolm King, Alexandra King, Christopher Mushquash, Nathan Oakes, Diane Redsky, Lisa Richardson, Robyn Rowe, Jamie Snook, and Jennifer Walker. *COVID-19 and Indigenous Health and Wellness: Our Strength Is in Our Stories*. Ottawa: Royal Society of Canada, 2020.

Ricoeur, Paul. *Time and Narrative*. 3 Vols. Translated by Kathleen McLaughlin and David Pellauer. Chicago: University of Chicago Press, 1984–88.

Rieff, David. *In Praise of Forgetting: Historical Memory and Its Ironies*. New Haven, CT: Yale University Press, 2016.

Riess, Helen, and Liz Neporent. *The Empathy Effect: Seven Neuroscience-Based Keys for Transforming the Way We Live, Love, Work, and Connect across Differences*. Louisville, CO: Sounds True, 2018.

Riha, Ortrun. "Subjektivität und Objektivität, Semiotik und Diagnostik: Eine Annäherung an den mittelalterlichen Krankheitsbegriff." *Sudhoffs Archiv* 80, no. 2 (1996): 129–49.

Riskin, Jessica. *The Restless Clock: A History of the Centuries-Long Argument over What Makes Living Things Tick*. Chicago: University of Chicago Press, 2016.

Risse, Guenter B. *Mending Bodies, Saving Souls: A History of Hospitals*. New York: Oxford University Press, 1999.

Rivera, Jason David, and DeMond Shondell Miller. "Continually Neglected: Situating Natural Disasters in the African American Experience." *Journal of Black Studies* 37, no. 1 (March 2007): 502–22.

Rizzolatti, Giacomo, and Leonardo Fogassi. "The Mirror Mechanism: Recent Findings and Perspectives." *Philosophical Transactions of the Royal Society of London Biological Sciences* 369, no. 1644 (June 2014): 1–12. https://doi.org/10.1098/rstb.2013.0420.

Robert, Voeks. "African Medicine and Magic in the Americas." *Geographical Review* 83, no. 1 (1993): 66–78.

Roberts, Dorothy E. "Abolish Race Correction." *Lancet* 397, no. 10268 (January 2021): 17–18.

———. *Fatal Invention: How Science, Politics, and Big Business Re-create Race in the Twenty-First Century*. New York: New Press, 2012.

———. *Killing the Black Body: Race, Reproduction, and the Meaning of Liberty*. New York: Vintage, 1999.

Rocher, Luc, Julien M. Hendrickx, and Yves-Alexandre de Montjoye. "Estimating the Success of Re-identifications in Incomplete Datasets Using Generative Models." *Nature Communications* 10, no. 3069 (2019): 1–9.

Roe, David, and Larry Davidson. "Self and Narrative in Schizophrenia: Time to Author a New Story." *Medical Humanities* 31 (2005): 89–94.

Rogaski, Ruth. *Hygienic Modernity: Meanings of Health and Disease in Treaty Port China*. Berkeley: University of California Press, 2004.

Ronell, Avital. *The Telephone Book: Technology, Schizophrenia, Electric Speech*. Lincoln: University of Nebraska Press, 1989.

Rose, Bird Deborah, Thom van Dooren, Matthew Chrulew, Stuart Cooke, Matthew Kearnes, and Emily O'Gorman. "Thinking through the Environment, Unsettling the Humanities." *Environmental Humanities* 1, no. 1 (2012): 1–5.

Rose, Geoffrey. "Sick Individuals and Sick Populations." *International Journal of Epidemiology* 30, no. 3 (June 1985): 32–38.

Rose, Nikolas. "Personalized Medicine: Promises, Problems and Perils of a New Paradigm for Healthcare." *Procedia—Social and Behavioral Sciences* 77 (2013a): 341–52.

———. "What Is Diagnosis For?" Lecture given at the Institute of Psychiatry Conference, June 4, 2013b. https://nikolasrose.com.

Rosen, David H., and Uyen Hoang. *Patient Centered Medicine: A Human Experience*. Oxford: Oxford University Press, 2017.

Rosen, George. *A History of Public Health*. Baltimore: Johns Hopkins University Press, 1958.

Rosen, Hannah. *Terror in the Heart of Freedom: Citizenship, Sexual Violence, and the Meaning of Race in the Postemancipation South*. Chapel Hill: University of North Carolina Press, 2009.

Rosenberg, Charles E. *The Care of Strangers: The Rise of America's Hospital System*. New York: Basic Books, 1987.

———. *The Cholera Years: The United States in 1832, 1849, and 1866*. Chicago: University of Chicago Press, 1962.

———. "Contested Boundaries: Psychiatry, Disease, and Diagnosis." *Perspectives in Biology and Medicine* 58, no. 1 (2015): 120–37.

———. "Disease in History: Frames and Framers." *Milbank Quarterly* 67, no. 1 (1989a): 1–15.

———. "Epilogue: Airs, Waters, Places. A Status Report." *Bulletin of the History of Medicine* 86, no. 4 (2012): 661–70.

———. *Explaining Epidemics and Other Studies in the History of Medicine*. Cambridge: Cambridge University Press, 1992.

———. "The Therapeutic Revolution: Medicine, Meaning, and Social Change in Nineteenth-Century America." In *The Therapeutic Revolution*, edited by Morris Vogel and Charles Rosenberg, 3–25. Philadelphia: University of Pennsylvania Press, 1979.

———. "The Tyranny of Diagnosis: Specific Entities and Individual Experience." *Milbank Quarterly* 80, no. 2 (2002): 237–60.

———. "What Is an Epidemic? AIDS in Historical Perspective 1989." *Daedalus* 11, no. 2 (Spring 1989b): 1–17.

———. "What Is Disease? In Memory of Owsei Temkin." *Bulletin of the History of Medicine* 77, no. 3 (2003): 491–505.

Rosenberg, Clifford. "The International Politics of Vaccine Testing in Interwar Algiers." *American Historical Review* 117, no. 3 (2012): 671–97.

Rosenberger, Bob. "When and How Did the Metaphor of the Computer 'Virus' Arise?" *Scientific American*, September 2, 1997. https://www.scientificamerican.com.

Ross, M. K., Wei Wei, and L. Ohno-Machado. "'Big Data' and the Electronic Health Record." *Yearbook of Medical Informatics* 9, no. 1 (2014): 97–104. https://doi.org/10.15265/IY-2014-0003.

Rotarangi, Stephanie, and Darryn Russell. "Social-Ecological Resilience Thinking: Can Indigenous Culture Guide Environmental Management?" *Journal of the Royal Society of New Zealand*: 39, no. 4 (2009): 209–13.

Rothberg, Michael. *Multidirectional Memory: Remembering the Holocaust in the Age of Decolonization*. Palo Alto, CA: Stanford University Press, 2009.

Rothkopf, David J. "When the Buzz Bites Back." *Washington Post*, May 11, 2003.

Rothman, David J. *Strangers at the Bedside: A History of How Law and Bioethics Transformed Medical Decision Making*. New York: Basic Books, 1991.

Rothman, Sheila M. *Living in the Shadow of Death: Tuberculosis and the Social Experience of Illness in American History*. Baltimore: Johns Hopkins University Press, 1994.

Rousseau, Jean-Jacques. *Émile*. London: Everyman, (1763) 1993.

Rubin, Gayle. "Thinking Sex: Notes for a Radical Theory of the Politics of Sexuality." In *Pleasure and Danger: Exploring Female Sexuality*, edited by Carole S. Vance, 267–319. Boston: Routledge & Kegan Paul, 1984.

Ruckenstein, Minna, and Natasha Dow Schüll. "The Datafication of Health." *Annual Review of Anthropology* 46, no. 1 (2017): 261–78. https://doi.org/10.1146/annurev-anthro-102116-041244.

Ruddick, Sara. *Maternal Thinking: Toward a Politics of Peace*. 1st digital print ed. Boston: Beacon, 2002.

Runsock, Andrea. *Vital Accounts: Quantifying Health and Population in Eighteenth-Century England and France*. Cambridge: Cambridge University Press, 2002.

Ruse, Michael. *Darwinism as Religion: What Literature Tells Us about Evolution*. New York: Oxford University Press, 2016.

Ryan, Frank. *Virolution*. Cork, Ireland: Collins, 2009.

Ryan, Marie Laure. "Aesthetics of Proliferation." In *World Building*, edited by Marta Boni, 31–46. Amsterdam: Amsterdam University Press, 2017.

Saks, Elyn R. *The Center Cannot Hold: My Journey through Madness*. New York: Hachette, 2007.

Samimian-Darash, Limor. "A Pre-event Configuration for Biological Threats: Preparedness and the Constitution of Biosecurity Events." *American Ethnologist* 36, no. 3 (2009): 478–91.

Samson, David R., and Charles L. Nunn. "Sleep Intensity and the Evolution of Human Cognition." *Evolutionary Anthropology* 24, no. 6 (2015): 225–37.

Sandel, Michael J. *The Case against Perfection*. Cambridge, MA: Belknap, 2009.

Sandler, Ronald. "Technology and Ethics." In *Ethics and Emerging Technologies*, edited by Ronald Sandler, 1–23. Basingstoke: Palgrave Macmillan, 2014.

Santana, Marie-Anne, and Barbara L. Dancy. "The Stigma of Being Named 'AIDS Carriers' on Haitian-American Women." *Health Care for Women International* 21, no. 3 (2000): 161–71.

Santos, Boaventura de Sousa. *The End of Cognitive Empire: The Coming of Age of Epistemologies of the South*. Durham, NC: Duke University Press, 2018.

Sartre, Jean-Paul. Preface to *The Wretched of the Earth*, by Frantz Fanon, xliii–lxii. New York: Grove, 1961.

Sass, Louis. *Madness and Modernism: Insanity in the Light of Modern Art, Literature and Thought*. Cambridge, MA: Harvard University Press, 1992.

Saunders, Barry. *CT Suite: The Work of Diagnosis in the Age of Noninvasive Body Cutting*. Raleigh, NC: Duke University Press, 2008.

Saunders, Harold. *A Public Peace Process: Sustained Dialogue to Transform Racial and Ethnic Conflicts*. New York: Springer International, 1999.

Saunders, John. "Validating the Facts of Experience in Medicine." In *Medical Humanities*, edited by Martyn Evans and Ilora G. Finlay, 223–36. London: BMJ, 2001.

Savarese, Ralph James. "Cognition." In *Keywords for Disability Studies*, edited by Rachel Adams, Benjamin Reiss, and David Serlin, 40–42. New York: New York University Press, 2015.

———. "Disability Studies and the Personal; or How You Can Learn to Stop Worrying and Love Neurodiversity." Neuroclastic. Accessed September 1, 2020. https://neuroclastic.com.

———. *Reasonable People: A Memoir of Autism and Adoption*. New York: Other Press, 2007.

Savarese, Ralph James, and Emily Thornton Savarese. "The Superior Part of Speaking." *Disability Studies Quarterly* 30, no. 1 (2010). https://dsq-sds.org.

Savulescu, Julian, and Guy Kahane. "The Moral Obligation to Create Children with the Best Chance at the Best Life." *Bioethics* 23, no. 5 (2009): 274–90.

Scarry, Elaine. *The Body in Pain: The Making and Unmaking of the World*. New York: Oxford University Press, 1985.

Schacter, Daniel L. *Searching for Memory: The Brain, the Mind, and the Past*. New York: Basic Books, 2008.

Schaff, Pamela B., Susan Isken, and Robert M. Tager. "From Contemporary Art to Core Clinical Skills: Observation, Interpretation, and Meaning-Making in a Complex Environment." *Academic Medicine* 86, no. 10 (2011): 1272–76.

Schell, Heather. "Outburst! A Chilling True Story about Emerging-Virus Narratives and Pandemic Social Change." *Configurations* 5, no. 1 (1997): 93–133.

Scheper-Hughes, Nancy. "Three Propositions for a Critically Applied Medical Anthropology." *Social Science & Medicine* 30, no. 2 (1990): 189–97.

Schiebinger, Londa L. "The Anatomy of Difference: Race and Sex in Eighteenth-Century Science." *Eighteenth-Century Studies* 23, no. 4 (Summer 1990): 387–405.

———. "Medical Experimentation and Race in the Eighteenth-Century Atlantic World." *Social History of Medicine* 26, no. 3 (2013): 364–82.

———. *Plants and Empire: Colonial Bioprospecting in the Atlantic World*. Cambridge, MA: Harvard University Press, 2004.

———. *Secret Cures of Slaves: People, Plants, and Medicine in the Eighteenth Century Atlantic World*. Palo Alto, CA: Stanford University Press, 2017.

Schivelbusch, Wolfgang. *The Railway Journey: The Industrialization and Perception of Time and Space*. Berkeley: University of California Press, 1986.

Schlich, Thomas. "Trauma Surgery and Traffic Policy in Germany in the 1930s: A Case Study in the Coevolution of Modern Surgery and Society." *Bulletin of the History of Medicine* 80, no. 1 (2006): 73–94.

Schlosberg, David. *Defining Environmental Justice: Theories, Movements, and Nature*. Oxford: Oxford University Press, 2007.

Schneider, Joseph, and Peter Conrad. *Deviance and Medicalization: From Badness to Sickness*. Philadelphia: Temple University Press, 1992.

Schnittker, Jason. *Unnerved: Anxiety, Social Change, and the Transformation of Modern Mental Health*. New York: Columbia University Press, 2021.

Schoepf, Grundfest Brooke. "AIDS, Sex and Condoms: African Healers and the Reinvention of Tradition in Zaire." *Medical Anthropology* 14, nos. 2–4 (1992): 225–42.

Schöne-Seifert, Bettina. "Harm." In *Encyclopedia of Bioethics*, edited by Bruce Jennings, 1381. Farmington Hills, MI: Macmillan, 2014.

Schuller, Kyla. *The Biopolitics of Feeling: Race, Sex, and Science in the Nineteenth Century*. Durham, NC: Duke University Press, 2018a.

—. "The Microbial Self: Sensation and Sympoiesis." *Resilience: A Journal of the Environmental Humanities* 5 (2018b): 51–67.

Schuller, Kyla, and Jules Gill-Peterson. "Introduction: Race, the State, and the Malleable Body." *Social Text* 38, no. 2 (June 2020): 1–17.

Scott, Daryl Michael. *Contempt and Pity: Social Policy and the Image of the Damaged Black Psyche, 1880–1996.* Chapel Hill: University of North Carolina Press, 1997.

Scott, David, and Sylvia Wynter. "The Re-enchantment of Humanism." *Small Axe: A Caribbean Journal of Criticism* 4, no. 2 (2000): 119–207.

Scott, Wilbur J. "PTSD in DSM-III: A Case in the Politics of Diagnosis and Disease." *Social Problems* 37, no. 3 (1990): 294–310.

Scull, Andrew. "Desperate Remedies: A Gothic Tale of Madness and Modern Medicine." *Psychological Medicine* 17, no. 3 (1987): 561–77. https://doi.org/10.1017/s0033291700025824.

Scully, Jackie Leach. *Disability Bioethics: Moral Bodies, Moral Difference.* Lanham, MD: Rowman & Littlefield, 2008.

Seaburn, David B., Diane Morse, Susan H. McDaniel, Howard Beckman, Jordan Silberman, and Ronald Epstein. "Physician Responses to Ambiguous Patient Symptoms." *Journal of General Internal Medicine* 20, no. 6 (2005): 525–30.

Seidel, Kathleen. *Neurodiversity Weblog* (blog). 2003. https://www.neurodiversity.com.

Selden, Steven. "Transforming Better Babies into Fitter Families: Archival Resources and the History of the American Eugenics Movement, 1908–1930." *Proceedings of the American Philosophical Society* 149, no. 2 (2005): 199–225.

Seltzer, Mark. "Wound Culture: Trauma in the Pathological Public Sphere." *October* 80 (1997): 3–26.

Selzer, Richard. *Letters to a Young Doctor.* New York: Simon & Schuster, 1982.

Sennett, Richard. *Flesh and Stone: The Body and the City in Western Civilization.* New York: W. W. Norton, 1994.

Serlin, David. *Replaceable You: Engineering the Body in Postwar America.* Chicago: University of Chicago Press, 2004.

Servitje, Lorenzo. *Medicine Is War: The Martial Metaphor in Victorian Literature and Culture.* Albany: SUNY Press, 2021.

Seth, Suman. *Difference and Disease: Medicine, Race, and the Eighteenth-Century British Empire.* Cambridge: Cambridge University Press, 2018.

Shah, Nayan H. *Contagious Divides: Epidemics and Race in San Francisco's Chinatown.* Berkeley: University of California Press, 2001.

Shah, Nigam H., and Jessica D. Tenenbaum. "The Coming Age of Data-Driven Medicine: Translational Bioinformatics' Next Frontier." *Journal of the American Medical Informatics Association* 19, no. e1 (2012): e2–e4. https://doi.org/10.1136/amiajnl-2012-000969.

Shakespeare, Tom. "Choices and Rights: Eugenics, Genetics and Disability Equality." *Disability & Society* 13, no. 5 (1998): 665–81.

—. "A Point of View: Happiness and Disability." BBC. June 1, 2014. https://www.bbc.com.

Shakespeare, Tom, Lisa Lezzoni, and Nora Groce. "Disability and the Training of Health Professionals." *Lancet* 374, no. 28 (2009): 1815–16.

Shapin, Steven, and Simon Schaffer. *The Leviathan and the Air-Pump: Hobbes, Boyle, and the Experimental Life.* Princeton, NJ: Princeton University Press, 1985.

Shapiro, Johanna, Jack Coulehan, Delese Wear, and Martha Montello. "Medical Humanities and Their Discontents: Definitions, Critiques, and Implications." *Academic Medicine* 84, no. 2 (February 2009): 192–98. https://escholarship.org.

Shapiro, Joseph P. *No Pity: People with Disabilities Forging a New Civil Rights Movement.* New York: Times Books, 1993.

Sharpe, Christina. *In the Wake: On Blackness and Being.* Durham, NC: Duke University Press, 2016.

Sharpe, Virginia Ashby, and Alan I. Faden. *Medical Harm: Historical, Conceptual and Ethical Dimensions of Iatrogenic Illness.* Cambridge: Cambridge University Press, 2001.

Shaw, Jennifer, and Darren Byler. "Cultural Anthropology." *Precarity*, September 13, 2016. https://culanth.org.

Shem, Samuel. *The House of God: A Novel.* New York: R. Marek, 1978.

Shephard, Ben. *A War of Nerves: Soldiers and Psychiatrists in the Twentieth Century.* Cambridge, MA: Harvard University Press, 2001.

Shklovsky, Viktor. "Art as Technique." In *Russian Formalist Criticism*, edited by Lee T. Lemon and Marion J. Reis, 18–28. Lincoln: University of Nebraska Press, (1917) 1965.

Showalter, Elaine. *The Female Malady: Women, Madness, and English Culture, 1830–1980.* New York: Pantheon, 1985.

Shuttleton, David E. *Smallpox and the Literary Imagination, 1660–1820*. Cambridge: Cambridge University Press, 2007.

Simmons, Dia T., Gavin C. Harewood, Todd H. Baron, Bret Thomas Petersen, Kenneth K. Wang, F. Boyd-Enders, and Beverly J. Ott. "Impact of Endoscopist Withdrawal Speed on Polyp Yield: Implications for Optimal Colonoscopy Withdrawal Time." *Alimentary Pharmacology & Therapeutics* 24, no. 6 (2006): 965–71.

Simpkin, Arabella L., and Ricahrd M. Schwartzstein. "Tolerating Uncertainty—the Next Medical Revolution?" *New England Journal of Medicine* 375, no. 8 (2016): 1713–15.

Sinclair, Jim. "Don't Mourn for Us: A Letter to Parents." 1993. https://www.autreat.com.

Singer, Merrill. "Interdisciplinarity and Collaboration in Responding to HIV and AIDS in Africa: Anthropological Perspectives." *African Journal of AIDS Research* 8, no. 4 (2009a): 379–87.

———. *Introduction to Syndemics: A Critical Systems Approach to Public and Community Health*. San Francisco: Jossey-Bass, 2009b.

Singer, T. Benjamin. "The Profusion of Things: The 'Transgender Matrix' and Demographic Imaginaries in US Public Health." *TSQ: Transgender Studies Quarterly* 2, no. 1 (2015): 58–76.

Sinha, Indra. *Animal's People*. New York: Simon & Schuster, 2007.

Sins Invalid. *Skin, Tooth, and Bone: The Basis of Movement Is Our People. A Disability Justice Primer*. 2nd ed. Berkeley, CA: Sins Invalid, 2019.

Sissom, Tom. "State Medical Board Investigates Use of Ivermectin to Fight Covid at Washington County Jail." *Arkansas Democrat Gazette*, August 27, 2021.

Slack, Paul. Introduction to *Epidemics and Ideas Essays on the Historical Perception of Pestilence*, edited by Terence Ranger and Paul Slack, 1–20. Cambridge: Cambridge University Press, 1992.

Smith, Barbara Herrnstein. "Narrative Versions, Narrative Theories." In *On Narrative*, edited by W. J. T. Mitchell, 209–32. Chicago: University of Chicago Press, 1981.

Smith, George Davey. "Epidemiology, Epigenetics and the 'Gloomy Prospect': Embracing Randomness in Population Health Research and Practice." *International Journal of Epidemiology* 40, no. 3 (2011): 537–62.

Smith, Linda Tuhiwai. *Decolonizing Methodologies: Research and Indigenous Peoples*. London: Zed Books, 2013.

Smith, Richard. "In Search of Non-diseases." *BMJ* 324, no. 7342 (2002): 883–85. https://doi.org/10.1136/bmj.324.7342.883.

Snorton, Riley C. *Black on Both Sides*. Minneapolis: University of Minnesota Press, 2017.

Snow, C. P. "The Two Cultures and the Scientific Revolution." Rede Lecture. Cambridge: Cambridge University Press, 1959.

Snowden, Frank. *Epidemics and Society: From the Black Death to the Present*. New Haven, CT: Yale University Press, 2020.

Snowden, Lonnie, and Genevieve Graaf. "The 'Undeserving Poor,' Racial Bias, and Medicaid Coverage of African Americans." *Journal of Black Psychology* 45, no. 3 (2019): 130–42.

"Social Science and Humanities Competencies." Northeastern Humanities Center, 2018. https://cssh.northeastern.edu.

Sokol, Joshua. "Meet the Xenobots, Virtual Creatures Brought to Life." *New York Times*, April 2020. https://www.nytimes.com.

Solomon, Harris. *Lifelines: The Traffic of Trauma*. Durham, NC: Duke University Press, 2022.

Sommerville, Siobhan B. *Queering the Color Line: Race and the Invention of Homosexuality in American Culture*. Durham, NC: Duke University Press, 2000.

Sontag, Susan. *AIDS and Its Metaphors*. New York: Farrar, Straus and Giroux, 1989.

———. *Illness as Metaphor*. New York: Farrar, Straus and Giroux, 1978.

Spade, Dean. *Normal Life: Administrative Violence, Critical Trans Politics, and the Limits of Law*. Brooklyn: South End Press, 2011.

Spiro, Howard. "The Medical Humanities and Medical Education." *JAMA* 295, no. 9 (2006): 997–98.

Spitzer, Robert L. "The Diagnostic Status of Homosexuality in DSM-III: A Reformulation of the Issues." *American Journal of Psychiatry* 138, no. 2 (1981): 210–17.

Spongberg, Mary. *Feminizing Venereal Disease: The Body of the Prostitute in Nineteenth-Century Medical Discourse*. New York: New York University Press, 1998.

Spurlin, William. "Queer Theory and Biomedical Practice: The Biomedicalization of Sexuality / The Cultural Politics of Biomedicine." *Journal of Medical Humanities* 40, no. 1 (August 3, 2018): 7–20.

Squier, Susan M. "Comics and Graphic Medicine as a Third Space for the Health Humanities." In *The Routledge Companion to Health Humanities*, edited by Paul Crawford, Brian Brown, and Andrea Charise, 60–65. London: Routledge, 2020.

———. "Comics in the Health Humanities: A New Approach to Sex and Gender Education." In *Health Humanities Reader*, edited by Therese Jones, Delese Wear, and Lester D. Friedman, 226–41. New Brunswick, NJ: Rutgers University Press, 2014.

Starr, Paul. *The Social Transformation of American Medicine.* New York: Basic Books, 1982.

Stearns, Justin K. *Infectious Ideas: Contagion in Premodern Islamic and Christian Thought in the Western Mediterranean.* Baltimore: Johns Hopkins University Press, 2011.

Stegenga, Jacob. "Measuring Harm." In *The Routledge Companion to Philosophy of Medicine*, edited by Miriam Solomon, Jeremy R. Simon, and Harold Kincaid, 342–52. New York: Routledge, 2017.

Stein, Jess. *The Random House College Dictionary.* New York: Random House, 1984.

Steinbock, Bonnie. "The Logical Case for 'Wrongful Life.'" *Hastings Center Report* 16, no. 2 (1986): 15–20.

Steinbock, Bonnie, and Ron McClamrock. "When Is Birth Unfair to the Child?" *Hastings Center Report* 24, no. 6 (1994): 15–21.

Steinbeck, John. *The Grapes of Wrath.* New York: Viking, 1939.

Steinecke, Anne, and Charles Terrell. "Progress for Whose Future? The Impact of the Flexner Report on Medical Education for Racial and Ethnic Minority Physicians in the United States." *Academic Medicine* 85, no. 2 (February 2010): 236–45.

Steingraber, Sandra. *Living Downstream: An Ecologist's Personal Investigation of Cancer and the Environment.* Cambridge, MA: Da Capo, 2010.

Stepan, Nancy Leys. *The Hour of Eugenics.* Ithaca, NY: Cornell University Press, 1996.

Stern, Alexandra Minna. "Cautions about Medicalized Dehumanization." *AMA Journal of Ethics* 23, no. 1 (2021): 64–69.

———. *Eugenic Nation.* Berkeley: University of California Press, 2015.

———. "STERILIZED in the Name of Public Health." *American Journal of Public Health* 95, no. 7 (2005): 1128–38. https://doi.org/10.2105/AJPH.2004.041608.

Stevens, Tina M. L. *Bioethics in America: Origins and Cultural Politics.* Baltimore: Johns Hopkins University Press, 2000.

Stevenson, Angus, and Christine Lindberg, eds. *New Oxford American Dictionary.* 3rd ed., s.v. "creativity." New York: Oxford University Press, 2010.

Stewart, Kearsley A., and Kelley K. Swain. "Global Health Humanities: Defining an Emerging Field." *Lancet* 388, no. 10060 (2016): 2586–87.

Stoddard Holmes, Martha, and Tod Chambers. "Thinking through Pain." *Literature and Medicine* 24, no. 1 (2005): 127–41.

Stoler, Ann Laura. *Along the Archival Grain: Epistemic Anxieties and Colonial Common Sense.* Princeton, NJ: Princeton University Press, 2009.

———. *Duress: Imperial Durabilities in Our Times.* Durham, NC: Duke University Press, 2016.

———. *Race and the Education of Desire: Foucault's* History of Sexuality *and the Colonial Order of Things.* Durham, NC: Duke University Press, 2000.

Strick, Simon. *American Dolorologies: Pain, Sentimentalism, Biopolitics.* Albany: SUNY Press, 2014.

Stuurman, Siep. "François Bernier and the Invention of Racial Classification." *History Workshop Journal* 50 (Autumn 2000): 1–21.

Sudan, Rajani. *The Alchemy of Empire: Abject Materials and the Technologies of Colonialism.* New York: Fordham University Press, 2016.

Sullivan, Garrett A. Jr. *Sleep, Romance and Human Embodiment: Vitality from Spenser to Milton.* Cambridge: Cambridge University Press, 2012.

Sundaram, Ravi. *Pirate Modernity: Delhi's Media Urbanism.* London: Routledge, 2009.

Sutherby, Kaitlin. *Oxfam Report on Global Poverty.* Nairobi: Oxfam, 2014. https://borgenproject.org.

Sze, Julie. *Environmental Justice in a Moment of Danger.* Berkeley: University of California Press, 2020.

———. *Noxious New York: The Racial Politics of Urban Health and Environmental Justice.* Cambridge, MA: MIT Press, 2007.

Tabb, Kathryn. "Should Psychiatry Be Precise? Reduction, Big Data, and Nosological Revision in Mental Health Research." In *Levels of Analysis in Psychopathology*, edited by Kenneth S. Kendler, Josef Parnas, and Peter Zachar, 308–34. Cambridge: Cambridge University Press, 2020.

Tabb, Kathryn, and Maël Lemoine. "The Prospects of Precision Psychiatry." *Theoretical Medicine and Bioethics* 42, no. 5/6 (December 2021): 193–210.

Tajima-Peña, Renee, dir. *No Más Bebés*. PBS, 2015. 1 hr., 19 min. https://www.pbs.org.

TallBear, Kim. "Genomic Articulations of Indigeneity." *Social Studies of Science* 43, no. 4 (2013): 509–33.

Tanner, Adam. *Our Bodies, Our Data: How Companies Make Billions Selling Our Medical Records*. Boston: Beacon, 2017.

Tarizzo, Davide. *Life: A Modern Invention*. Translated by Mark William Epstein. Minneapolis: University of Minnesota Press, 2017.

Tasca, Cecilia, Mariangela Rapetti, Mauro Giovanni Carta, and Bianca Fadda. "Women and Hysteria in the History of Mental Health." *Clinical Practice & Epidemiology in Mental Health* 8 (2012): 110–19. https://doi.org/10.2174/1745017901208010110.

Taylor, Ashley, and Lauren Shallish. "The Logic of Bio-Meritocracy in the Promotion of Higher Education Equity." *Disability & Society* 34, nos. 7–8 (2019): 1200–1223.

Taylor, Dorceta E. "American Environmentalism: The Role of Race, Class and Gender in Shaping Activism, 1820–1995." In *Environmental Sociology: From Analysis to Action*, edited by Leslie King and Deborah McCarthy, 87–106. Lanham, MD: Rowman & Littlefield, 2005.

Taylor, Robert B. "Please Don't Call Me 'Provider.'" *American Family Physician* 63, no. 12 (2001): 2340–43.

Teachman, Bethany A., Dean McKay, Deanna M. Barch, Mitchell J. Prinstein, Steven D. Hollon, and Dianne L. Chambless. "How Psychosocial Research Can Help the National Institute of Mental Health Achieve Its Grand Challenge to Reduce the Burden of Mental Illnesses and Psychological Disorders." *American Psychologist* 74, no. 4 (2018): 415–31.

Temkin, Owsei. *The Double Face of Janus and Other Essays in the History of Medicine*. Baltimore: Johns Hopkins University Press, 1977.

Terry, Jennifer. *Attachments to War: Biomedical Logics and Violence in Twenty-First-Century America*. Durham, NC: Duke University Press, 2017.

Thacker, Eugene. *After Life*. Chicago: University of Chicago Press, 2010.

Thibault, George E. "Humanism in Medicine: What Does It Mean and Why Is It More Important Than Ever?" *Academic Medicine* 94, no. 8 (2019): 1074–77.

Thomison, J. B. "Primum non nocere." *Southern Medical Journal* 80, no. 2 (February 1987): 149–50.

Thompson, Evan. "Introduction to the Revised Edition." In *The Embodied Mind*, edited by Francisco J. Varela, Evan Thompson, and Eleanor Roch, xvii–xxxiv. Cambridge, MA: MIT Press, 2016.

Thompson, Helen. *Fictional Matter: Empiricism, Corpuscles, and the Novel*. Philadelphia: University of Pennsylvania Press, 2016.

Thompson, Kurt. "What Is Poverty?" ReviseSociology. July 2011. https://revisesociology.com.

Thornber, Karen Laura. *Global Healing. Literature, Advocacy, Care*. Leiden: Brill/Rodopi, 2020.

"Through the Magic Glass." *Harper's Bazaar* 13, no. 16 (April 1880): 245.

Tierney, Kathleen J., and Barbara Baisden. *Crisis Intervention Programs for Disaster Victims: A Source Book and Manual for Smaller Communities*, 1977. *Disaster Research Center*. https://udspace.udel.edu.

Tilley, Helen. *Africa as a Living Laboratory: Empire, Development, and the Problem of Scientific Knowledge, 1870–1950*. Chicago: University of Chicago Press, 2011.

Timmermann, Carsten. "Not Moribund at All! An Historian of Medicine's Response to Richard Horton." Somatosphere. August 2014. http://somatosphere.net.

Titchener, Edward Bradford. *Lectures on the Experimental Psychology of the Thought-Process*. New York: Macmillan, 1909.

Todd, Zoe. "An Indigenous Feminist's Take on the Ontological Turn: 'Ontology' Is Just Another Word for Colonialism." *Journal of Historical Sociology* 29, no. 1 (2016): 4–22.

Todorov, Tzvetan. *The Poetics of Prose*. Translated by Richard Howard. Ithaca, NY: Cornell University Press, 1977.

Tognotti, Eugenia. "Lessons from the History of Quarantine, from Plague to Influenza A." *Emerging Infectious Diseases* 19, no. 2 (2013): 254.

Tomes, Nancy. *The Gospel of Germs: Men, Women, and the Microbe in American Life.* Cambridge, MA: Harvard University Press, 1998.

———. *Remaking the American Patient: How Madison Avenue and Modern Medicine Turned Patients into Consumers.* Chapel Hill: University of North Carolina Press, 2016.

Tone, Andrea. *The Age of Anxiety: A History of America's Turbulent Affair with Tranquilizers.* New York: Basic Books, 2009.

Topol, Eric. "Why Doctors Should Organize." *New Yorker*, August 5, 2019. https://www.newyorker.com.

Treichler, Paula A. "AIDS, Gender, and Biomedical Discourse: Current Contests for Meaning." In *AIDS: The Burdens of History*, edited by Elizabeth Fee and Daniel M. Fox, 190–234. Berkeley: University of California Press, 1988.

Treitel, Corinna. *Eating Nature in Modern Germany: Food, Agriculture, and Environment, 1870–2000.* Cambridge: Cambridge University Press, 2017.

Trent, James W. *Inventing the Feeble Mind: A History of Intellectual Disability in the United States.* New York: Oxford University Press, 2017.

Tronto, Joan C. *Moral Boundaries: A Political Argument for an Ethic of Care.* New York: Routledge, 2015.

Trostle, James A. *Epidemiology and Culture.* Cambridge: Cambridge University Press, 2005.

Trungpa, Chogyam. *True Perception: The Path of Dharma Art.* Boulder, CO: Shambhala, 2008.

Trzeciak, Stephen and Anthony Mazzarelli. *Compassionomics: The Revolutionary Scientific Evidence That Caring Makes a Difference.* Pensacola, FL: Studer Group, 2019.

Tsevat, Rebecca K., Anoushka A. Sinha, Kevin J. Gutierrez, and Sayantani DasGupta. "Bringing Home the Health Humanities: Narrative Humility, Structural Competency, and Engaged Pedagogy." *Academic Medicine* 90, no. 11 (2015): 1462–65.

Tulving, Endel. "Are There 256 Different Kinds of Memory?" In *The Foundations of Remembering: Essays in Honor of Henry L. Roediger, III*, edited by J. S. Nairn, 39–52. New York: Psychology Press, 2007.

Tutton, Richard. *Genomics and the Reimagining of Personalized Medicine.* Farnham, UK: Ashgate, 2014.

Tyler, Imogen. *Stigma: The Machinery of Inequality.* London: Zed Books, 2020.

Ulrich, Laurel. *A Midwife's Tale: The Life of Martha Ballard, Based on Her Diary, 1785–1812.* New York: Vintage, 1990.

UN General Assembly. *International Covenant on Economic, Social and Cultural Rights.* United Nations, 1966.

———. "United Nations Declaration on the Rights of Indigenous Peoples." *UN Wash* 12 (2007): 1–18.

———. "United Nations Plan of Action on Disaster Risk Reduction for Resilience." United Nations, 2017.

———. *Universal Declaration of Human Rights.* United Nations, 1948.

US Centers for Medicare and Medicaid Services. "How Can I Pay for Nursing Home Care?" Medicare.gov. 2020. https://www.medicare.gov.

US National Library of Medicine. "Big Data MeSH Descriptor Data." MeSH Browser. January 2019. https://meshb.nlm.nih.gov.

van der Geest, Sjaak, Susan Reynolds White, and Anita Hardon. "The Anthropology of Pharmaceuticals: A Biographical Approach." *Annual Review of Anthropology* 25, no. 1 (1996): 153–78.

van der Schaaf, Marieke, Arthur Bakker, and Olle ten Cate. "When I Say . . . Embodied Cognition." *Medical Education* 53, no. 3 (2019): 219–20.

van de Wiel, Lucy. "The Time of the Change: Menopause's Medicalization and the Gender Politics of Aging." *International Journal of Feminist Approaches to Bioethics* 7, no. 1 (2014): 74–98.

van Dijck, Jose. "Datafication, Dataism and Dataveillance: Big Data between Scientific Paradigm and Ideology." *Surveillance & Society* 12, no. 2 (2014): 197–208. https://doi.org/10.24908/ss.v12i2.4776.

van Middendorp, Joost J., Gonazalo M. Sanchez, and Alywn L. Burridge. "The Edwin Papyrus: A Clinical Reappraisal of the Oldest Known Document on Spinal Injuries." *European Spine Journal* 19, no. 11 (2010): 1815–23.

Van Schaik, Katharine. "'Taking' a History." *JAMA* 304, no. 11 (September 2010): 1159–60.

Varela, Francisco. "The Emergent Self." In *The Third Culture*, edited by John Brockman, 209–22. New York: Touchstone, 1995.

Varela, Francisco J., Evan Thompson, and Eleanor Rosch. *The Embodied Mind: Cognitive Science and Human Experience*. Rev. ed. Cambridge, MA: MIT Press, 2017.

Varlik, Nükhet. *Plague and Empire in the Early Modern Mediterranean World: The Ottoman Experience, 1347–1600*. Cambridge: Cambridge University Press, 2015.

Vaughan, Megan. *Curing Their Ills: Colonial Power and African Illness*. Cambridge: Polity, 1991.

Veysey, Laurence R. *The Emergence of the American University*. Chicago: University of Chicago Press, 1965.

Vitale, Francesco. *Biodeconstruction: Jacques Derrida and the Life Sciences*. Translated by. Mauro Senatore. Albany: SUNY Press, 2018.

Vora, Kalindi. *Life Support: Biocapital and the New History of Outsourced Labor*. Minneapolis: University of Minnesota Press, 2015.

Vyas, Darshali A., Leo G. Eisenstein, and David S. Jones. "Hidden in Plain Sight—Reconsidering the Use of Race Correction in Clinical Algorithms." *New England Journal of Medicine* 389, no. 9 (2020): 874–82.

Wachtler, Caroline, Susanne Lundin, and Margareta Troein. "Humanities for Medical Students? A Qualitative Study of a Medical Humanities Curriculum in a Medical School Program." *BMC Medical Education* 6, no. 16 (2006). https://doi.org/10.1186/1472-6920-6-16.

Wacquant, Loic. *Punishing the Poor: The Neoliberal Government of Social Insecurity*. Durham, NC: Duke University Press, 2009.

Waddington, Ivan. "The Movement toward the Professionalization of Medicine." *British Medical Journal* 301, no. 6754 (October 1990): 688–90. https://www.ncbi.nlm.nih.gov.

Waddington, Keir, and Martin Willis. "Pharmacology, Controversy, and the Everyday in Fin-de-Siècle Medicine and Fiction." In *Literature and Medicine*, vol. 2, *The Nineteenth Century*, edited by Andrew Mangham and Clark Lawlor, 135–53. Cambridge: Cambridge University Press, 2021.

Wahlert, Lance, and Autumn Fiester. "Queer Bioethics: Why Its Time Has Come." *Bioethics* 26, no. 1 (2012): ii–iv.

Wailoo, Keith. *Dying in the City of the Blues: Sickle Cell Anemia and the Politics of Race and Health*. Chapel Hill: University of North Carolina Press, 2001.

———. *Pain: A Political History*. Baltimore: Johns Hopkins University Press, 2014.

Wajcman, Judy. *Feminism Confronts Technology*. University Park: Penn State University Press, 1991.

Wald, Priscilla. "Blood and Stories: How Genomics Is Rewriting Race, Medicine and Human History." *Patterns of Prejudice* 40 (2006): 303–33.

———. *Contagious: Cultures, Carriers, and the Outbreak Narrative*. Durham, NC: Duke University Press, 2008.

———. "Cultures and Carriers: 'Typhoid Mary' and the Science of Social Control." *Social Text* 52/53 (1997): 181–214.

———. "Pandemics and the Politics of Planetary Health." In *The Edinburgh Companion to the Politics of American Health*, edited by Martin Halliwell and Sophie A. Jones, 601–17. Edinburgh: Edinburgh University Press, 2022.

Walker, Nick. "Neurodiversity: Some Basic Terms and Definitions." Neuroqueer. 2014. https://neuroqueer.com.

Wallis, Faith. "Signs and Senses: Diagnosis and Prognosis in Early Medieval Pulse and Urine Texts." *Social History of Medicine* 13, no. 2 (2000): 265–78. https://doi.org/10.1093/shm/13.2.265.

Warner, John Harley. *Against the Spirit of System: The French Impulse in Nineteenth-Century American Medicine*. Baltimore: Johns Hopkins University Press, 2003.

———. "The History of Science and the Sciences of Medicine." *Osiris* 10 (1995): 164–93.

———. "The Humanising Power of Medical History: Responses to Biomedicine in the 20th Century United States." *Medical Humanities* 37 (2011): 91–96.

Warner, Michael. *The Trouble with Normal: Sex, Politics, and the Ethics of Queer Life*. Cambridge, MA: Harvard University Press, 1999.

Washington, Harriet A. *Medical Apartheid: The Dark History of Medical Experimentation of Black Americans from Colonial Times to the Present*. New York: Anchor, 2006.

———. *A Terrible Thing to Waste: Environmental Racism and Its Assault on the American Mind*. New York: Little, Brown Spark, 2019.

Watego, Chelsea, Lisa J. Whop, David Singh, Bryan Mukandi, Alissa Macoun, George Newhouse, Ali Drummond, Amy

McQuire, Janet Stajic, Helena Kajlich, and Mark Brough. "Black to the Future: Making the Case for Indigenist Health Humanities." *International Journal of Environmental Research and Public Health* 18, no. 8704 (2021): 1–10.

Watkins, Katie. "Life Expectancy in Houston Can Vary up to 20 Years Depending on Where You Live." Houston Public Media. 2019. https://www.houstonpublicmedia.org.

Weaver, Richard M. *The Ethics of Rhetoric*. Battleboro, VT: Echo Point Books & Media, 1953.

Weed, Kym. "Microbial Perspectives: Mark Twain's Imaginative Experiment in Ethics." *Literature and Medicine* 37, no. 1 (2019): 219–40.

Weheliye, Alexander G. *Habeas Viscus: Racializing Assemblages, Biopolitics, and Black Feminist Theories of the Human*. Durham, NC: Duke University Press, 2014.

Weiner, Dora, and Michael Sauter. "The City of Paris and the Rise of Clinical Medicine." *Osiris* 18 (2003): 23–42.

Weir, Robert F. "The Morality of Physician-Assisted Suicide." *Law, Medicine and Health Care* 20, nos. 1–2 (1992): 116–26.

Weizman, Eyal. *Forensic Architecture: Violence at the Threshold of Detectability*. Cambridge, MA: MIT Press, 2017.

Wellmon, Chad. *Organizing Enlightenment: Information Overload and the Invention of the Modern Research University*. Baltimore: Johns Hopkins University Press, 2015.

Wertz, Richard W., and Dorothy C. Wertz. "Notes on the Decline of Midwives and the Rise of Medical Obstetricians." In *The Sociology of Health and Illness: Critical Perspectives*, edited by Peter Conrad and Rochelle Kern, 165–83. New York: St. Martin's Press, 1981.

West, C. P., L. N. Dyrbye, and T. D. Shanafelt. "Physician Burnout: Contributors, Consequences and Solutions." *Journal of Internal Medicine* 283, no. 6 (2018): 516–29.

Wexler, Laura. *Tender Violence: Domestic Visions in the Age of U.S. Imperialism*. Chapel Hill: University of North Carolina Press, 2000.

Wheeler, Roxann. *The Complexion of Race: Categories of Difference in Eighteenth-Century British Culture*. Philadelphia: University of Pennsylvania Press, 2001.

Whitehead, Anne. *Medicine and Empathy in Contemporary British Fiction: A Critical Intervention in Medical Humanities*. Edinburgh: Edinburgh University Press, 2017.

Whitehead, Anne, and Angela Woods. Introduction to *The Edinburgh Companion to the Critical Medical Humanities*, edited by Anne Whitehead, Angela Woods, Sarah Atkinson, Jane Macnaughton, and Jennifer Richards, 1–26. Edinburgh: Edinburgh University Press, 2018.

Whittaker, Maxine. "How Infectious Diseases Have Shaped Our Culture, Habits and Language." Conversation. July 12, 2017. https://theconversation.com.

Whorton, James. *Nature Cures: The History of Alternative Medicine in America*. Oxford: Oxford University Press, 2002.

Wiegman, Robyn. *Object Lessons*. Durham, NC: Duke University Press, 2012.

Williams, Donna. *Nobody Nowhere*. New York: Crown, 1992.

———. *Somebody Somewhere*. New York: Crown, 1994.

Williams, Jeffrey. "The New Humanities: Once-Robust Fields Are Being Broken Up and Stripped for Parts." *Chronicle Review*, November 14, 2019. https://www-chronicle-com.ezproxy.neu.edu.

Williams, Raymond. *Keywords: A Vocabulary of Culture and Society*. New York: Oxford University Press, 1976.

———. *Marxism and Literature*. Oxford: Oxford University Press, 1977.

Williams, William Carlos. *The Doctor Stories*. New York: New Directions, 1984.

Willig, Carla. "Cancer Diagnosis as Discursive Capture: Phenomenological Repercussions of Being Positioned within Dominant Constructions of Cancer." *Social Science & Medicine* 73, no. 6 (2011): 897–903.

Willsher, Kim. "Vaccine Scepticism in France Reflects Dissatisfaction with Political Class." *Guardian*, January 11, 2021. https://www.theguardian.com.

Wilson, Elizabeth A. *Psychosomatic: Feminism and the Neurological Body*. Durham, NC: Duke University Press, 2004.

———. "The Work of Antidepressants: Preliminary Notes on How to Build an Alliance between Feminism and Psychopharmacology." *BioSocieties* 1, no. 1 (2006): 125–31.

Wilson, Harold. *The War on World Poverty*. London: Gollancz, 1953.

Wilson, Shawn. *Research Is Ceremony: Indigenous Research Methods*. Halifax, NS: Fernwood, 2008.

Winner, Langdon. "Technologies as Forms of Life." In *Epistemology, Methodology, and the Social Sciences*, edited by Robert S. Cohen and Marx X. Wartofsky, 249–63. Boston: Kluwer Academic, 1983.

Winter, Alison. *Memory: Fragments of a Modern History*. Chicago: University of Chicago Press, 2012.

Winter, Jay. *Sites of Memory, Sites of Mourning: The Great War in European Cultural History*. Cambridge: Cambridge University Press, 1995.

Wolf-Meyer, Matthew. *The Slumbering Masses: Sleep, Medicine, and Modern American Life*. Minneapolis: University of Minnesota Press, 2012.

Woods, Angela. "Rethinking Patient Testimony in the Medical Humanities: Schizophrenia Bulletin's First Person Accounts." *Journal of Literature and Science* 6, no. 1 (2013): 38–54.

———. *The Sublime Object of Psychiatry: Schizophrenia in Clinical and Cultural Theory*. Oxford: Oxford University Press, 2011.

Woods, Angela, Ben Alderson-Day, and Charles Fernyhough, eds. *Voices in Psychosis: Interdisciplinary Perspectives*. Oxford: Oxford University Press, 2022.

Woodward, Kathleen. *Statistical Panic: Cultural Politics and Poetics of the Emotions*. Durham, NC: Duke University Press, 2009.

Wool, Zoë. *After War: The Weight of Life at Walter Reed*. Durham, NC: Duke University Press, 2015.

Worboys, Michael. *Spreading Germs: Disease Theory and Medical Practice in Britain, 1865–1900*. Cambridge: Cambridge University Press, 2000.

World Health Organization. *Global Health Observatory (GHO) Data: Life Expectancy*. Geneva: World Health Organization, 2020a. https://www.who.int.

———. *Health Systems That Meet the Needs of Older People*. Geneva: World Health Organization, 2020b. https://www.who.int.

———. *The ICD-10 Classification of Mental and Behavioural Disorders: Clinical Descriptions and Diagnostic Guidelines*. Geneva: World Health Organization, 1992.

———. "A World at Risk: Annual Report on Global Preparedness for Health Emergencies." Global Preparedness Monitoring Board. September 2019. https://www.gpmb.org.

World Medical Association. "Human Experimentation: Code of Ethics of the World Medical Association—Declaration of Helsinki." *British Medical Journal* 2, no. 5402 (1964): 177.

Wynter, Sylvia. "The Ceremony Found: Towards the Autopoetic Turn/Overturn, Its Autonomy of Human Agency and Extra-Territoriality of Self-Cognition." In *Black Knowledges, Black Struggles: Essays in Critical Epistemology*, edited by Jason R. Ambroise, 184–252. Liverpool: Liverpool University Press, 2015.

———. "Unsettling the Coloniality of Being/Power/Truth/Freedom: Towards the Human, after Man, Its Overrepresentation—an Argument." *New Centennial Review* 3, no. 3 (2003): 257–337.

Yach, Derek, and Douglas Bettcher. "The Globalization of Public Health, I: Threats and Opportunities." *American Journal of Public Health* 88, no. 5 (1998): 735–44.

Yancy, Clyde W. "COVID-19 and African Americans." *JAMA* 323, no. 19 (2020): 1891–92.

Yetish, Gandhi, Hillard Kaplan, Michael Gurven, Brian Wood, Herman Pontzer, Paul R. Manger, Charles Wilson, Ronald McGregor, and Jerome M. Siegel. "Natural Sleep and Its Seasonal Variations in Three Pre-industrial Societies." *Current Biology* 25 (2015): 2862–68. https://doi.org/10.1016/j.cub.2015.09.046.

Young, Allan. *The Harmony of Illusions: Inventing Post-traumatic Stress Disorder*. Princeton, NJ: Princeton University Press, 1995.

Young, Dean. *The Art of Recklessness: Poetry as Assertive Force and Contradiction*. Minneapolis: Graywolf, 2010.

Young, James. *The Texture of Memory: Holocaust Memorials and Meanings*. New Haven, CT: Yale University Press, 1993.

Yoshino, Kenji. *Covering: The Hidden Assault on Our Civil Rights*. New York: Random House, 2006.

zedkat. "The Vertigo of Explaining the Inexplicable." 2021. https://zedkat.wordpress.com.

Zhan, Mei. "Civet Cats, Fried Grasshoppers, and David Beckham's Pajamas: Unruly Bodies after SARS." *American Anthropologist* 107, no. 1 (March 2005): 31–42.

Zinsser, Hans. *Rats, Lice and History*. Boston: Little, Brown, 1935.

Zolnoori, Maryam, Joyce E. Balls-Berry, Tabetha A. Brockman, Christi A. Patten, Ming Huang, and Lixia Yao. "A Systematic Framework for Analyzing Patient-Generated Narrative Data: Protocol for a Content Analysis." *JMIR Research Protocols* 8, no. 8 (2019): 3914. https://doi.org/10.2196/13914.

Zook, Matthew, Solon Barocas, danah boyd, Kate Crawford, Emily Keller, Seeta Peña Gangadharan, Alyssa Goodman et al. "Ten Simple Rules for Responsible Big Data Research." *PLoS Computational Biology* 13, no. 3 (2017): e1005399. https://doi.org/10.1371/journal.pcbi.1005399.

Zunshine, Lisa, ed. "Who Is He to Speak of My Sorrow?" In "Special Issue on Cognitive Approaches to Comparative Literature," edited by Lisa Zunshine. Special issue, *Poetics Today* 41, no. 2 (June 2020): 223–41.

About the Editors

Sari Altschuler is Associate Professor of English and the founding director of Health, Humanities, and Society at Northeastern University. She is the author of *The Medical Imagination: Literature and Health in the Early United States* (University of Pennsylvania Press, 2018) and currently at work on a monograph about disability and citizenship in the early United States.

Dr. Jonathan M. Metzl is the Frederick B. Rentschler II Professor of Sociology and Psychiatry and the Director of the Department of Medicine, Health, and Society at Vanderbilt University. He is the winner of the 2020 Robert F. Kennedy Human Rights Book Award, and notable books include *The Protest Psychosis*, *Prozac on the Couch*, *Against Health: How Health Became the New Morality* (Beacon Press, 2011), and *Dying of Whiteness: How the Politics of Racial Resentment Is Killing America's Heartland* (Basic Books, 2019).

Priscilla Wald is the R. Florence Brinkley Professor of English at Duke University and author of *Constituting Americans: Cultural Anxiety and Narrative Form* (Duke University Press, 1995) and *Contagious: Cultures, Carriers, and the Outbreak Narrative* (Duke University Press, 2008). She is currently at work on a monograph entitled *Human Being after Genocide*.

About the Contributors

Rachel Adams is a professor of English at Columbia University. Her most recent book is *Raising Henry: A Memoir of Motherhood, Disability, and Discovery*.

Aziza Ahmed is a professor of law and the R. Gordon Butler Scholar in International Law at Boston University. She is the author of the forthcoming book *Risk and Resistance: How Feminists Transformed the Law and Science of AIDS*.

Robert A. Aronowitz is the Walter H. and Leonore C. Annenberg Professor in the Social Sciences and a professor of history and the sociology of science at the University of Pennsylvania. He is the author of *Risky Medicine: Our Quest to Cure Fear and Uncertainty*.

Michael Barthman is a poet, musician, and emergency physician at Tséhootsooí Medical Center on the Navajo Nation. His poems have appeared in *Synapsis*, *Paper Darts*, and Vita Brevis Press, and he is currently working on his latest collection of poetry.

Jay Baruch is an emergency physician, writer, and professor of emergency medicine at Alpert Medical School of Brown University, where he is the director of the medical humanities and bioethics scholarly concentration. He is the author of *Tornado of Life: A Doctor's Journey through Constraints and Creativity in the ER*.

John Basl is an associate professor of philosophy in the department of philosophy and religion at Northeastern University and the associate director of the Northeastern Ethics Institute leading AI- and data-ethics initiatives. He is the author of *The Death of the Ethic of Life*.

Catherine Belling is an associate professor of medical education (medical humanities and bioethics) at Northwestern University Feinberg School of Medicine. She is the author of *A Condition of Doubt: The Meanings of Hypochondria*.

Michael Blackie is an associate professor of health humanities in the Department of Medical Education at the University of Illinois, Chicago. He is the co-editor of *From Reading to Healing: The Use of Literature to Teach Professionalism*.

Amy Boesky is a professor of English and directs the minor in medical humanities, health, and culture at Boston College. She is the author of *What We Have* and editor of *The Story Within: Personal Essays on Genetics and Identity*.

Allan M. Brandt is the Amalie Moses Kass Professor of the History of Medicine at Harvard University. He is the author of *The Cigarette Century: The Rise, Fall, and Deadly Persistence of the Product That Defined America*.

David Cantor is a researcher at the Instituto de Desarrollo Económico y Social (IDES), Buenos Aires, Argentina. He is a co-editor with Edmund Ramsden of *Stress, Shock, and Adaptation in the Twentieth Century*.

Todd Carmody is a writer, researcher, and strategy consultant. He is the author of *Work Requirements: Race, Disability, and the Print Culture of Social Welfare*.

Sara Jensen Carr is an assistant professor of architecture and program director for the master of design in sustainable urban environments at Northeastern University. She is the author of *The Topography of Wellness: How Health and Disease Shaped the American Landscape*.

Pratik Chakrabarti is the National Endowment for the Humanities Cullen Chair in History and Medicine at the University of Houston. He is the author of *Inscriptions of Nature: Geology and the Naturalization of Antiquity*.

Tod S. Chambers is an associate professor of medical education (medical humanities and bioethics) and of Medicine at Northwestern University Feinberg School of Medicine. He is the author of *The Fiction of Bioethics*.

James Chappel is the Gilhuly Family Associate Professor of History at Duke University. He is the author of *Catholic Modern: The Challenge of Totalitarianism and the Remaking of the Church* (Harvard University Press, 2018). He is working on a history of old age in the American Century.

Rita Charon is a general internist and literary scholar at Columbia University. She is a professor and chair of the Department of Medical Humanities and Ethics and co-author of *The Principles and Practice of Narrative Medicine*.

Ed Cohen is a professor of women's gender and sexuality studies. His most recent books are *A Body Worth Defending: Immunity, Biopolitics, and the Apotheosis of the Modern Body* (Duke University Press, 2009) and *On Learning to Heal, or What Medicine Doesn't Know* (Duke University Press, 2023).

Peter Cryle is a professor emeritus of intellectual history at the University of Queensland. He is a co-author with Elizabeth Stephens of *Normality: A Critical Genealogy*.

Gwen D'Arcangelis is an associate professor and the director of the gender studies program at Skidmore College in New York. D'Arcangelis is the author of *Bio-Imperialism: Disease, Terror, and the Construction of National Fragility*.

Sayantani DasGupta is a senior lecturer in the graduate program in narrative medicine, the Center for the Study of Ethnicity and Race, and the Institute for Comparative Literature and Society, all at Columbia University. She is the co-author of *The Principles and Practice of Narrative Medicine*.

Michele Marie Desmarais is a Métis, Dakota, and settler poet and scholar from the lands now known as Canada. An associate professor in religious studies at the University of Nebraska at Omaha, Dr. Desmarais is the author of *owlmouth* and co-author of "From the Ground Up: Indigenizing Medical Humanities and Narrative Medicine."

Lisa Diedrich is a professor of women's, gender, and sexuality studies at Stony Brook University. She is the author of *Indirect Action: Schizophrenia, Epilepsy, AIDS, and the Course of Health Activism*.

Samuel Dubal was a physician and assistant professor of anthropology at the University of Washington. He was the author of *Against Humanity: Lessons from the Lord's Resistance Army*.

René Esparza is an assistant professor of women, gender, and sexuality studies at Washington University in St. Louis. He is the author of the forthcoming manuscript *From Vice to Nice: Race, Sex, and the Gentrification of AIDS*.

Erica Fretwell is an associate professor of English at the University at Albany, SUNY. She is the author of *Sensory Experiments: Psychophysics, Race, and the Aesthetics of Feeling*.

Rosemarie Garland-Thomson is a Hastings Center Fellow and senior advisor and a professor emerita of English and bioethics at Emory University. She is the author of *Staring: How We Look*.

Pamela K. Gilbert is the Albert Brick Professor of English at the University of Florida. Her most recent book is *Victorian Skin: Surface, Self, History*.

Martin Halliwell is a professor of American thought and culture at the University of Leicester. He is the author of *American Health Crisis: One Hundred Years of Panic, Planning, and Politics* (2021) and co-editor of *The Edinburgh Companion to the Politics of American Health* (2022).

Percy C. Hintzen is a professor emeritus of African diaspora studies at the University of California, Berkeley. He is the author of the forthcoming volume *Reproducing Domination: On the Caribbean Postcolonial State*.

Rana Hogarth is an associate professor of history at the University of Illinois at Urbana-Champaign. She is the author of *Medicalizing Blackness: Making Racial Difference in the Atlantic World, 1780–1840* (University of North Carolina Press, 2017)

Heather Houser's most recent book is *Infowhelm: Environmental Art and Literature in an Age of Data* (Columbia University Press, 2020). She is the Mody C. Boatright Regents Professor in American and English Literature at the University of Texas at Austin.

Regina Emily Idoate (Cherokee Nation) is a population health scientist and assistant professor in the Department of Health Promotion in the College of Public Health at the University of Nebraska Medical Center.

Deborah Jenson, professor of romance studies and global health at Duke University, is the founding co-director of the Duke Health Humanities Lab and co-editor of *Unconscious Dominions: Psychoanalysis, Colonial Trauma, and Global Sovereignty*.

David S. Jones is the Ackerman Professor of the Culture of Medicine at Harvard University. He is the author of *Broken Hearts: The Tangled History of Cardiac Care*.

Jaymelee Kim is an associate professor of forensic sciences at the University of Findlay.

Erin Gentry Lamb is the Carl F. Asseff, MD, MBA, JD, Designated Professor in Medical Humanities; the faculty lead of the Humanities Pathway; and an associate professor of bioethics at Case Western Reserve University School of Medicine. She is the co-editor of *Research Methods in Health Humanities*.

Lisa M. Lee is the associate vice president of research and innovation and a professor of population health sciences at Virginia Tech. She writes about bioethics, public health ethics, and teaching ethics.

Sandra Soo-Jin Lee is a professor of medical humanities and ethics and the director of the Division of Ethics at Columbia University. She is a co-editor of *Revisiting Race in a Genomic Age*.

Martha Lincoln is an assistant professor of medical and cultural anthropology at San Francisco State University. She is the author of *Epidemic Politics in Contemporary Vietnam: Public Health and the State*.

John Lwanda, an honorary senior research fellow in the School of Social and Political Sciences and Institute of Health and Wellbeing at Glasgow University, is the author of *Politics, Culture and Medicine in Malawi: Historical Continuities and Ruptures with Special Reference to HIV/AIDS*.

Lisa Lynch is a professor of media and communications at Drew University. She is the author, most recently, of *Native Advertising: Advertorial Disruptions in the Twenty-First Century News Space*.

Christos Lynteris is a professor of medical anthropology at the University of St Andrews. His most recent book is *Visual Plague: The Emergence of Epidemic Photography* (MIT Press, 2022).

Annika Mann is an associate professor of English in the School of Humanities, Arts, and Cultural Studies at Arizona State University. She is the author of *Reading Contagion: The Hazards of Reading in the Age of Print*.

Alexa Miller is the founder of Arts Practica and a co-creator of Harvard Medical School's elective *Training the Eye: Improving the Art of Physical Diagnosis*. She has taught at Wellesley College, Brandeis University, and Quinnipiac.

Justine S. Murison is an associate professor of English at the University of Illinois at Urbana-Champaign. She is the author of *The Politics of Anxiety in Nineteenth-Century American Literature* (Cambridge University Press, 2011).

Kirsten Ostherr is the Gladys Louise Fox Professor of English and Director of the Medical Humanities program at Rice University. She is the author of *Cinematic Prophylaxis: Globalization and Contagion in the Discourse of World Health* and *Medical Visions: Producing the Patient through Film, Television, and Imaging Technologies*.

Robert Peckham was the director of the Centre for the Humanities and Medicine at the University of Hong Kong, where he was also the chair of history and the M. B. Lee Professor in the Humanities and Medicine from 2009 to 2021. He is the author of *Epidemics in Modern Asia* (2016) and *Fear: An Alternative History of the World* (forthcoming, 2023).

David N. Pellow is the Dehlsen Chair and Distinguished Professor of Environmental Studies at the University of California, Santa Barbara. His teaching, research, and activism focus on environmental justice in the US and globally. His books include *What Is Critical Environmental Justice?* and *Garbage Wars: The Struggle for Environmental Justice in Chicago*. He has served on the boards of directors of Greenpeace USA and International Rivers.

Anne Pollock is a professor of global health and social medicine at King's College London. She is the author of

Sickening: Anti-Black Racism and Health Disparities in the United States.

Benjamin Reiss is the Samuel Candler Dobbs Professor and Chair of the English department at Emory University. He is the author of *Wild Nights: How Taming Sleep Created Our Restless World.*

Ronald Sandler is a professor of philosophy and the director of the Ethics Institute at Northeastern University. He is the author of *Environmental Ethics: Theory in Practice, Food Ethics: The Basics, The Ethics of Species,* and *Character and Environment.*

Ralph James Savarese is a professor of English at Grinnell College. His most recent book is *See It Feelingly: Classic Novels, Autistic Readers, and the Schooling of a No-Good English Professor.*

Cristobal Silva is an associate professor of English at UCLA. He is the author of *Miraculous Plagues: An Epidemiology of Early New England Narrative.*

Harris Solomon is the Fred W. Shaffer Associate Professor of Cultural Anthropology at Duke University. He is the author of *Lifelines: The Traffic of Trauma.*

Maura Spiegel is the co-director of the Division of Narrative Medicine in the Department of Humanities and Ethics at the Columbia University Vagelos College of Physicians and Surgeons. She is a co-author of *The Principles and Practice of Narrative Medicine.*

Elizabeth Stephens is an associate professor of cultural studies at the University of Queensland and founder of the Australasian Health and Medical Humanities

Network. She is a co-author, with Peter Cryle, of *Normality: A Critical Genealogy.*

Kathryn Tabb is an assistant professor of philosophy at Bard College. She works in the history and philosophy of medicine, medical ethics, and moral psychology.

Matthew A. Taylor is an associate professor in the Department of English and Comparative Literature at the University of North Carolina at Chapel Hill. He is the author of *Universes without Us: Posthuman Cosmologies in American Literature.*

Jane F. Thrailkill teaches US literature and health humanities at the University of North Carolina at Chapel Hill. She is a founding director of UNC's health humanities lab (HHIVE) and author of *Philosophical Siblings: Varieties of Playful Experience in Alice, William, and Henry James.*

Helen Tilley is an associate professor of history and has a courtesy appointment in the Pritzker School of Law at Northwestern University. She is the author of *Africa as a Living Laboratory: Empire, Development, and the Problem of Scientific Knowledge, 1870–1950.*

Nancy Tomes is a Distinguished Professor of History at Stony Brook University. She is the author of *Remaking the American Patient: How Madison Avenue and Modern Medicine Turned Patients into Consumers.*

Corinna Treitel is a professor of History and co-founder of the medical humanities minor at Washington University in St. Louis. She is the author of *Eating Nature in Modern Germany: Food, Agriculture, and Environment, 1870–2000.*

Keir Waddington is a professor of history and co-director of the Science Humanities Initiative at Cardiff

University. He is the author of *An Introduction to the Social History of Medicine: Europe since 1500*.

Kym Weed is a teaching assistant professor of English and comparative literature at the University of North Carolina at Chapel Hill, where she is also the co-director of the HHIVE Lab and graduate programs in Literature, Medicine, and Culture. Her writings on health humanities and nineteenth-century science and literature have appeared in *Journal of Medical Humanities* and *Literature and Medicine*.

Deborah F. Weinstein is an associate professor of American studies and the director of the Science, Technology, and Society Program at Brown University. She is the author of *The Pathological Family: Postwar America and the Rise of Family Therapy*.

Martin Willis is a professor of English literature and co-director of the ScienceHumanities Initiative at Cardiff University. He is the author of *Vision, Science and Literature, 1870–1920* and editor of the *Journal of Literature and Science*.

Angela Woods is a professor of medical humanities and the director of the UK's first Institute for Medical Humanities at Durham University. She is the author of *The Sublime Object of Psychiatry: Schizophrenia in Clinical and Cultural Theory*.

Kathleen Woodward is the Lockwood Professor in the Humanities and a professor of English at the University of Washington, where she directs the Simpson Center for the Humanities. She is the author of *Statistical Panic: Cultural Politics and Poetics of the Emotions*.